Recent Results in Cancer Research 110

Recent Results in Cancer Research

P. Schlag   P. Hohenberger
U. Metzger   (Eds.)

Combined
Modality Therapy
of Gastrointestinal
Tract Cancer

With 105 Figures and 122 Tables

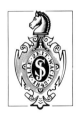

Springer-Verlag
Berlin Heidelberg New York
London Paris Tokyo

Professor Dr. Peter Schlag
Dr. Peter Hohenberger
Chirurgische Klinik, Klinikum der Universität Heidelberg
Im Neuenheimer Feld 110, 6900 Heidelberg, FRG

Priv. Doz. Dr. Urs Metzger
Departement Chirurgie, Universitätsspital Zürich
Rämistraße 100, 8091 Zürich, Switzerland

ISBN 3-540-18610-7 Springer-Verlag Berlin Heidelberg New York
ISBN 0-387-18610-7 Springer-Verlag New York Berlin Heidelberg

Library of Congress Cataloging-in-Publication Data
Combined modality therapy of gastrointestinal tract cancer/
P. Schlag, P. Hohenberger, U. Metzger (eds.)
p. cm. - (Recent results in cancer research; 110)
Includes index.
ISBN 0-387-18610-7 (U.S.):
1. Gastrointestinal system - Cancer - Adjuvant treatment.
I. Schlag, P. (Peter), 1948- . II. Hohenberger, P. (Peter),
1953- . III. Metzger, U. (Urs), 1945- . IV. Series.
[DNLM: 1. Combined Modality Therapy. 2. Gastrointestinal
Neoplasms - therapy. W1   RE106P   v. 110 / WI   149   C731]
RC261.R35   vol. 110   [RC271.A35]   616.99'4   s - dc   19
[616.99'406]   DNLM/DLC   88-4517

© Springer-Verlag Berlin Heidelberg 1988
Printed in Germany

Typesetting, printing, and binding: Appl, Wemding
2125/3140-543210

Foreword

Modern surgical oncology is characterized by multimodal therapy. In recent years numerous therapeutic approaches of pre-, peri-, intra- and postoperative treatment have been investigated with regard to their use in combination with surgical intervention.

It now is time to analyze and to define the state of our knowledge. For tumors of the gastrointestinal tract there are several encouraging therapeutic approaches, such as preoperative chemotherapy in esophageal and perioperative chemotherapy in colon cancer. For some special tumors, like anal carcinoma, we have clearly defined combined therapies which even now must be viewed as standard treatment.

It is also time to demonstrate the results of several clinical studies that have been conducted within the last few years that combined surgical efforts with pre- or postinterventional chemotherapy or radiotherapy. It is necessary to evaluate whether these trials contribute to progress in oncological therapy.

The editors of this volume – surgeons at the university hospitals of Heidelberg and Zürich – must be given the merit of achieving these goals. It was especially appropriate for the Department of Surgery in Heidelberg, in close cooperation with the Comprehensive Cancer Center Heidelberg/ Mannheim, to prepare a review of our present knowledge of surgical oncology as it is in the tradition of attempting to combine different therapeutic approaches to cancer therapy. Surgeon Vincenz Czerny was the first to found an institute for cancer research and therapy, in 1906 in Heidelberg. At this time two similar hospitals were already in existence, the

Roswell Park Memorial Institute in Buffalo (USA) and the Morosoff Clinic in Moskow. And it was the surgeon K. H. Bauer from Heidelberg who established the German Cancer Research Center in 1962. Thus the Gastrointestinal Tract Cancer Cooperative Group of the EORTC discussed their experiences in a location that represents both a long tradition and an awareness of our responsibility.

Ch. Herfarth
Professor of Surgery
Head, Department of Surgery
University of Heidelberg
Director, Comprehensive Cancer Center
Heidelberg/Mannheim

Preface

The EORTC (European Organization for Research and Treatment of Cancer) Gastrointestinal Tract Cancer Cooperative Group, founded in 1972, is devoted to clinical research in the combined modality treatment of gastrointestinal tract cancer. To date, the group has conducted 30 multicenter clinical trials, 13 of which have been completed and reported in various cancer journals. Five studies are closed to patient entry but follow-up still continues, and 12 trials are currently open to patient entry. More than 3500 patients have been entered so far in these studies with an annual entry rate of 300–350 patients.

Why collaborative research in oncology? Collaborative research is needed when a problem is too big to be tackled or solved by a single center. Many problems in oncology are so difficult that the simple rule of "two know more than one" or "two can do more than one" certainly applies. Individual medical centers are dominated by one or a few outstanding people, which tends to narrow one's vision and precludes the emergence of alternative ideas. Multicenter collaboration promotes the comparison of different viewpoints, which is a condition for progress. Apart from the intellectual aspects there is the obvious advantage of pooling resources and facilities. Even if a single center is sufficiently large to perform its own study, the results which emerge after several years have to be repeated by other centers before they can be generally accepted. In publication policy, there is an obvious bias to select and publish positive results. In cancer treatment, however, negative results may be of similar clinical value and it is obvious that multicenter trials are more suitable for sharing the risk of producing and publishing negative results.

Beside the regular semiannual meetings, the EORTC Gastrointestinal Tract Cancer Cooperative Group organizes review sessions every 3 years, where up to date information is given on the different aspects of combined modality treatment in gastrointestinal tract cancer. Analysis of the current EORTC trials is supplemented by state-of-the-art lectures from extramural experts.

This volume summarizes selected papers, which were presented during the recent EORTC-GI Group Conference in Heidelberg. The editor's wish is to give a topical survey on pre-, peri- and post-operative chemotherapy and radiotherapy, both in the adjuvant situation and for the treatment of advanced disease. In addition, new preclinical and experimental data relevant to the clinical situation are included.

Hopefully, this volume will further stimulate preclinical and clinical research in the treatment of the most common solid malignancy, the gastrointestinal tract tumor. Through combined efforts, surgeons, radiotherapists, and medical oncologists will achieve progress step-by-step.

Heidelberg/Zürich, February 1988   P. Schlag
                                                      P. Hohenberger
                                                      U. Metzger

Contents

List of Contributors*

Achterrath, W. *198*[1]
Adloff, M. *101*
Adolph, J. *281*
Arnaud, J.P. *101, 130, 181*
Bechstein, W.O. *65*
Beersiek, F. *111*
Bengmark, S. *74, 178*
Berger, M.R. *286*
Berrod, J.L. *130*
Beuningen, D. van *274*
Bignami, P. *164*
Bischoff, H. *286*
Bleiberg, H. *21, 181*
Blijham, G.H. *207*
Blöcher, G. *111*
Bozzetti, F. *164*
Bruckner, R. *130*
Buyse, M. *1, 21, 36, 101, 130*
Calciati, A. *219*
Camelot, G. *130*
Cartei, G. *36*
Chiarion-Sileni, V. *196*
Civalleri, D. *175*
Cocconi, G. *212*
Comandone, A. *219*
Dalesio, O. *1, 21, 130, 181*
De Besi, P. *196*
De Lisi, V. *212*

Delvaux, G. *181*
Denecke, H. *134*
Depadt, G. *181*
Di Costanzo, F. *212*
Dittrich, C. *44*
Dobrowsky, E. *140*
Dobrowsky, W. *140*
Doci, R. *164*
Duez, N. *1, 21, 36, 101, 130, 181*
Eibl-Eibesfeldt, B. *187*
Eigler, F.-W. *111, 274*
Eisenhut, M. *281*
Ekberg, H. *178*
Erhard, J. *111*
Fielding, J.W.L. *57*
Fink, U. *198*
Fiorentino, M.V. *196*
Flowerdew, A. *150*
Fornasiero, A. *36*
Fosser, V. *196*
Freund, U. *168*
Funovics, J. *44*
Gall, F.P. *79*
Garzon, F.T. *286*
Gennari, L. *164*
Georgi, P. *281*
Gerard, A. *130, 181*

---

* The address of the principal author is given on the first page of each contribution.
[1] Page on which contribution begins.

Gez, E. *52*
Gignoux, M. *1, 21*
Gillét, M. *1*
Grecchi, G. *219*
Groß, D. *168*
Gross, E. *274*
Gruenagel, H.H. *168*
Guimaraes dos Santos, J. *36*
Gunderson, L.L. *119*
Haegele, P. *21*
Halama, H. *111*
Heintz, J.P. *21*
Herfarth, C. *14*
Herrmann, R. *14*
Hofbauer, F. *44*
Jacob, J.H. *21*
Jakesz, R. *44*
James, R.D. *104*
Jeppsson, B. *178*
Jung, G.M. *21*
Kimmig, B. *281*
Köckerling, F. *79*
Kummermehr, J. *187*
La Ciura, P. *219*
La Grotta, G. *219*
Lauchart, W. *65*
Laugier, A. *130*
Lehner, B. *14*
Leonardi, F. *212*
Leria, G. *219*
Lise, M. *36, 181*
Loo, J. van de *198*
Loygue, J. *130*
Metzger, U. *95, 130*
Meyer, H.-J. *198*
Meyer, J. *198*
Mlynek, M.-L. *274*
Molzahn, E. *168*
Morabito, A. *164*
Muggianu, M. *175*
Namer, A. *21*
Nasca, S. *21*
Neuhaus, P. *65, 198*
Niebel, W. *111*
Nier, H. *111*
Nigra, E. *219*
Nitti, D. *36, 181*

Nobile, M.T. *175*
Nordlinger, B. *101*
Overgaard, J. *244*
Overgaard, M. *244*
Paccagnella, A. *196*
Paillot, B. *1, 21*
Papillon, J. *114, 146*
Pector, J.C. *101, 181*
Pene, F. *130*
Peracchia, A. *196*
Percivale, P.L. *175*
Peretz, T. *52*
Persson, B. *178*
Pichlmayr, R. *65*
Preusser, P. *198*
Puntis, M.C.A. *178*
Raeth, U. *14*
Rainer, H. *44*
Razzi, S. *175*
Reiner, G. *44*
Repetto, M. *175*
Ried, M. *111*
Ringe, B. *65*
Roloff, R. *134*
Roth, A. *30*
Roussel, A. *1, 21*
Savagno, L. *196*
Schalhorn, A. *187*
Schemper, M. *44*
Scherer, E. *111*
Schiessel, R. *44*
Schlag, P. *1, 14, 181*
Schmähl, D. *286*
Schulz, U. *111*
Schwarz, V. *14*
Simoni, G. *175*
Sindelar, W.F. *226*
Soldani, M. *212*
Starlinger, M. *44*
Storz, V. *187*
Streffer, C. *274*
Sugarbaker, P.H. *254*
Sulkes, A. *52*
Tatarek, R. *175*
Taylor, I. *150*
Tonato, M. *212*
Toso, S. *196*

Combined Therapy in Esophageal Cancer

The Value of Preoperative Radiotherapy in Esophageal Cancer: Results of a Study by the EORTC*, **

M. Gignoux, A. Roussel, B. Paillot, M. Gillet, P. Schlag, O. Dalesio, M. Buyse, and N. Duez***

Service de Chirurgie Digestive, C.H.U. Côte de Nacre, 14040 Caen, France

Attempts to combine radiation therapy and surgery in operable patients with carcinoma of the esophagus started 30 years ago. The first reported surgical series showed a low rate of resectability and a high postoperative mortality. Results of radiation therapy alone were also disappointing in the long run, especially in patients who appeared to be excellent operative risks with small localized tumors. The rationale for a combined approach was that X-ray therapy could bring about a reduction of tumor activity and bulk, an improvement in nutritional state through the restoration of the ability to swallow, a reduction of transplantability of the tumor, and a curative effect on periesophageal regional disease, which is not treated well by surgery. On the other hand, surgery often allowed an extended resection, clearing residual foci or distant esophageal wall extension. The limitation of a combined approach is the toxicity of the preoperative radiation, which must be mild enough to allow surgery to proceed without excessive delay or increased mortality. Numerous radiotherapy schedules were tried using different fields, doses, and fractionations, most of them in nonrandomized studies. Two prospective randomized trials have recently been reported. The final results of a third prospective trial, run by the E.O.R.T.C*, will be presented.

Review of the Literature

Historical Studies

A comparative analysis of historical studies (Table 1) is made difficult by the frequent lack of data concerning the staging of the tumor, the delay between radiation and surgery, the toxicity and the morbidity of radiation, and the number of patients at risk for long-term evaluation.

---

   * European Organisation for Research and Treatment of Cancer.
  ** Adapted from: Gignoux M, Roussel A, Paillot B, Gillet M, Schlag P, Favre J-P, Dalesio O, Buyse M, Duez N (1987) The value of preoperative radiotherapy in esophageal cancer: results of a study of the EORTC. World J Surg 11: 426–432 with permission.
 *** We thank Mrs. R. Pitois for typing the manuscript.

Table 1. Data from historical studies on preoperative radiotherapy

	Dose (Gy)	Interval	No. of patients	Operable	Resectable	Op. mortality	C.R.	Alive at 2 years	Alive at 5 years
Goodner [1] (1956–1966)	45 4.6 wks	–	85	59	47	7	7	–	3
Doggett et al. [3] (1970)	50–60 4–5 wks	4–6 wks	42	29	24	8[b]	4	5	–
Akakura et al. [8] (1963–1968)	50–60 4–6 wks	2–4 wks	–	117	96	20[b]	49	–	(25% patients at risk?)
Nakayama [5] (1957–1964)	20–25 4–5 days	3–5 days	–	–	161	7[b]	–	–	3 of 8 at risk
Parker et al. [2] (1962–1967) [16] (1967–1975)	45 3–4 wks. "	1–8 wks "	138	47	41 75	13[b] 14[b]	5 10	17 –	9 7
Marks et al. [4] (1960–1973)	45 3–4 wks	4–8 wks	332	137	101	18[b]	3	23	14 (median survival 25.5 mos. in resected)
van Andel et al. [15] (1970–1978)	40 4 wks	4–6 wks	–	133	81	17	–	–	(21% of resected)
Kelsen et al. [22] (1965–1979)	40–60[a] 4–6 wks	2–4 wks	76	66	41	8	–	–	(5% overall)
Sugimachi et al. [9] (1972–1983)	25–30 3–4 wks	–	–	–	104	6[b]	15	–	(16.7% of resected)

a 20 Gy × 5 days in 19 patients.
b Resected cases.

Doses, Fractionation, and Toxicity. The first studies [1] used a long-term fractionated radiation, about 45 Gy in 4 weeks, and surgery was performed after a 4- to 8-week period of recovery, sometimes later [2]. High doses of up to 50-60 Gy were tested in Stanford and by Akakura, but they led to an unacceptable toxicity (12% lethality) [3]. An analysis of the available reports (Table 1) shows that surgery had to be canceled for as many as 50% of irradiated patients. However, in most series the staging and the evaluation of operability were done at the end of the radiation period, not before. Complications related to radiation necrosis (hemorrhages, perforations, fistulas) have been reported. Radiation pneumonitis in 5% of survivors was mentioned only in the series of Marks et al. [4]. A different approach, consisting of short-term concentrated radiation, was advocated by Nakayama and Kinoshita on the basis of its high antitumor effect observed in mice [5]. Surgery was performed after a few days. This method was not used frequently, except in Europe, where it was usually administered in ten fractions for 12 days [6, 7].

Resectability. Five studies (Table 1) reported that esophageal resection could be performed in 37.5% of preoperatively irradiated patients, or in 75% of patients submitted for surgery. Akakura et al. reported a resectability rate of 82% after radiotherapy, compared with 39.5% in a former control group, but these results point to the need for confirmation in prospective trials. Severe adherences around the cancer due to connective fibrosis were encountered after 50-60 Gy radiation [8].

Operative Mortality. In the recorded data, the mean rate of postoperative deaths was 12.5% in patients submitted to surgery, 14.5% in resected patients. Great disparities exist between the series: the mortality was 22.5% among resected patients in earlier Western studies, whereas it was only 4%-6% in two Japanese studies [5, 9]. These rates were not different from those observed for surgery alone at the same time in the same countries. Nevertheless, radiation doses beyond 50 Gy [3, 8] were followed by increased mortality (21% for Akakura et al. over 13% the control group). Pulmonary complications were more frequent in preoperatively irradiated patients [9].

Tumor Response. A beneficial effect on dysphagia and on the esophagograms was noted in several studies, but a precise evaluation could be made only on resected specimens [10]. In Western studies using 40-50 Gy the complete response (CR) rate was about 10%. Japanese studies showed a high rate of markedly effective responses, correlated to radiation dosage: 49/96 after 50-60 Gy [8], 16/49 after 40 Gy [11], 15/104 after 25-30 Gy [9]. Compared with control groups, less infiltration of adventitia and resected stumps and less mediastinal lymph node involvement were noted by Akakura et al. [8]. Long-term survival was significantly better in responders, but this observation is known to be subject to potential selection bias.

Long-term Results. Survival results were disappointing. The 37.5% 5-year survival rate in resected patients assessed by Nakayama and Kinoshita [5] was based on only eight patients at risk, and Nakayama's last report indicated a 5-year survival of only 15.8% [12]. Of all patients included in the literature, 4.6% were alive at 5 years, 10.5% of patients receiving surgery and of resected patients about 15%.

The question is whether combined treatment is better than surgery alone: an improved survival rate of 25% over 13.5% was reported by Akakura et al. [8] over two consecutive time periods, whereas other simultaneous studies offered identical [9] or even worse [13] results. A better survival experience in Rotterdam [5] could be due to a high proportion of women (one-third) in that series. Concentrated radiation appeared to be better in the series of Kelsen et al. [12], but they had a small ample. Distant progression was common [3, 14] and more frequent in irradiated patients, contrary to local recurrences, which were less frequent [8]. Overall, long-term results of the combined treatment appeared to be better than those of radiation alone in a priori operable patients [4, 15, 16].

Prospective Studies

In the French study [6] (see Table 2) a high dose of concentrated radiation was administered before surgery to 67 patients, whereas 57 received surgery alone. There was no difference between the two groups of patients, either in the resection rate or in operative mortality (22.5% in the radiation group versus 33.5% in the control group). The pretreatment clinical staging in the two groups was not specified (ten of the 57 patients in the control group were not operated on at all). Excluding postoperative deaths, long-term survival was identical. The mean survival following all exploratory procedures was better in the control group (8.2 months versus 4.5 months), suggesting that this intensive regimen may have contributed to the unusually short survival for the combined-modality patients [17].

The Chinese study [18] concerned two groups of 83 (pretreated) and 77 patients. Radiation was delivered in ten fractions over 4 weeks, and surgery was performed after a rest interval of 2–3 weeks. Operative mortality was low. The resectability rate was not significantly modified. The rate of lymph node metastases was 21.5% in irradiated patients versus 30.4% in the control group. Although in half of the cases the anastomotic site was within the field of preoperative radiation, the incidence of anastomotic leakage for the radiation group was not higher than that for the group treated by surgery alone. No information was available on the long-term survival of the whole group, and the slight improvement at 5 years in the combined-modality group was not significant.

The EORTC Study

Material and Methods. This prospective randomized trial[1] was conducted by nine European institutions.[2] Patients of both sexes who fulfilled the following criteria

[1] Supported in part by a grant from the National Cancer Institute, Bethesda, MD, USA.
[2] Centre H. Becquerel, Rouen (B. Paillot, A. Kunlin, J. Heintz); C. H. U. Besançon (M. Gillet, G. Camelot, J. F. Bosset, G. Mantion); C. H. U. Caen (M. Gignoux, P. Segol, P. Marchand); C. F. B. Caen (A. Roussel, J. M. Ollivier); C. H. U. Dijon (H. Viard, J. P. Favre, J. P. Horiot); C. M. C. Strasbourg (M. Adloff, J. P. Arnaud, G. M. Jung); University of Heidelberg (P. Schlag); Institut Bordet, Brussels (A. Gerard, J. C. Pector, J. Henry); EORTC Data Center, Brussels (O. Dalesio, M. Buyse, N. Duez).

Table 2. Data from prospective studies on preoperative radiotherapy

	No. of patients	included	Dose (Gy)	Interval	Operable	Resectable	Op. mortality	C.R.	Alive at 5 years
Launois et al. [6] (1973–1976)	124	{ 67	39–45 8–12 days	<8 days	62	47	14	1	(9.5% of resected)[a]
		{ 57	–	–	47	33	11	–	(11.5% of resected)[a]
Huang et al. [18] (1977–1982)	160	{ 83	40 4 wks	2–3 wks	83	79	3	unknown	10 of 22 at risk
		{ 77			77	69	3	–	4 of 16 at risk
EORTC (1976–1982)	208	{ 102	33 12 days	<8 days	97	75	24	2	(10% overall) 16% of resected
		{ 106	–	–	106	87	19	–	9% overall 10% of resected

[a] Postoperative survival.

were eligible: a squamous cell carcinoma of the esophagus located at least 20 cm from the dental line, no previous treatment for the lesion, no other synchronous cancer, no presumed visceral metastasis, no presumed mediastinal involvement such as laryngeal palsy or tracheobronchial invasion (T_1–T_2 according to the American Joint Committee for Cancer Staging). Some tumors with mediastinal extensions at T_3 but without invasion of adjacent viscera were included. The preoperative evaluation included a complete clinical examination with special attention to weight loss and general condition as measured by the Karnofsky index. Patients with morbid conditions such as senility, severe pulmonary insufficiency or infection, cardiac abnormalities, hepatic damage, impaired renal function, or severe denutrition (weight loss of 20%) were excluded. Radiological evaluation included esophagography and CT-scanning or ultrasonography of the liver. Endoscopic evaluation required esophagoscopy, laryngoscopy and bronchoscopy if the lesion was located between 20 and 35 cm from the dental line. Thoracic CT-scanning, azygography, bone scanning and laparoscopy were optional. Radiotherapy was performed in ten fractions over 12 days, up to a total dose of 3300 rads, by linear accelerator. Two anterior and posterior fields were used on a mediastinal volume including 5 cm of the esophagus above and below the tumor. Patients in both groups of the study were submitted to an intensive preoperative preparation, including nutritional support by the enteral route in as much as this was possible; special attention was given to dental care and thoracic physiotherapy. Surgery was performed within 8 days after the completion of radiotherapy. A one-stage procedure was recommended. The esophagus was resected at least 5 cm away from the tumor margin, and lymph node dissection to the celiac, paratracheal, and paraesophageal regions was routinely carried out. Esophageal replacement was done with stomach or intestinal interposition. Tumors located above the aortic or azygos arch required a subtotal esophagectomy with cervical anastomosis. After surgery patients were classified as curative or palliative cases. Resection was considered curative if there was no macroscopic or microscopic evidence of residual tumor (including biopsies of adhesions) in the celiac and mediastinal areas and no invasion of the proximal esophageal stump. The trial was initially intended only for patients with a so-called curative resection. Because of the high rate of unpredictable palliative resections, all the randomized patients were followed up carefully every 3 months during the first year and every 6 months thereafter. Survival curves and disease-free curves were calculated from the date of randomization and were compared using the log-rank test.

Two hundred and twenty-nine patients were randomized into two groups: group I (115 patients) received preoperative radiation and group II (114 patients) received surgery alone. Of the 229 patients, 15 were ineligible because of inadequate staging prior to randomization, eight in group I and seven in group II. The reasons for exclusion were extraesophageal spread in nine cases, associated cancer in one, inaccurate preoperative biopsy in three, and associated disease in two. Two other patients did not receive the planned radiotherapy and no data were available on four cases. The remaining 208 patients were fully evaluable: 102 in group I and 106 in group II. There were 199 men and nine women; the median age was 55 years (range: 33–73). Tumor staging and tumor level were similar for the two groups (Table 3).

Table 3. Comparison of tumor staging and tumor level for the two groups

		Group I (combined treatment)	Group II
Clinical stage			
	T_1	26	33
	T_2	69	66
	T_3	6	3
	(Unknown)	(1)	(4)
Level			
	Upper	24	24
	Middle	44	43
	Lower	30	35
	(Unknown)	(4)	(4)

Table 4. Surgical procedure according to treatment group

	Group I (combined treatment)	Group II
Surgery canceled	5	–
Exploratory procedure	22 (5)[a]	19 (2)
Palliative resection	27 (11)	26 (6)
Curative resection	48 (8)	61 (11)
Total	102	106

[a] Numbers in parentheses refer to operative deaths.

Results. Tolerance to radiotherapy was reported as good in 87, moderate in nine, and bad in three. Four patients had progression or complications during radiotherapy (two mediastinal fistulas, one digestive hemorrhage leading to death, and one severe esophagitis). The median time between the end of the radiotherapy and surgery was 4.8 days (range: 2–17). Five patients were not operated on at all; all of them had received radiotherapy (two refusals, two progressions, one esophagitis). This left 203 patients who were operated on (Table 4). No resection was performed in 41 patients with local or distant extension (20%), 53 patients (26%) underwent a resection considered palliative by the surgeon, and resection was considered curative in 109 cases (54%). There is no difference between the two treatment groups in terms of resectability or curability. Among the 162 resected patients, a one-stage procedure with gastric transposition was used in 160, coloplasty in one, and a two-stage procedure in one. The anastomosis was intrathoracic in 116 and cervical in 46; among the 41 nonresected patients, a bypass procedure was performed in 14 and an endoprosthesis was implanted in two. The postoperative mortality (calculated within the whole hospital stay) was similar in both treatment groups (17% in nonresected cases, 32% after palliative resection, 17.4% after curative resection; Table 4). The median postoperative stay (22 days) and the causes of postoperative deaths (six pulmonary complications in group I versus eight in group II) did not differ between the two treatments.

The pathological analysis of resected specimens showed no significant difference between the two treatment groups with regard to lymph node invasion or penetration of the tumor (Table 5). In the group receiving radiotherapy, two superficial tumors had been sterilized while ten patients had a modified irradiated epithelioma. The rates of lymph node invasion were 56% in group I and 58.2% in group II.

After a mean follow-up time of 3.6 years, 25 patients are alive, 15 in group I and ten in group II. The mean overall survival was similar for patients of both groups, being 49 weeks and 48 weeks respectively (Fig. 1). The type of surgical procedure was the most significant prognostic factor ($P=0.001$): the 5-year actuarial survival was 3% after palliative resection (mean survival 39 weeks versus 37 weeks), 21%

Table 5. Depth of invasion

	Palliative resections		Curative resections	
	Group I	Group II	Group I	Group II
Mucosa	–	–	3	2
Submucosa	1	–	4	10
Muscularis propria	4	1	17	19
Beyond M. propria	22	25	23	30
(unknown)	–	–	(1)	–

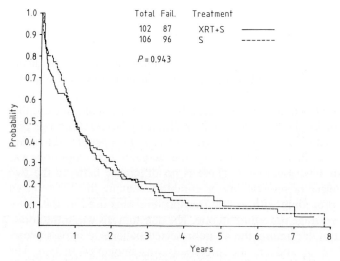

Fig. 1. Overall survival by treatment group

after curative resection (90 weeks versus 93 weeks) (Fig. 2). For curative resections without lymph node involvement, the mean survival was 76 weeks in group I and 111 weeks in group II, but long-term results were similar (Fig. 3). With regard to the local extent of the tumor, the two treatment groups showed no difference between any of their subgroups, except perhaps for the 20 patients with mucosal and submucosal growths: mean survival was 142 weeks versus 99 weeks ($P=0.33$) (Fig. 4). A slight benefit was also observed in upper-third lesions: nine patients in group I and 13 in group II had a curative resection and the mean survival was 161 weeks and 97 weeks respectively ($P=0.04$) (Fig. 5).

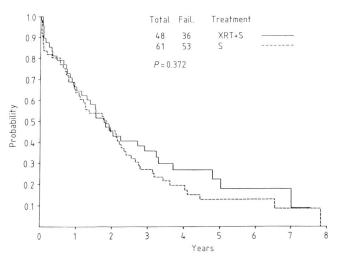

Fig. 2. Curative resections: survival by treatment group

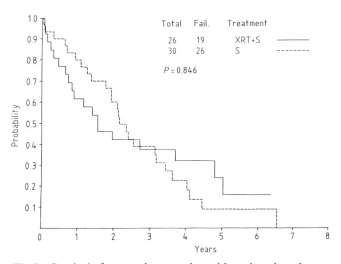

Fig. 3. Survival after curative resection without lymph node invasion

commending preoperative radiation as a routine procedure. This approach could be beneficial for carefully selected patients, but the question is whether identical results could not be obtained by radiation alone in these patients. Postoperative radiation in patients with resectable disease is most appropriate with regard to the assessment of extension, but it presents some disadvantages (lower radiosensitivity of ischemic tissues, presence of the transplant). Radiation is able to eradicate microscopic disease in the neck and mediastinum and to enhance local control [20] but without evident improvement in overall survival. The suggestion of benefit for patients without nodal metastases [21] was not confirmed in the preliminary results from a French randomized trial (Association Universitaire de Recherche en Chirurgie, unpublished data).

Approaches using both local and systemic therapy have recently been reviewed [22]. Combinations of chemotherapy and radiation prior to surgery, with the intent of enhancing the effectiveness of radiation and acting against disseminated disease, are limited by the lack of very effective regimens in esophageal cancer and by the toxicity of these treatments prior to surgery. Although preliminary results are encouraging, these approaches must still be considered experimental.

References

1. Goodner JT (1969) Surgical and radiation treatment of cancer of the thoracic esophagus. Am J Roentgenol Radium Ther Nucl Med 105: 523–528
2. Parker EF, Gregorie HB (1976) Carcinoma of the esophagus. Long-term results. JAMA 235: 1018–1020
3. Doggett RLS, Guernsey JM, Bagshaw A (1970) Combined radiation and surgical treatment of carcinoma of the thoracic esophagus. Front Radiat Ther Oncol 5: 147–154
4. Marks RM, Scruggs HJ, Wallace KM (1976) Preoperative radiation therapy for carcinoma of the esophagus. Cancer 38: 84–89
5. Nakayama K, Kinoshita Y (1974) Surgical treatment combined with preoperative concentrated irradiation. JAMA 227: 178–181
6. Launois B, Delarue D, Campion JP et al. (1981) Preoperative radiotherapy for carcinoma of the esophagus. Surg Gynecol Obstet 153: 690–692
7. Beaulieux J, Benhaim R, Boulez J et al. (1981) Traitement du cancer de l'oesophage thoracique. Intérêt de la cobaltothérapie et de la chimiothérapie post-opératoire. Nouv Presse Med 10: 1633–1641
8. Akakura I, Nakamura Y, Kakegawa T et al. (1970) Surgery of carcinoma of the esophagus with preoperative radiation. Chest 57: 47–56
9. Sugimachi K, Matsufuji H, Kai H et al. (1986) Preoperative irradiation for carcinoma of the esophagus. Surg Gynecol Obstet 162: 174–176
10. Japanese Society of Esophageal Diseases (1976) Guidelines for the clinical and pathological studies on carcinoma of the esophagus. Jpn J Surg 6: 79–86
11. Morita K, Takagi I, Watanabe M et al. (1985) Relationship between the radiologic features of esophageal cancer and the local control by radiation therapy. Cancer 55: 2668–2676
12. Nakayama K (1979) My experience in the management of esophageal cancer. Int Surg 64: 7–11
13. Skinner DB (1983) En-bloc resection for neoplasms of the esophagus and cardia. J Thorac Cardiovasc Surg 85: 59–71
14. Kelsen DP, Ahuja DP, Hopfan S et al. (1981) Combined-modality therapy of esophageal carcinoma. Cancer 48: 31–37

15. van Andel JG, Dees J, Dijkhuis CM et al. (1979) Carcinoma of the esophagus. Results of treatment. Ann Surg 190: 684–689
16. Parker EF, Gregorie HB, Prioleau WH et al. (1982) Carcinoma of the esophagus. Observations of 40 years. Ann Surg 195: 618–622
17. Hancock SL, Glatstein E (1984) Radiation therapy of esophageal cancer. Semin Oncol 11: 144–158
18. Huang GJ, Gu XZ, Wang LJ et al. (1986) Experience with combined pre-operative irradiation and surgery for carcinoma of the esophagus. GANN Monogr 31: 159–164
19. Gunnlaugsson GH, Wychulis AR, Roland C, Ellis FH Jr et al. (1970) Analysis of the records of 1657 patients with carcinoma of the esophagus and cardia of the stomach. Surg Gynecol Obstet 130: 997–1005
20. Kasai M, Mori S, Watanabe T (1978) Follow-up results after resection of thoracic esophageal carcinoma. World J Surg 2: 543–551
21. Pearson JG (1969) The value of radiotherapy in the management of esophagus cancer. Br Med J 105: 500–511
22. Kelsen D, Bains M, Hilaris B et al. (1984) Combined-modality therapy in esophageal cancer. Semin Oncol 11: 169–177

Preoperative (Neoadjuvant) Chemotherapy in Squamous Cell Cancer of the Esophagus

P. Schlag, R. Herrmann, U. Raeth, B. Lehner, V. Schwarz, and
C. Herfarth

Chirurgische Klinik, Klinikum der Universität Heidelberg, Im Neuenheimer Feld 110,
6900 Heidelberg, FRG

Even after radical tumor resection less than 15% of the patients with esophageal cancer are alive 5 years after surgery [2, 4, 5]. Moreover, local tumor removal is possible only in some of the patients. There have been many efforts to search for ways of improving the treatment results in esophageal cancer [10]. These include surgical techniques [11, 14] as well as combined treatment modalities [3, 8, 15]. Nevertheless, the results obtained have been rather negative. This is due to a still high percentage of primarily unresectable tumors, early metastases, and a high local relapse rate. Preoperative chemotherapy seems to be a promising new strategy [13, 16]. The objective of neoadjuvant chemotherapy is to bring about tumor regression and thereby improve resectability. The risk of tumor spread during surgery should also be decreased by devitalization of the tumor cells. Already existing micrometastases, which cause metastases later on, should be destroyed as well. Even if the theoretical aspects of this therapy seem very attractive, the question remains whether this kind of treatment is feasible at all in patients with cancer of the esophagus. On the one hand, these patients mostly suffer multimorbidity and so may not tolerate this approach. On the other hand, it has to be taken into consideration that short- or long-term side effects of preoperative chemotherapy may impair surgery. In the following report we therefore present our own experiences with a phase-II study evaluating preoperative chemotherapy in esophageal cancer. By comparing these results with those reported in the literature it should be possible to clarify the current impact of this treatment modality for the primary therapy of esophageal cancer.

Material and Methods

Patients eligible for the trial had biopsy-proven, untreated and nonmetastatic squamous cell carcinoma of the esophagus. The preoperative workup included esophagography, endoscopy, chest roentgenography and computerized tomography (CT). Normal serum electrolytes, blood urea nitrogen, and creatinine levels were required prior to study entry, as well as a white blood cell count of $4000/mm^3$ and a platelet count of $100000/mm^3$ prior to starting chemotherapeutic treatment.

From March 1983 through October 1986 106 patients with squamous cell carcinoma of the esophagus were referred to the Department of Surgery, University of Heidelberg (FRG). Forty-three patients had metastatic tumors or were not operable and could therefore not participate in the trial (Fig. 1). Among the other 58 patients only 42 fulfilled the following inclusion criteria for the study: age less than 68 years, Karnofsky-performance status > 70%, no concomitant cancer in the history, no prior chemo- or radiation therapy, and informed consent of the patient.

The chemotherapy was administered according to a modification of a protocol described by Kelsen et al. [8]. The operative therapy should be performed 2 weeks after the second cycle of combination chemotherapy with cis-platin, vindesine, and bleomycin (Fig. 2). Side effects of the chemotherapy were evaluated according to the WHO scale. After completing chemotherapy, each patient was reevaluated

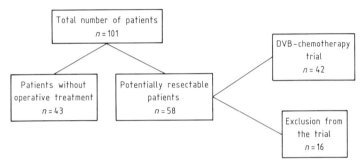

Fig. 1. Selection of patients for preoperative DVB-chemotherapy (cisplatin, vindesine and bleomycin) in cancer of the esophagus

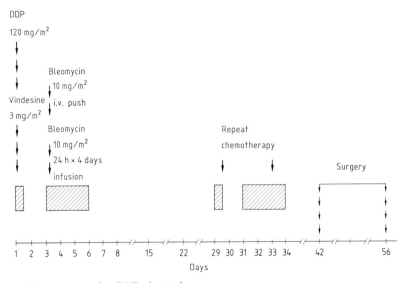

Fig. 2. Protocol for preoperative DVB-chemotherapy

by esophagogram, chest roentgenogram, and comparison of CT scans. Response to the preoperative chemotherapy was classified as follows:

- "Progression" was defined as increase of the primary tumor by more than 25% or appearance of metastases regardless of a response by the primary lesion.
- "No change" was defined as stable disease according to the patient's subjective or objective condition on comparing pre- and postchemotherapy status.
- "Minor response" was defined as an improvement in the subjective symptoms, in particular as related to dysphagia, whenever an objective tumor regression could not be documented unequivocally by the methods described.
- "Major response" was classified as a clear-cut 50% measurable reduction of tumor size measured by barium swallow and/or endoscopy.
- "Complete remission" was defined as a disappearance of all symptoms and signs of disease and no tumor in histology.

For tumors localized in the distal third of the esophagus a standard abdomino-thoracic esophagectomy was done and for tumors of the mid and upper third the thoracoabdominocervical approach was chosen. Dissection of celiac lymph nodes and posterior mediastinectomy including lymphadenectomy of the paraesopha-geal and paratracheal nodes was compulsory. Restoration of the gastrointestinal continuity was achieved in all cases by means of interposing the stomach. In the abdominothoracic approach the stomach was pulled up into the old bed of the esophagus and intrathoracic anastomosis was carried out. In the thoracoabdomino-cervical approach a left-sided cervical anastomosis was performed after the stomach had been pulled up behind the sternum. Postoperative follow-up was performed with all patients every 3 months. Survival rate and disease-free interval were analyzed using the Kaplan-Meier method [6] and for statistical analysis the log-rank test was performed [12].

Results

The number and severity of chemotherapy-induced side effects are shown in Tables 1 and 2. Severe side effects were relatively rare. Nevertheless, in three cases preoperative chemotherapy had to be discontinued – twice because of severe hematologic side effects and once because of nephrotoxicity. The most common side effects were nausea and vomiting, as expected, and partial or complete alopecia.

According to the chosen criteria for response, complete tumor remission was seen in two patients. However, these two were patients with clinical T1 tumors less than 3 cm in length. Partial remission was seen in 17 patients. In these cases there was no correlation with the clinical T stage of the primary tumor. Eight patients profited at least subjectively from therapy without showing clear tumor regression by objective measurements (minor response). Tumor size was stable in five patients as compared with their prechemotherapeutic status. These five include three patients for whom chemotherapy had to be discontinued before the end of the second cycle because of severe side effects. In ten patients chemotherapeutic treatment had no influence on further tumor growth. In four patients there was a clear progression even during the first cycle of chemotherapy, so that therapy was

Table 1. Side effects of preoperative chemotherapy in esophageal cancer (42 patients)

	WHO Grade				
	0	1	2	3	4
Alopecia	0	6	11	25	0
Fever with drug	28	7	7	–	–
Diarrhea	30	8	4	–	–
Stomatitis	38	3	1	–	–

Table 2. Toxic effects of preoperative chemotherapy in esophageal cancer (42 patients)

	WHO Grade				
	0	1	2	3	4
Leukocytes	16	11	10	3	4
Thrombocytes	20	10	7	3	2
Blood creatinine	33	5	3	–	1

Table 3. Response to preoperative chemotherapy and operative procedure

	Type of surgery		
	Curative (n=22)	Palliative (n=14)	Explorative (n=4)
Progression	2	5	3
No change	2	4	–
Minor response	4	2	1
Major response	12	3	–
Complete remission	2	–	–

stopped after the first cycle and surgery was performed without delay. Thus, nine patients were operated on after the first cycle of chemotherapy and 33 patients were ready for surgery after the second cycle, according to the study protocol. Two of these patients with tumor localization in the proximal third of the esophagus refused surgery after partial response to chemotherapy because surgery would have meant esophagolaryngectomy for them. These two patients were treated with further chemotherapy and consecutive radiotherapy; they died 8 and 35 months after their diagnosis.

Thus, 40 of 42 patients treated with chemotherapy underwent surgical therapy. In 36 of the 40 patients tumor resection was possible (resectability rate 90%). Based on the histologic workup of the operative specimen, surgery was judged to be curative in 22 patients and palliative in 14. The resectability rate was higher in the group of patients who responded to preoperative chemotherapy (Table 3).

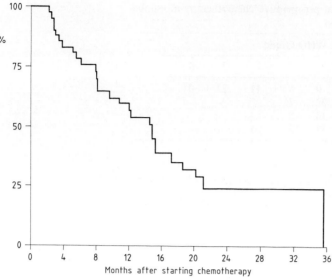

Fig. 3. Survival of the 42 patients participating in the study

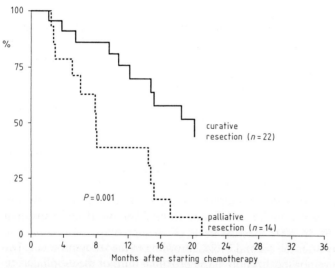

Fig. 4. Survival of palliatively and curatively resected patients

Postoperative mortality in the resection group was 4/36 (11%). The median survival for all patients treated in the trial from the time of diagnosis was 16 months
(Fig. 3). Curatively operated patients had a significantly longer survival than palliatively operated patients did (Fig. 4). There is also a significant difference in the
survival time for the resected patients who responded to chemotherapy compared
with the patients who did not (Fig. 5).

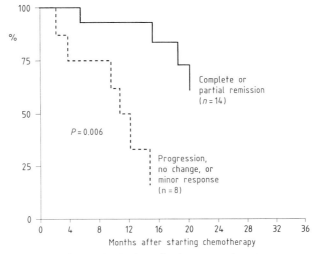

Fig. 5. Survival of curatively resected patients who had received preoperative chemotherapy according to tumor response

Discussion

Promising results of preoperative chemotherapy in esophageal cancer have already been published by Kelsen and co-workers [7, 8] and by Carey et al. [1]. There are differences between the trials according to patient selection, the operative approach, and the chosen chemotherapeutic regimen. While our study used a combination chemotherapy modified after Kelsen et al., Carey et al. combined *cis*-platin with 5-FU. The effect of the latter chemotherapy was also investigated in combination with preoperative radiotherapy [9]. In the first Wayne State University study [15] radiotherapy was evaluated in combination with 5-FU and mitomycin C. Radiotherapy was generally administered at doses of 30 Gy in both trials [9, 15]. The rate of side effects was tolerable in all of these studies and was identical to what we observed. The rate of partial response in these trials was 50%, approximately the same as we had. With combined preoperative chemotherapy and radiotherapy, however, there might be a higher rate of complete remissions, but this seems to be accompanied by a higher rate of postoperative complications and an increased postoperative mortality [9]. Experiences with preoperative chemotherapy to date in patients with cancer of the esophagus can be summarized as follows: With preoperative chemotherapy it is possible in 50% of cases to obtain a reduction of tumor size and sometimes even complete tumor remission. The rate of complete remissions might be increased by combining radiotherapy and chemotherapy preoperatively. There is no increased postoperative complication rate with preoperative chemotherapy in esophageal cancer if patients are carefully selected. On the other hand, this is a limitation of preoperative chemotherapy, and results could therefore be biased by patient selection. Furthermore, the question of whether preoperative treatment might increase the rate of resectable tumors could not be answered definitively according to the design of a phase-II study. It is also not clear whether the improved survival time of the patients in our trial is due to the preoperative treatment or to patient selection. Therefore, a final conclusion regarding the benefit of preoperative chemotherapy can be made only by performing a phase-III study; this is now underway.

References

1. Carey RW, Hilgenberg AD, Wilkins EW, Choi NC, Mathisen DJ, Grillo H (1986) Preoperative chemotherapy followed by surgery with possible postoperative radiotherapy in squamous cell carcinoma of the esophagus: evaluation of the chemotherapy component. J Clin Oncol 4: 697–701
2. DeMeester TR, Levin B (eds) (1985) Cancer of the esophagus. Grune and Stratton, New York
3. Gignoux M, Roussel A, Paillot B, Gillet M, Schlag P, Dalesio A, Buyse M, Duez N (1987) The value of preoperative radiotherapy in esophageal cancer. World J Surg 11: 426–432
4. Giuli R (ed) (1984) Cancer of the esophagus. Maloine, Paris
5. Huang GJ, K'ai WY (eds) (1984) Carcinoma of the esophagus and gastric cardia. Springer, Berlin Heidelberg New York Tokyo
6. Kaplan EL, Meier P (1958) Nonparametric estimation for incomplete observations. J Am Stat Assoc 53: 457–481
7. Kelsen DP (1984) Chemotherapy of esophageal cancer. Semin Oncol 11: 159–168
8. Kelsen P, Bains M, Hilaris B, Martini N (1984) Combined modality therapy of esophageal cancer. Semin Oncol 11: 169–177
9. Leichman L, Steiger Z, Seydel HG, Vaitkevicius VK (1984) Combined preoperative chemotherapy and radiation therapy for cancer of the esophagus: The Wayne State University, Southwest Oncology Group and Radiation Therapy Oncology Group Experience. Semin Oncol 11: 178–185
10. Linder F, Belsey R, Ong GB, Richard CA, Siewert JR, Skinner DB, Dietz R, Hissen W (1982) Panel discussion on treatment of oesophageal carcinoma. Langenbecks Arch Chir 357: 237–257
11. Orringer MB, Sloan H (1978) Esophagectomy without thoracotomy. J Thorac Cardiovasc Surg 76: 643
12. Peto R (1978) Clinical trial methodology. Biomedicine 28: 24–36
13. Ragaz J, Band PR, Goldie JH (eds) (1986) Preoperative (neoadjuvant) chemotherapy. Recent results in cancer research, vol 103. Springer-Verlag, Berlin Heidelberg New York Tokyo
14. Skinner DB (1984) Surgical treatment for esophageal carcinoma. Semin Oncol 11: 136–143
15. Steiger Z, Franklin R, Wilson RF, Leichman L, Seydel H, Loh JJK, Vaishampayan G, Knechtges T, Asfaw I, Dindogru A, Rosenberg JC, Buroker T, Torres A, Hoschner D, Miller P, Pietruk T, Vaitkevicius V (1981) Eradication and palliation of squamous cell carcinoma of the esophagus with chemotherapy, radiotherapy, and surgical therapy. Thorac Cardiovasc Surg 82: 713–719
16. Wagener DJT, Blijham GH, Smeets JBE, Wils JA (eds) (1985) Primary chemotherapy in cancer medicine. Liss, New York

Controlled Clinical Trial for the Treatment of Patients with Inoperable Esophageal Carcinoma: A Study of the EORTC Gastrointestinal Tract Cancer Cooperative Group

A. Roussel, J. H. Jacob, P. Haegele, G. M. Jung, B. Paillot, J. P. Heintz, M. Gignoux, S. Nasca, A. Namer, H. Bleiberg, M. Buyse, O. Dalesio, and N. Duez

Centre Francois Baclesse, Route de Lion-sur-Mer, 14021 Caen Cedex, France

Radiotherapy is the usual treatment for inoperable esophageal carcinoma. Results published before 1976, when this trial was begun were very modest, except for those of Pearson [1]. The 1-year survival rate varies from 15% to 30%, and 5-year survival rates were about 5% [2–7].

Few attempts were made to combine chemotherapy with radiotherapy in this type of lesion. Only bleomycin [8–10] seemed to give a better local response, but no impact on the duration of survival was demonstrated. Moreover, the high toxicity (mediastinal necrosis, pulmonary sclerosis) observed discouraged further utilization. Other drugs, e.g., methylhydrazine [11], tested in association with radiotherapy did not show better results. No randomized trial was published or was being carried out.

In 1975, Roussel [2] published the results of two historical series of patients treated with radiotherapy alone (116 patients) or with radiotherapy preceded by a short administration of methotrexate (144 patients). Survival rates at 1, 3, and 5 years were 23%, 4%, and 2.5% respectively in the group treated with radiotherapy alone and 33.5%, 9%, and 5% in the group treated with the combination of methotrexate and radiotherapy. Based on these results, the EORTC GI Tract Cooperative Group began a randomized study in 1976 to compare the efficacy of methotrexate administered before radiotherapy (MTX + RT) with that of radiotherapy alone (RT).

Material and Methods

Patient Population. Patients with histologically proven squamous cell carcinoma of the esophagus who were nonoperable or refused surgery were eligible for this trial. Patients with fistula or tracheal invasion (compression and edema were accepted) or with visceral or nodal metastases apart from supraclavicular nodes were ineligible. In addition, patients had to be aged 75 or less, with no history of cancer or concomitant affection which could influence the survival and no previous antitumor treatment. Patients with more than 25% weight loss and patients for whom a regular follow-up was judged impossible were not eligible for this trial, neither

Recent Results in Cancer Research, Vol. 110
© Springer-Verlag Berlin · Heidelberg 1988

were patients with infection or with abnormal hematological, renal, or hepatic tests (WBC count < 3500, platelet count < 100000, prothrombine < 50%, urea > 0.70 g in spite of hydroelectrolytic reequilibration, creatinine > 15 mg, creatinine clearance < 60 ml/min). The workup just before randomization included a complete clinical examination; renal, hepatic, and blood counts; roentgenograms of the esophagus and the thorax; an esophageal endoscopy (with biopsy) and a bronchial endoscopy; a laryngoscopy (direct or indirect); and a scintigraphy and/or echotomography and/or laparoscopy.

Treatment Modalities

Radiotherapy. Radiotherapy was given at the same dose and schedule in both treatment groups and was to be started 8–12 days after the end of chemotherapy in the MTX + RT group and on the day of randomization in the RT group. The treatment included irradiation of the lesion and the surrounding nodes in two modalities, depending on the location of the tumor: (a) upper third – irradiation of the superior part of the mediastinum and right and left supraclavicular nodes, at a dose of 40.50 Gy, raised to 56.25 Gy on the tumor site alone; (b) median and lower third – irradiation of the inferior two thirds of the mediastinum and the celiac nodes at a dose of 40.50 Gy, raised to 56.25 Gy on the tumor site alone.

The first part of the irradiation was done in 18 fractions of 2.25 Gy (5 fractions/ week), anterior and posterior field. The complement to the tumor site was delivered in an X-shaped field (2 cm around the lesion) in seven fractions of 2.25 Gy, for a total dose of 56.25 Gy in 25 fractions (5 weeks).

Chemotherapy. Methotrexate was administered subcutaneously every 6 h for 4 days (a total of 16 injections). At the beginning of the trial the dose was 0.5 mg/ 10 kg/injection; it was modified during the trial to 1.5 mg/m²/injection. This modification of the protocol was done in order to follow the general international method of prescription, which prevents overmedication in patients with high weight, since the reference to body weight implies a quicker increase of the dose as compared with body surface. Hematological counts were to be done every 48 h until the 10th day after treatment, and continued if there were signs of aplasia.

Follow-up

Patients were to be followed up every 2 months during the first year, every 3 months during the second year, and every 6 months thereafter. The follow-up included a complete clinical examination, roentgenograms of the thorax and the esophagus, and a complete biological workup.

Randomization

Patients were randomized by telephone at the Data Center. A randomized block design, stratifying by institution, was used to assign the corresponding treatment.

End Points

The main end points of the study were survival and time to progression.

Statistical Methods

Survival and time-to-progression curves were calculated, taking as the starting point the date of randomization and using the Kaplan-Meier technique [12]. Comparisons of the curves were performed by the log-rank test [13]. A Cox proportional-hazard model was adjusted in order to investigate the simultaneous effect of the different variables on the duration of survival.

Results

From May 1976 to January 1982, 170 patients were randomized in the trial by seven institutions. Ninety percent of the total accrual was made by four of these institutions. Nine patients were found to be ineligible for the trial, the reasons being the existence of distant metastases and abnormal values of blood parameters, preventing treatment. For four patients no data were available, two patients refused treatment and were lost to follow-up shortly thereafter, two patients died just after randomization and before receiving any treatment, one patient was taken off the study to undergo surgery, and for two patients the radiotherapy was inadequate (Table 1).

Treatment groups were well balanced with respect to age, sex, performance status, histology, nodal extent, type of feeding, and weight loss, as shown in Table 2.

Toxicity

Hematological toxicity was reported without grading and without distinguishing among the different counts. However, severe cases were carefully documented. Of the 76 patients receiving methotrexate, hematological toxicity was reported in 29 (38%); six of these were detailed as severe pancytopenia. These severe episodes led to death in one case, caused cessation of the chemotherapy in one case, and

Table 1. Non-evaluability by treatment group

	MTX + XRT	XRT	Total
Ineligible	3	6	9
No data available	2	2	4
Refused treatment	2	–	2
Early death	–	2	2
Inadequate radiotherapy	–	3	3
Total	7	13	20

Table 2. Patient characteristics by treatment group

	MTX + XRT	XRT	Total
Sex *(n)*			
male	75	69	144
female	2	4	6
Age (years)			
median	60	63	62
range	41–78	31–74	31–78
Karnofsky			
median	80	80	80
range	50–100	50–100	50–100
Histology			
well differentiated	28	26	54
poorly differentiated	34	37	71
anaplastic	8	4	12
Supraclavicular nodes *(n)*			
no	75	68	142
yes	3	3	6
Distance superior border to dental arcade (cm)			
median	26	26	26
range	15–33	18–38	15–38
Weight loss (%)			
median	10	9	10
range	0–30	0–23	0–30
Feeding *(n)*			
oral	72	69	141
solid	19	23	42
chopped-up	34	31	65
liquid	19	15	34
nonoral	4	3	7
nasoesophageal	2	1	3
abdominal	2	2	4

precluded the radiotherapy in another. Cutaneous-mucosa reactions (skin, mucositis, and esophagitis) to methotrexate were reported in 14 cases; five of them were severe, and in two cases this was the reason for stopping chemotherapy.

A severe hepatic reaction led to discontinuation of the administration of methotrexate but did not prevent radiotherapy being given.

Other toxicities were reported in nine patients (13%): fever (5), articular pain (2; chemotherapy had to be discontinued in one case), nausea (1), and weakness (1).

Tolerance to radiotherapy was similar in both treatment groups, and the number of complications was comparable. Nine cases of esophagitis were reported (five in MTX + RT, one severe, and four in RT). Deterioration of the general condition during RT was observed in 13 patients of the MTX + RT group (three severe, one leading to cessation of RT), and in 15 patients of the RT group (five severe, one requiring cessation of RT). Four esophagotracheal fistulas were observed (one in the

MTX + RT group and three in the RT group, one of these appearing immediately after treatment). Esophageal burns were reported once in each group (this led to cessation of treatment in the RT group).

One patient in the MTX + RT group had a skin infection (zona) and another a severe cutaneomucosa reaction. One patient died of respiratory trouble in the RT group; this patient had suffered from respiratory problems before randomization. One patient treated only by radiotherapy died of a non-confirmed myelopathy 10 months after radiotherapy.

Survival

Of the 150 evaluable patients, 142 were reported dead. Table 3 shows the causes of death according to treatment group. Six of the eight patients still alive had been treated with MTX + RT and two with RT. No difference was detected in the duration of survival according to the treatment assigned (Fig. 1). Median survival was 9 months for the MTX + RT group and 8 months for the RT group. The 1- and

Table 3. Cause of death by treatment group

Cause of death	MTX + XRT	XRT
Malignant disease	72	70
Toxicity	1	1
Infection	6	4
Associated chronic disease	–	2
Other	9	7
Unknown	8	4

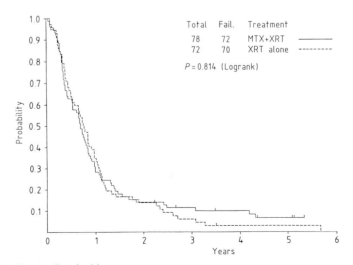

Fig. 1. Survival by treatment group

3-year survival rates are 31% and 12% respectively for MTX + RT and 35% and 6% for RT.

A comparison including all randomized patients for whom some data on survival were available showed essentially the same results.

Progression

Table 4 gives the type of progression by treatment group. For 21 patients no progression was detected, either because they were alive and free of disease at the time of the analysis or because they died of other causes (toxicity, infection, other disease) before a progression was observed. Nine patients died of unknown causes and are considered in the curves as progressing at the date of death. For 117 patients the type of progression was recorded; it was only local in 54% of the cases, only metastatic in 21% of the cases, and simultaneously local and metastatic in 21%.

Time-to-progression curves were constructed for all the types of progression together and for local progression and development of distant metastases separately. Eight percent of the progressions as well as 50% of the metastases occurred during the first year. No significant difference was detected between treatment group for any of these parameters.

Feeding

The mode of feeding is a good measure of the intensity of dysphagia. It has been reported for 114 patients at the time of randomization (Table 2). To evaluate the benefit of the treatments in terms of feeding possibilities, the mode of feeding just before treatment has been compared with the mode of feeding 1 month after treatment. In 30% of the cases there was a degeneration and in 70% of the cases the feeding could be thickened or stayed unchanged. No difference can be observed between the two treatment groups.

Table 4. Type of progression by treatment group

	MTX + XRT	XRT	Total
Local progression	35	28	63
Distant metastases	12	13	25
Both local and distant	11	18	29
Type unknown	1	2	3
No progression and cause of death unknown	6	3	9
No progression	13	8	21
Total	78	72	150

Prognostic Factors

Several factors were analyzed in order to detect those that discriminate groups with different prognoses.

Sex, age, and location of the tumor were not found to be of prognostic importance for the duration of survival. The survival of patients with anaplastic tumors is somewhat shorter than that of moderate and well differentiated tumors; the difference, however, is not significant ($P=0.08$). The Karnofsky performance status and the weight loss before treatment were found to be of prognostic importance. Patients with a performance status under 70 had a shorter survival ($P=0.003$) as did patients with a loss of more than 10% of their normal weight ($P=0.002$, Fig.2). The cutting point at 10% weight loss was adopted after we had calculated death rates in smaller subgroups and regrouped those with similar death rates. The advantage of patients with low weight loss can still be observed in terms of time to progression ($P=0.036$) and especially in the time to develop distant metastases ($P=0.007$).

A Cox proportional-hazard model was adjusted in order to test the relative importance of the variables for the duration of survival. Using a step-down procedure, factors adding no significant discrimination were excluded from the model. Two variables were retained in the model, in decreasing order of importance: the weight loss and the performance status.

It has to be mentioned that a comparison by treatment group of the subgroups of patients with less than 10% weight loss showed a significant advantage for the combined-treatment group in terms of time progression ($P=0.034$, Fig.3). The advantage was of borderline significance for the development of distant metastases ($P=0.08$). However, no difference was seen in the survival. Comparisons by treatment in the group of patients with more than 10% weight loss showed no difference for any of the end points.

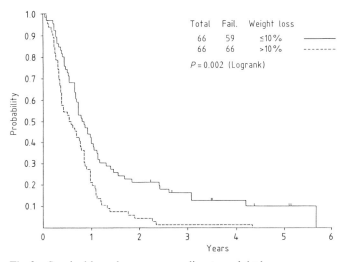

Fig. 2. Survival by subgroups according to weight loss

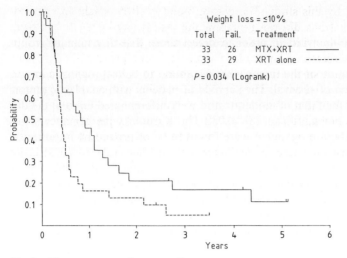

Fig. 3. Time to progression according to treatment group

Discussion

Chemotherapy was well tolerated overall; it had to be stopped in eight cases and precluded radiotherapy in two cases. It is impossible to determine whether the only death during treatment can be ascribed to hematologic toxicity due to methotrexate or was the result of bone marrow invasion.

Radiotherapy was also well tolerated, the only death under radiotherapy being due to major preexistant respiratory trouble. It is unlikely that the three esophagotracheal fistulas reported were due to local necrosis if the dose given is taken into consideration. They were more likely due to the undetected invasion of the mucosa or submucosa of the tracheobronchial tree.

The duration of survival was similar in both treatment groups and is comparable to that of the series treated with MTX + RT reported by Roussel [3].

The survival rates depend on several characteristics of the population. It is therefore very difficult to compare different results in the literature since selection criteria are often poorly delineated. The review by Earlam and Cunha-Melo [14] shows that the proportion of patients for whom a palliative treatment is possible varies in the different series from 20% to 100%, and the survival rates at 1 and 5 years vary from 8% to 50% and from 0% to 21% respectively. These differences are certainly related to the proportion of patients with visceral or distant-node invasion. The trial reported here excluded patients with metastatic involvement. Only supraclavicular nodes were included, since their evolution may be controlled by radiotherapy.

Micro- and macroscopic characteristics of the tumor did not appear to play an important prognostic role, neither did the sex or age of the patients. Only the general condition of the patients, as measured by the performance status and the loss of weight, had an impact on survival.

The importance of weight loss had already been pointed out by Roussel [15] and has been confirmed by this study. The cutting point of 10% weight loss is proposed, as smaller divisions did not represent the results any better. It has been shown [16, 17] that malnutrition is correlated with tumor extent and, in particular, with metastatic involvement. This could explain the poor prognosis of patients with great weight loss. A small loss of weight might be an indicator of the absence of metastases, and only in these patients could the addition of chemotherapy be of benefit, as suggested by the results.

It is recommended that future studies take into account the importance of weight loss as a factor of prognosis and that stratification by this factor should be routinely done.

References

1. Pearson JG (1971) The value of radiotherapy in the management of squamous esophageal cancer. Br J Surg 58: 794-798
2. Roussel A (1975) Bilan des cancers de l'oesophage traites au centre Francois Baclesse depuis 1964. Ouest Med 28 (6): 381-386
3. Verhaege M, Rohart J, Adenis L, Demaille A, Lequint A, Vankemel B, Delloitte M (1971) Possibilites et resultats de la radiotherapie dans les cancers de l'oesophage (a propos de 300 cas en 10 ans). Presse Med 79: 236
4. Pierquin B, Wanbersie A, Tubiana M (1966) Cancer of thoracic oesophagus: two series of patients treated by 22 mv betatron. Br J Radiol 39: 189-192
5. Marcial VA, Tome JM, Ubinas J, Bosh A, Correa JN (1966) Esophageal cancer: the role of radiation therapy. Radiology 87: 231-239
6. Lederman M (1966) Carcinoma of esophagus with special reference to upper third. Part I. Clinical considerations. Br J Radiol 39: 193-197
7. Leborgne R, Leborgne F, Bartocci L (1963) Cancer of the esophagus: results of radiotherapy. Br J Radiol 36: 806-811
8. Kolaric K et al. (1976) Therapy of advanced oesophageal cancer with bleomycin, irradiation and combination of bleomycin with irradiation. Tumori 62 (3): 255-262
9. Okamoto T et al. (1972) Systemic chemotherapy of esophageal cancer. Jpn J Cancer Clin [Suppl]: 370-374
10. Soga J, Fujimaki M, Kawaguchi M et al. (1971) Bleomycin and irradiation effects on the esophageal carcinoma: a preliminary historical evaluation. Acta Med Biol 19 (2): 119-136
11. Robillard J, Couedic Y (1967) Resultats compares de 80 cas de cancers de l'oesophage traites soit par telecobalt soit par association telecobalt-methylhydrazine. J Radiol Electrol 48: 867-871
12. Kaplan EL, Meier P (1958) Nonparametric estimation from incomplete observations. J Am Stat Assoc 53: 457-481
13. Mantel N (1966) Evaluation of survival data and two new rank order statistics arising into consideration. Cancer Chemother Rep 50: 163-170
14. Earlam R, Cunha-Melo JR (1980) Oesophageal squamous cell carcinoma. II. A critical review of radiotherapy. Br J Surg 67: 457-461
15. Roussel A (1979) Le pronostic du cancer de l'oesophage. Gaz Med France 86 (37): 4361-4369
16. Belghiti J, Langonnet F, Wessely JY, Fekete F (1981) Faut-il corriger la denutrition des malades ayant un cancer de l'oesophage ou du cardia en periode pre-operatoire? Nouv Presse Med 10 (27): 2273-2279
17. Paillot B, Bodenes P, Czervichow P (1985) Facteurs pronostiques des cancers epidermoides de l'oesophage. Gastroenterol Clin Biol 9 (2b): 68 A

Combination of Chemotherapy and Irradiation: A New Approach in the Treatment of Locally Advanced Esophageal Cancer

A. Roth

Central Institute for Tumors and Allied Diseases, I Lica 197, 41000 Zagreb, Yugoslavia

In an attempt to improve the conservative treatment of inoperable esophageal cancer we began 10 years ago to use the combined chemo-radiotherapy approach. Before conducting clinical trials we investigated the interaction of cytostatics and radiation in vitro on various cell lines.

Before presenting the results of our new study of inoperable esophageal cancer using epirubicin and radiation, I will briefly outline the results of our earlier studies.

Three prospective controlled studies were performed, using cytostatics alone and a combination of cytostatics and radiotherapy for 103 patients with inoperable esophageal cancer. Study A included bleomycin alone and a combination of bleomycin and radiation, study B adriamycin and the combination of adriamycin with radiation, and study C was a combination chemotherapy (bleomycin and adriamycin) versus bleomycin and adriamycin and radiation. The treatment schedules are presented in Table 1. In study A, of 15 patients treated with bleomycin alone, four responded to treatment with a response rate ($>50\%$ tumor regression) of 26% (Table 2). Combining bleomycin with radiation in 24 patients, response was observed in 15, giving a response rate of 62%. The difference in response was statistically significant ($P<0.01$). In study B, 18 patients were treated with adriamycin alone and six patients responded to treatment, so that the response rate was 33%. With the combined-treatment modality of adriamycin plus radiation, response was observed in 60% of the patients treated, i.e., nine of 15 patients responded to treatment, with a statistically significant difference in treatment results ($P<0.05$). Study C consisted of a combination of bleomycin and adriamycin in 16 patients, with three responders and a response rate of 19%. Combined treatment with these two drugs plus radiation resulted in nine responders among 15 patients, a response rate of 60%. The difference in treatment results was also statistically significant ($P<0.01$). All but two of the complete responses were observed in combined-treatment modalities. Remissions obtained by single-agent treatment or by combination chemotherapy were of short duration (2–3 months), while the remission in combined-treatment modalities lasted 9–11 months. Combined-treatment modalites also showed markedly prolonged patient survival compared with chemotherapy alone. The results of these studies showed that cytostat-

Table 1. Treatment schedules

Study A	
Bleomycin	15 mg/m^2 body surface i.v. twice a week – total dose 200–350 mg
Bleomycin + radiation	10 mg/m^2 body surface i.v. twice a week (total dose 180–250 mg) simultaneously with radiation (3800–4400 R Betatron, Siemens)
Study B	
Adriamycin	40 mg/m^2 body surface i.v. daily, 2 days – total 6 cycles with a rest period of 3 weeks between cycles
Adriamycin + radiation	40 mg/m^2 body surface i.v. daily, 2 days – 3 cycles simulta- neously with radiation (3800–4400 R Betatron, Siemens)
Study C	
Bleomycin	15 mg/m^2 body surface i.v. daily, day 1, 4
Adriamycin	40 mg/m^2 body surface i.v. daily, days 2, 3 Total 5–6 cycles administered with 3-week rest periods between cycles
Bleomycin	15 mg/m^2 body surface i.v. daily, days 1, 4
Adriamycin	30 mg/m^2 body surface i.v. daily, days 2, 3
Irradiation	3600–4000 rad (42 MeV Betatron, Siemens) 2 cycles of chemotherapy given simultaneously with radiation plus a 3rd cycle 1 month after radiation was completed

Table 2. Results of treatment, three prospective controlled studies

	Number of patients	Complete remission (100%)	Partial remission (>50%)	Response rate
Bleomycin	15	1	3	4/15 (26%)
				P<0.01
Bleomycin + radiation	24	6	9	15/24 (62%)
Adriamycin	18	1	5	6/18 (33%)
				P<0.05
Adriamycin + radiation	15	4	5	9/15 (60%)
Bleomycin + adriamycin	16	–	3	3/16 (19%)
				P<0.01
Bleomycin + adriamycin + radiation	15	3	6	9/15 (60%)

ics alone, even in combination chemotherapy, produced a lower antitumor activity in esophageal cancer than did the combination of these drugs with radiation.

The antitumor activity of 5-fluorouracil (5-FU), combined either with bleomycin or adriamycin plus radiation, was studied in another controlled randomized clinical trial. Sixty-one previously untreated inoperable esophageal cancer patients entered the study, and 56 have been evaluated: 58 male and three female patients with a mean age of 57 years (range 37–74). Modality A consisted of a combination

Table 3. Results of treatment, controlled randomized clinical trial

Treatment modality	Weight loss	Complete response (100%)	Partial response (>50%)	Stable disease (0%–50%)	Progression	Response rate
5-Fluorouracil	<10%	8 (61%)	3	2	0	11/13 (85%)
+						
Bleomycin	>10%	3 (20%)	7	3	2	10/15 (67%)
+						
Radiation	Total	11 (39%)	10 (36%)	5	2	21/28 (75%)
5-Fluorouracil	<10%	1	7	3	0	8/11 (73%)
+						
Adriamycin	>10%	1	9	2	5	10/17 (59%)
+						
Radiation	Total	2 (8%)	16 (57%)	5	5	18/28 (64%)

of 5-FU (10 mg/kg i.v. 2×weekly, 4 weeks) and bleomycin (10 mg/m^2 i.v. 2×weekly, 4 weeks) which was given concurrently with radiation (3600–4000 cGy, 1000 cGY weekly). In modality B the combination of 5-FU (same dose) and adriamycin (30 mg/m^2 i.v., days 1, 2, 23, and 24) was administered with the same schedule and dosage of radiation. Seventy-five percent of the patients (21/28) have responded to treatment (CP + PR) with modality A, with 11 complete and ten partial responses. With modality B, response was recorded in 64% of patients (18/28), with two complete and 16 partial responses (Table 3). The difference in complete responses (39% vs 8%) was statistically significant ($P<0.05$). The median remission duration for complete responders was 12 months with modality A (range 6–18 months) and 6.8 months with modality B (range 3–10 months). All the responses occurred in patients with squamous cell carcinoma, except for one partial response in a case of adenocarcinoma. As far as the age is concerned (<55 vs >55 years), no significant difference in response rate was found (67% vs 71%). More favorable results were observed in the group of patients with <10% weight loss (79% vs 63%). Toxicity was moderate (myelosuppression, cardiotoxicity).

The interaction of 4-epi-doxorubicin (4-epi-DX) and irradiation has not been studied either; however, being aware of the synergistic activity of ADM and irradiation, we recently studied the effect of 4-epi-DX and radiation on V-79 hamster lung cells in vitro [1, 2]. The results showed a synergistic mode of action when the cells were treated with a subtoxic drug concentration and a fixed (7 Gy) radiation dose. These experimental results, and the clinical experience acquired through the use of ADM and irradiation, provided the stimulus for a pilot clinical trial on the combination of 4-epi-DX and irradiation in inoperable locoregionally advanced squamous cell esophageal cancer.

Patients and Methods

Thirty-eight patients (30 men and eight women), 36 to 75 years old (mean age 60 years), entered the study during 1984. All suffered from locoregionally ad-

Table 4. Patient characteristics

Patients entered *(n)*	38
Patients evaluable *(n)*	33
Mean age (years)	60
Male	30
Female	3
Weight loss	
> 10%	20
< 10%	13
Location of the tumor in the esophagus	
Upper third	3
Middle third	20
Lower third	10
Filling defects (X ray)	
< 5 cm	5
5–8 cm	20
> 8 cm	8
Histology	
Squamous cell	30
Adenocarcinoma	1
Anaplastic (squamous cell)	2

vanced inoperable tumors, however, without distant metastases. The tumor was localized in the middle third of the esophagus in 20 patients and in the lower or upper third in the remainder. Thirty-three patients completed the treatment program and were evaluable. They included 30 squamous cell carcinomas, two anaplastic (squamous cell) carcinomas, and one adenocarcinoma. The roentgenographic filling defect was up to 5 cm long in five patients and 5–8 cm long in 20, and in eight the length of the esophagus segment involved in the tumor exceeded 8 cm. A weight loss exceeding 10% of body weight was recorded in 20 patients; in the other 13 cases the weight loss was less than 10% (Table 4).

Before treatment, biopsy samples were obtained by esophagoscopy, and all the tumors were confirmed. Pretreatment examinations also included routine blood, liver, and kidney tests, chest roentgenography with tomography of the mediastinum, and bronchoscopy. Esophagoscopy and roentgenography were repeated at the end of therapy. Patients older than 75 years and patients with heart, liver, or kidney failure weren excluded from the study.

The patients were irradiated in two opposite thoracic fields (42 MeV Betatron, Siemens) with a daily dose of 200 cGy, i.e., 1000 cGy weekly; the total radiation dose was 3600–4000 cGy. 4-Epi-doxorubicin was administered concurrently at a daily dose of 50 mg/m^2 on days 1, 2, 22, and 23. The drug was injected through a running infusion tube.

All the toxic side effects were monitored regularly. ECGs were performed before treatment and once a week during therapy.

Table 5. Pilot study of 4-epi-doxorubicin + irradiation in locoregionally advanced esophageal cancer, Central Institute for Tumors, Zagreb

Patients entered in the study	No. of evaluable patients	Complete response	Partial response	Stable disease	Progres- sion	Response rate
38	33	11	12	6	4	22/33 (70%)

Median remission duration = 9 + months (CR 14 + months)

Table 6. Endoscopic and histologic findings 3 months after the end of treatment

Total number of patients	Histology: negative Endoscopy: negative	Histology: positive Endoscopy: negative	Histology: positive Endoscopy positive
33	8 (24%)	3	22

Table 7. Response according to weight loss (4-epi-doxorubicin + irradation in esophageal cancer)

Weight loss	Complete response	Partial response	Stable disease	Progres- sion	Response rate
<10%	7	8	3	2	15/20 (75%)
>10%	4	4	3	2	8/15 (53%)

$P < 0.05$

Results

The results showed a pronounced antitumorigenic activity of 4-epi-DX plus radiation (Table 5), since 11 complete and 12 partial remissions were achieved with a response rate of 70% (23/33). In addition, in six patients minor regression (stable disease) was observed, whereas in four cases the disease progressed. Endoscopic and histologic findings following treatment are compared in Table 6. In eight patients the endoscopy and biopsy specimens were negative, in three patients endoscopy was negative but the biopsy material positive (all the 11 were complete clinical responders), and in 22 cases (partial responders, stable disease, progression) both endoscopy and biopsy material were positive. The median duration of remission was 9 + months (14 + months in complete responders) over an average observation period of 18 months.

Analysis of some prognostic factors (tumor localization, length of filling defect, and weight loss) which might affect the outcome of therapy showed that only weight loss influenced the results ($P < 0.05$). Patients with a weight loss of less than 10% presented a higher response rate and longer remission (Table 7).

Toxic side effects (Table 8) were mainly radiation mucositis and retrosternal pain in all the patients, occurring 10-12 days after the start of treatment. The mucositis symptoms disappeared completely 15-20 days after the end of therapy. Leukopenia was pronounced in nine patients (27%). No thrombocytopenia was

Table 8. Toxic side effects (33 patients)

	Grade				
	I	II	III	IV	
Alopecia	–	2	8	23	(100%)
Mucositis with retrosternal pain	5	13	15	–	(100%)
Leukopenia	5	3	1	–	(27%)
Thrombocytopenia	–	–	–	–	
ECG changes	2	1	–	–	(9%)
Cardiac failure	–	–	–	–	

observed. Alopecia was present in all cases: grades II and III in 10 and grade IV in 23 patients. Tracheobronchial fistulae were not observed. Insofar as cardiotoxicity is concerned, there was not a single case of heart failure. In three patients ventricular extrasystoles were temporarily pronounced on ECG records during treatment. On examination of these patients 3 months after the end of treatment, the changes were found to have disappeared.

Discussion

The combination of 4-epi-DX with irradiation in a pilot study of 33 patients with inoperable esophageal cancer clinically confirmed the experimental data on the synergistic antitumorigenic action of this combined approach. The objective response observed in 70% of patients is encouraging, considering the well-known chemo- and radioresistance of such tumors. It should also be noted that the toxicity of this treatment mode was mild and tolerable. The combined approach may also prove to be relevant as an adjuvant prior to surgery to improve the resectability rate, since only multimodality treatment may be expected to improve the still very poor results achieved by surgery alone.

To close, I would like to stress the advantages of chemo-radiotherapy in correlation with radiotherapy alone. These are:

1. Higher response rate (50%–80%)
2. Higher proportion of complete responses (up to 40%)
3. Longer remission duration (8–15 months)
4. Lower radiation dosage (3200–4000 cGy)
5. Better tolerance of treatment (less toxicity)
6. Prolongation of survival (?)

References

1. Bistrović M, Nagy B, Maričić Ž, Kolarić K (1978) Interaction of adriamycin and radiation in combined treatment of L-mice cells. Eur J Can 14: 411–414
2. Ban J, Bistrović M, Maričić Ž, Kolarić K (1986) Combined treatment of 4-epi doxorubicin and radiation on hamster lung cell. Tumori 72: 339–344

Phase-III Clinical Trial of Adjuvant FAM2 (5-FU, Adriamycin and Mitomycin C) vs Control in Resectable Gastric Cancer: A Study of the EORTC Gastrointestinal Tract Cancer Cooperative Group

M. Lise, D. Nitti, M. Buyse, G. Cartei, A. Fornasiero, J. Guimaraes dos Santos, and N. Duez

Istituto di Patologia Chirurgia 1a, Universita degli Studi di Padova, Via Giustiniani 2, 35100 Padova, Italy

Despite a reported decrease in incidence, gastric carcinoma remains a major oncologic problem in Western Europe. Surgery is at present the only hope for cure. The 5-year survival after curative surgery is about 40% for stage 2 and 20% for stage 3.

Gastric carcinoma is a chemosensitive cancer; however, only a few anticancer drugs have shown some effectiveness as single agents. Several protocols of combination chemotherapy were proposed between 1974 and 1980 for the treatment of advanced gastric cancer. Among them, the FAM regimen of McDonald et al. became the most popular, with a reported response rate of 42%–55% and mild toxicity [1–3]. A modification of the FAM regimen, with increased doses and reduced intervals between them, was tested in Padova from 1977 to 1982 and was reported as having a 60% response rate [4]. The same group also used FAM2 as an adjuvant treatment for 25 patients with curatively resected gastric cancer. Toxicity was acceptable, with only one case of grade-4 toxicity for platelets. Treated patients showed a better actuarial survival at 4 years than a similar group of patients who had had surgery alone in a non-randomized comparison [5]. On these grounds, a phase-3 clinical trial of adjuvant FAM2 was accepted by the EORTC in 1982. As the study is still open to patient entry, the aim of this paper is to present only toxicity data and an analysis of prognostic factors.

Methods

Patients who have undergone "curative" resection of histologically proven gastric adenocarcinoma are included in the study. Only stage-2 and stage-3 tumors, according to the UICC staging, are considered eligible. Patients must be under 70 years of age, with a performance status of 0–2 according to the WHO scale, with the possibility of follow-up and declared acceptance of therapy.

Patients with coexistent malignant disease are excluded from the study, as are patients with UICC stage-1 tumors or obvious distant metastases. Also excluded

Recent Results in Cancer Research, Vol. 110
© Springer-Verlag Berlin·Heidelberg 1988

Table 1. The EORTC protocol of adjuvant FAM2 in gastric cancer

Stratification

According to UICC staging system:

- Stage 2
- Stage 3

R A N D O M I Z A T I O N

→ No further treatment

↘ FAM2

FAM2 regime							
Drugs (mg/m^2)	1	2	3	22	23	24	days
5-FU 400	X	X	X	X	X	X	
ADM 40		X			X		
MMC 10	X						
Recycle from day 43 (7 cycles) then							
5-FU 800	X	X	X	X	X	X	
MMC 10	X						
For 1 cycle							

are patients with carcinoma of the cardia, previous chemo- and/or radiotherapy, cardiac disease, active infection, or other pathologies for which systemic chemotherapy is contraindicated.

Before randomization patients are stratified in two categories according to their UICC stage. Chemotherapy is to be started 3 weeks after surgery. 5-fluorouracil, adriamycin and mitomycin C are increased by 30%, 77%, and 33% respectively in comparison with the original FAM regimen, mainly by reducing the intervals of treatment (Table 1). Progressive parameters of hematologic toxicity, evaluated at day 1 and day 22, are used when necessary to calculate lower doses of chemotherapeutic agents. The end points of the protocol are to detect a significant improvement in overall survival and disease-free intervals in these patients compared with those who are treated by surgery alone. A total of about 300 evaluable patients are needed to complete the study.

Results

Two hundred and twenty-one patients have entered the study so far, from seven different countries and 27 institutions. Patients are evenly distributed between treatment (112) and control groups (109), but there is a clear prevalence of stage-3 (158) over stage-2 cases (63).

Table 2. Percentage of patients with hematologic toxicity on day 22 by degree of severity

Severity grade (WHO)	WBC		PLT		HB	
	(No./ml)	(%)	(No./ml)	(%)	(g/100 ml)	(%)
1	3000–4000	40	75 000–100 000	11	9.5–10.9	29
2	2000–3000	19	50 000– 75 000	10	8.0– 9.4	3
3	1000–2000	5	25 000– 50 000	3	6.5– 7.9	5
4	<1000	–	<25 000	2	<6.5	–
	Total	64		26		37

Table 3. Percentage of patients with non-hematologic toxicity by degree of severity

Severity grade (WHO)	Nausea/ vomiting	Diarrhea	Mucositis	Hair	Skin	Neuro- logic	Hemor- rhage	Cardiac	Other
1	29	14	30	16	5	8	2	5	19
2	30	5	3	27	3	–	–	–	11
3	11	–	5	24	–	–	–	2	3
4	2	–	2	–	–	–	–	–	–

Table 4. Prognostic factors related to patient characteristics

Prognostic factor	Levels	Number of patients	Survival (P-value)	Disease-free interval (P-value)
Age (years)	Up to 49	29	0.65	0.67
	50–59	52		
	60 and over	62		
Sex	Male	95	0.90	0.75
	Female	53		
Weight loss	5% or less	52	0.35	0.33
	Over 5%	34		
	Over 10%	57		
Performance status	Grade 0 (normal)	103	0.33	0.63
	Grade 1 (ambulatory)	34		
	Grade 2–3 (disabled)	6		

Data are available for 79 of the 112 patients receiving chemotherapy. These 30% have completed the treatment; 54% have received six or more cycles and 67% four or more cycles. For the 45 patients that have been withdrawn from the study the median number of cycles was 4.4.

Chemotherapy had to be reduced in 35% of patients and postponed in 25%, mainly because of hematologic toxicity. This was manifested in the WBC in 64% of patients, in platelets in 26%, and in the Hb in 37%. In only two patients was grade-4 toxicity for platelets registered (Table 2). Nausea and vomiting were re-

Table 5. Prognostic factors related to tumor characteristics

Prognostic factor	Levels	Number of patients	Survival (P-value)	Disease-free interval (P-value)
Tumor location	Upper third	15	0.09	n/a
	Middle third	26		
	Lower third	94		
	Upper + middle	3		
	Lower + middle	20		
	All three	6		
	Linitis plastica	5		
Tumor stage	Stage II	43	0.06	0.15
	Stage III	107		
Primary tumor	T1	5	0.005	0.008
	T2	74		
	T3	55		
	T4	14		
Lymph nodes	N0	43	< 0.001	0.02
	N1	46		
	N2	50		
	N3	7		
Histopathologic grading	High diff.	44	0.03	0.02
	Medium diff.	38		
	Low diff.	59		
	Undefined diff.	3		
Ming's classification	Expansive	21	0.52	0.11
	Infiltrative	68		

ported at least once in 72% of patients, hair loss in 67%, and mucositis in 40% (Table 3). Severe non-hematologic toxicity was present in 2% of cases with nausea and vomiting and in 2% with mucositis. No cases of death from toxicity or cases of severe irreversible toxicity were reported.

Reasons for withdrawal from the study before completion of treatment were: intercurrent death (5%), loss to follow-up (3%), refusal of treatment (19%), toxicity (22%), relapse (32%), protocol violation (3%), and ineligibility (6%).

An analysis of prognostic factors shows no difference in survival for sex, presurgical age, weight loss, or performance status (Table 4). With regard to the characteristics of the tumor (Table 5), differences in survival are emerging for T penetration, lymph nodal status, and grading. No significant differences have yet been found for tumor stage, tumor location, or histologic subtypes according to Ming's classification.

The median overall survival for all cases at 3 years is 50% (Fig. 1), with 40 months median survival rate for stage 2 and 28 months for stage 3 (Fig. 2). The median disease-free survival rate at 3 years for all cases is 40% (Fig. 3).

With regard to the type of surgery, the trend is towards better results with subtotal gastrectomy (Fig. 4).

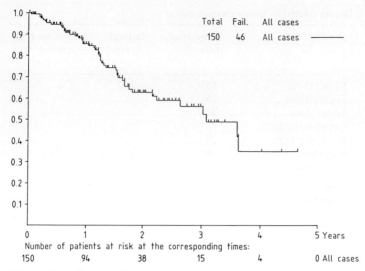

Fig. 1. Overall survival

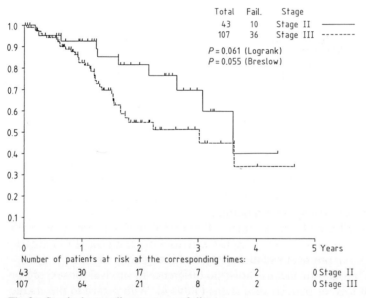

Fig. 2. Survival according to stage of disease

Discussion

The problem of whether adjuvant chemotherapy is of any benefit in the treatment of gastric cancer is still wide open. Conflicting results have been obtained so far in Western countries. In a recent controlled clinical study of the GITSG, patients who underwent postsurgical adjuvant chemotherapy with 5-FU and methyl-

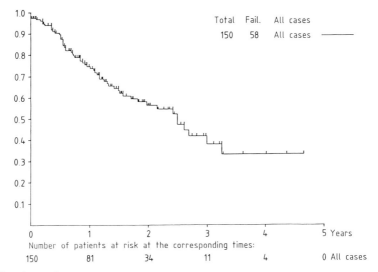

Fig. 3. Disease-free interval

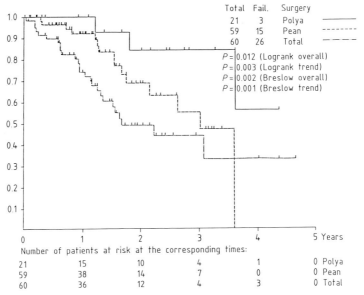

Fig. 4. Survival according to type of surgery. *Polya*, subtotal gastrectomy with gastrojeju-nostomy; *Pean*, subtotal gastrectomy with gastroduodenostomy

CCNU had a survival rate of 44% compared with the 26% survival rate of patients treated with surgery alone [6]. However, these results were not confirmed in similar studies carried out by the VASOG [7] and the ECOG [8]. Other trials conducted in England [9] and Germany [10] using 5-FU plus mitomycin C and 5-FU plus BCNU respectively showed no advantage for patients treated with adjuvant chemotherapy. On the other hand, recent Japanese studies [11, 12], most frequently using mitomycin C and 5-FU, seem to demonstrate the efficacy of adjuvant chemotherapy after radical surgery. It is not clear whether these contrasting results are due to the impact of earlier diagnosis, to different criteria for patient selection, or to other factors. In Japan, unlike in Western countries, most adjuvant chemotherapy trials are begun in the perioperative period, several of them using intraperitoneal drug administration. It has been suggested that these procedures would allow better control of residual microscopic disease, especially in the lymph nodes and on the peritoneum, when the total tumor burden is smallest [13]. In any case, both these results and this hypothesis require further confirmation.

The FAM chemotherapeutic regimen became widely popular in the 1970s. Although its efficacy has been questioned recently [14], this combination is probably the most widely used for the treatment of advanced gastric cancer in Western countries. Unfortunately, it is also often used as an adjuvant without proof of its effectiveness.

One prospective study with the adjuvant FAM regimen was recently completed by the IATGC with the coordination of Dr. Schein [15]. Preliminary results, after a median follow-up of 36 months, seem to indicate a positive trend in disease-free survival in favor of the patients treated with FAM. However, a longer follow-up is needed before more definitive conclusions can be drawn.

The goal of the FAM2 protocol is to improve the efficacy of the treatment by increasing the chemotherapeutic dose. It is obviously too early to determine the possible therapeutic advantages of FAM2 in this protocol. Thus far, we can say that the increased doses of the three agents undoubtedly cause more toxicity, although this remains fairly constant in the three cycles. Mainly because of the hematologic toxicity, chemotherapy had to be reduced or postponed in a significant number of patients. However, the average length of treatment is 6 months, currently considered an adequate period for adjuvant therapy in other types of cancer. It remains to be seen if the increased toxicity is a reasonable price to pay for a still undefined therapeutic advantage.

Given the scarcity of available data in this field and the conflicting results which have emerged so far, it is especially important that this study be completed. Furthermore, a careful analysis of prognostic factors may show whether there is any difference in response to treatment among different subgroups of patients.

References

1. MacDonald JS, Schein PS, Wooley PV, et al. (1980) 5-Fluorouracil, doxorubicin, mitomycin C (FAM) combination chemotherapy for advanced gastric cancer. Ann Intern Med 93: 533
2. Bitran JD, Desser RK, Kozzloff MF, et al. (1979) Treatment of metastatic pancreatic and gastric adenocarcinoma with fluorouracil, adriamycin and mitomycin C (FAM). Cancer Treat Rep 36: 2049
3. Panettiere PJ, Heiburn L (1981) Experience with two treatment schedules in combination chemotherapy of advanced gastric carcinoma. In: Carter S, Crooke S (eds) Mitomycin C: current status and new developments. Flam Academic, Orlando, pp 145–157
4. Fornasiero A, Cartei G, Daniele O, Fosser V, Fiorentino M (1982) FAM2 regimens in disseminated gastric cancer. Eur Soc Med Onc 8: 74

5. Cartei G, Fornasiero A, Daniele O, Favretti F, Nitti D, Lise M, Fiorentino M (1982) Adjuvant FAM after radical surgery in gastric carcinoma. Abstract, 1st Eur Soc Surg Oncol, p 101
6. The Gastrointestinal Tumor Study Group (1982) Controlled trial of adjuvant chemotherapy following curative resection for gastric cancer. Cancer 49: 1116
7. Higgins GA, Amadeo JH, Smith DE, et al. (1983) Efficacy of prolonged intermittent therapy with combined 5-FU and methyl-CCNU following resection for gastric carcinoma. A Veterans Administration Surgical Oncology Group report. Cancer 52: 1105
8. Engstrom PF, Lavin PT, Douglass HO jr, et al. (1985) Postoperative adjuvant 5-fluorouracil plus methyl-CCNU therapy for gastric cancer patients. Eastern Cooperative Oncology Group Study (EST 3275). Cancer 55: 1868
9. Fielding JWL, Fagg SL, Jones BG, et al. (1983) An interim report of a prospective, randomized, controlled study of adjuvant chemotherapy in operable gastric cancer. British Stomach Cancer Group. World J Surg 7: 390
10. Schlag P, Schreml W, Gaus W, et al. (1982) Adjuvant 5-fluorouracil and BCNU chemotherapy in gastric cancer: 3-year results. In: Mathé G, Bonadonna G, Salmon S (eds) Adjuvant therapies of cancer. Recent results in cancer research, vol. 80. Springer-Verlag, Berlin Heidelberg New York, p 277
11. Inokuchi K, Hattori T, Taguchi T, et al. (1984) Postoperative adjuvant chemotherapy for gastric carcinoma. Analysis of data on 1805 patients followed for 5 years. Cancer 53: 2393
12. Akiyoshi T, Kawaguchi M, Arinaga S, et al. (1984) A trial of adjuvant combination chemoimmunotherapy for stage-III carcinoma of the stomach. J Surg Oncol 26: 86
13. Douglass HO jr (1985) Gastric cancer: overview of current therapies. Semin Oncol 12: 57
14. Cullinan SA, Moertel CG, Fleming TR, et al. (1985) A comparison of three chemotherapeutic regimens in the treatment of advanced pancreatic and gastric carcinoma: fluorouracil vs fluorouracil and doxorubicin vs fluorouracil, doxorubicin, and mitomycin. JAMA 253: 2061
15. Schein PS, Coombes RC, Chilvers C (1986) A controlled trial of FAM (5-FU – doxorubicin – mitomycin) chemotherapy as adjuvant treatment for resected gastric carcinoma: an interim report. Proc American Society of Clinical Oncology, no 308

The Effect of Adjuvant Chemotherapy in Gastric Carcinoma Is Dependent on Tumor Histology: 5-Year Results of a Prospective Randomized Trial

R. Jakesz, C. Dittrich, J. Funovics, F. Hofbauer, H. Rainer, G. Reiner, M. Schemper, R. Schiessel, and M. Starlinger

I. Chirurgische Klinik, Universität Wien, Alser Straße 4, 1090 Wien, Austria

Gastric carcinoma is decreasing in incidence in Western Europe and the United States. However, this disease is still a major cause of cancer death [1]. Extended surgical procedures over the past 20 years have not profoundly altered the poor outcome of patients with gastric carcinoma [2]. This fact indicates that surgery alone may not be enough to control the disease. In 1978 we began a prospective randomized, one-center trial to determine, whether postoperative treatment with mitomycin C (MMC), 5-fluorouracil (5-FU), and cytosine-arabinoside (Ara-C) given for three courses could substantially improve the overall survival of patients treated by curative resection for gastric carcinoma. The regimen employed had been shown to be the most effective chemotherapy combination at the time the study started [3]. At a median follow-up of 5 years we found no significant effect of adjuvant chemotherapy on overall survival compared with an untreated control group. However, in a retrospective subgroup analysis we observed a significant improvement in the overall survival of patients with the intestinal tumor type, but no effect in patients with mucocellular carcinoma. We therefore believe that there is a selective effect of adjuvant chemotherapy in patients with gastric carcinoma with intestinal type of tumors.

Methods

Patients

Between 1978 and 1982, 102 patients with histologically proven adenocarcinoma of the stomach were entered in the trial after curative resection. Patients who had not sufficiently recovered by the end of 6 weeks postoperatively were excluded from the study. Further causes for ineligibility were age over 75, previous chemotherapy, other malignant diseases, serious medical or emotional problems, early stomach cancer (T_1, involvement of mucosa or submucosa exclusively), gastric cancer with peritoneal seedings, and microscopic tumor involvement of the resection line. Fifteen patients refused treatment after they had given their informed consent. Thus, results are available from 87 cases. The median observation time

Recent Results in Cancer Research, Vol. 110
© Springer-Verlag Berlin · Heidelberg 1988

was 5 years. Patients were followed up every 3 months with a complete physical examination, and blood chemistry was performed every 6 months. Additional follow-up investigations were done if indicated by the clinical course. Patients were followed up until death; no patient was lost to follow-up.

Criteria for recurrence were histologic proof or evidence of metastases on roentgenogram or CT-scan.

Surgical Procedures

In all patients a curative resection was defined as removal of all visible tumor by an en-bloc technique with removal of adjacent organs and tissues. In every patient lymph nodes around the celiac axis were removed and investigated by frozen section intraoperatively. Standard lymphadenectomy included all perigastric lymph nodes, nodes around the celiac axis, and the hepatoduodenal ligament.

In addition, the lesser and greater omentum were removed. Based on the operative specimen tumor stage, nodal involvement and type of tumor histology (intestinal type, mucocellular type) were recorded.

Stratification and Randomization

Patients who were sufficiently recovered from the surgical procedure were stratified prospectively according to the pathological tumor stage (T_2, T_3, T_4), nodal involvement (negative, positive) and tumor histology (intestinal, mucocellular type).

After giving informed consent, eligible patients were randomly allocated by the method of Pocock and Simon [4] to one of the following three groups:

1. Untreated controls
2. Chemotherapy
3. Chemoimmunotherapy

Chemotherapy consisted in the administration of 100 mg Ara-C orally on day 1. 2 mg/m^2 mitomycin C and 500 mg/m^2 5-FU i.v. was given on day 1 to day 4. Three cycles of this chemotherapy regimen were administered at 6-week intervals.

In the third group an identical chemotherapy protocol was combined with the administration of an unspecific immunostimulant OK-432 every 3 weeks after chemotherapy.

Drug doses were modified according to nadir platelet and leukocyte counts.

Statistical Evaluation

Survival functions were estimated according to the method of Kaplan and Meier [5]. Univariate analyses of various prognostic factors were based on Mantel's test [6].

Cox's proportional-hazard regression served to delineate factors independently effecting survival [7].

Table 1. Characteristics of 87 evaluable patients

	Number	(%)
Tumor stage		
T$_2$	25	(29)
T$_3$	37	(42)
T$_4$	25	(29)
Lymph node status		
N negativ	39	(45)
N positiv	48	(55)
Histology		
Intestinal	46	(53)
Mucocellular	41	(47)
Tumor localization		
Cardia	15	(17)
Corpus	35	(40)
Antrum	30	(34)
Gastric stump	7	(9)
Surgical procedure		
Distal resection	33	(38)
Proximal resection	8	(9)
Total gastrectomy	20	(23)
Extended total gastrectomy	26	(30)

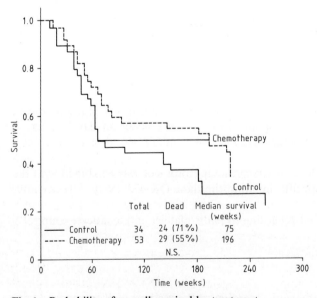

	Total	Dead	Median survival (weeks)
Control	34	24 (71%)	75
Chemotherapy	53	29 (55%)	196
N.S.			

Fig. 1. Probability of overall survival by treatment

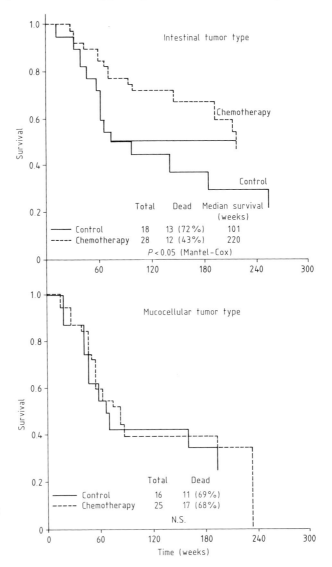

Fig. 2. Effect of treatment in patients with T_2 and T_3 and patients with T_4 lesions

Since survival data of patients treated with chemotherapy and chemoimmunotherapy showed identical behavior, we pooled these two groups together and compared them with the untreated controls.

Results

A total of 87 patients were evaluable; 54 were male and 33 female. The median age was 66 years, with a range from 36 to 75 years. Further patient characteristics are given in Table 1.

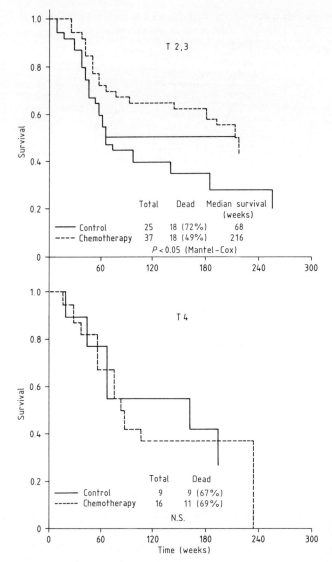

Fig. 3. Probability of overall survival by treatment and tumor histology

All Patients

During our observation period 53 patients (61%) have died. In Fig. 1 survival curves of patients treated with chemotherapy and controls are shown. Prognostic criteria in these two groups of patients were analyzed and proved to be reasonably well balanced. At 5 years we found a survival rate of 45% for patients treated with chemotherapy compared with 29% for the control group. This difference was not statistically significant. However, the median survival of 196 weeks for patients treated with chemotherapy seems to be much longer than that of 75 weeks for the control group.

Table 2. Significance of prognostic factors in the Cox model (all factors included), with Mantel's test and estimated median survival by the levels of the factors

Variables	P value		Estimated median suvival (in weeks)		
	Cox	Mantel			
Stage of primary tumor	0.0001	0.001	T_2 > 144	T_3 66	T_4 84
Lymph node status	0.15	0.08	N_+ 80	N_- 196	
Tumor histology	0.03	0.04	Intestinal 196	Mucocellular 72	
Adjuvant chemotherapy	0.1	0.13	Therapy 196	Control 75	

Table 3. Type of recurrence in all patients in relation to tumor histology

Type of recurrence	Type of histology	
	Intestinal	Mucocellular
Local	5	2
Peritoneal carcinosis	1	16 (70%)
Liver metastases	13 (68%)	4
Other	0	1
	$P < 0.0005$ (Pearson's χ^2)	

Subset Analysis

Tumor Stage. In a retrospective analysis we evaluated the effect of therapy by tumor stage (Fig. 2). In patients with T_2 and T_3 lesions we found a beneficial effect in the overall survival for patients treated with chemotherapy ($P < 0.05$). However, we did not find any impact on the survival rate of patients with T_4 lesions when treated with chemotherapy. It should be noted, of course, that the patient numbers are rather small in both groups.

Tumor Histology. Analyzing the relation between tumor histology and the relative effect of chemotherapy, we found a significantly higher survival rate in patients with the intestinal type treated with chemotherapy compared with untreated controls (Fig. 3). The median survival of these patients was prolonged to 220 weeks as compared with 101 in the control group. For patients with mucocellular carcinoma chemotherapy does not seem to influence survival.

Prognostic Factors. In a Cox regression analysis we investigated prognostic criteria in our patient material (Table 2). Tumor stage was found to be the most important prognostic parameter ($P < 0.001$), and the second most important was tumor histology ($P < 0.03$). Only these two parameters exhibited a significant influence on the overall survival of patients.

Finally, the type of tumor histology was correlated with the site of tumor recurrence (Table 3). In patients with intestinal tumors the majority (68%) developed liver metastases as the first sign of recurrence, whereas peritoneal carcinosis was the predominant form of recurrence in patients with mucocellular carcinoma (70%). This difference was shown to be statistically highly significant ($P < 0.0005$).

Discussion

In accordance with most other reports from Europe and the United States our results demonstrate no benefit of postoperative adjuvant chemotherapy in patients with gastric carcinoma.

The Gastrointestinal Tumor Study Group (GITSG) [8] was the only institution – aside from several Japanese groups – to demonstrate that combination chemotherapy exhibited superior results in the adjuvant setting. Unfortunately, two almost identical trials did not confirm this result [9, 10]. Furthermore, in a very recent report the most effective combination chemotherapy in metastatic gastric carcinoma to date (5-FU, doxorubicin, MMC) used in the adjuvant situation failed to show a significant improvement in the overall survival [11].

However, our results raise an important point: We found an obvious effect of adjuvant chemotherapy in patients with the intestinal tumor type and no effect in patients with the mucocellular type.

The adjuvant treatment prevented the occurrence of liver metastases in several patients with the intestinal tumor type, but it did not influence the incidence of peritoneal carcinosis as the most important form of recurrence in patients with mucocellular carcinoma. These results are in agreement with those of Imanaga and Nakazato [12], who used MMC as a single-drug chemotherapy. Unfortunately, these authors did not differentiate between the intestinal and the mucocellular tumor type. One possible explanation for the lack of efficacy of adjuvant systemic treatment in preventing peritoneal carcinosis might be an insufficient level of cytotoxic drugs to kill tumor cells in the peritoneal cavity. Jitsuka and co-workers [13] have shown a 30% occurrence of free cancer cells in the peritoneal cavity when the primary tumor invaded the serosa and a 65% incidence when the tumor invaded other organs. The viability of free cancer cells was high, but it could be remarkably suppressed by intraperitoneal administration of MMC. Therefore, our current adjuvant protocol employing local intraperitoneal delivery of cytotoxic drugs seems to be a reasonable way of addressing this point.

However, it must be noted that the number of patients in our study is rather small, and that the evaluation of a different effect of adjuvant chemotherapy in these two histological tumor types was done in a retrospective fashion. Since this is, to our knowledge, the first report which addresses a different effect of adjuvant chemotherapy in patients with different histological types of gastric carcinoma, results of further prospective randomized trials employing similar chemotherapy regimens and differentiation of similar histological tumor types have to be awaited before definite conclusions can be drawn.

References

1. Haenszel W (1958) Variation in incidence of and mortality from stomach cancer with particular reference to the United States. JNCI 21: 213–262
2. Buchholtz TW, Welch CE, Malt RA (1978) Clinical correlates of resectability and survival in gastric carcinoma. Ann Surg 188: 711–715
3. Ota K, Kunita S, Nishimura A (1972) Combination therapy with mitomycin C (CNSC-26980), 5-fluorouracil (NSC-19883), and cytosine arabinoside (NSC-63878) for advanced cancer in man. Cancer Chemother Rep 56: 373–385
4. Pocock SJ, Simon R (1975) Sequential treatment assignment with balancing for prognostic factors in the controlled clinical trial. Biometrics 31: 103–115
5. Kaplan EL, Meier P (1958) Nonparametric estimation from incomplete observations. J Am Stat Assoc 53: 457–481
6. Mantel N (1966) Evaluation of survival data and two new rank-order statistics arising in its consideration. Cancer Chemother Rep 50: 163–170
7. Cox DR (1972) Regression models and life tables. J R Stat Soc B 34: 187–220
8. The Gastrointestinal Tumor Study Group (1982) Controlled trial of adjuvant chemotherapy following curative resection for gastric cancer. Cancer 49: 1116–1122
9. Higgins GA, Amadeo JH, Smith DE, Humphrey EW, Keehn RJ (1983) Efficacy of prolonged intermittent therapy with combined 5-FU and methyl-CCNU following resection for gastric carcinoma. Cancer 52: 1105–1112
10. Engstrom PF, Lavin PT (1984) Adjuvant fluorouracil plus methyl-CCNU for resected gastric cancer: EST 3275. In: Jones SE, Salmon SE (eds) Adjuvant therapy of cancer IV. Grune and Stratton, New York, pp 449–455
11. Schein PS, Coombes RG, Chilvers C (1986) A controlled trial of FAM (5-FU, doxorubicin, and mitomycin C) chemotherapy as adjuvant treatment for resected gastric carcinoma. Proc. American Society of Clinical Oncology, no. 308
12. Imanaga H, Nakazato H (1977) Results of surgery for gastric cancer and effect of adjuvant mitomycin C on cancer recurrence. World J Surg 1: 213–221
13. Jitsuka Y, Kaneshima S, Tanida O, Takeuchi T, Koga S (1979) Intraperitoneal free cancer cells and their viability in gastric cancer. Cancer 44: 1476–1480

Combined 5-Fluorouracil and Radiation Therapy Following Resection of Locally Advanced Gastric Carcinoma: A 5-Years Follow-up

E. Gez, A. Sulkes, T. Peretz, and Z. Weshler

Department of Oncology, Hadassah University Hospital, Jerusalem 91120, Israel

The prognosis for patients with gastric carcinoma is poor; the overall 5-year survival is about 12% [1]. Surgery remains the mainstay of treatment for gastric carcinoma, and the results depend on the extent and penetration of the tumor into the stomach wall and the involvement of the regional lymph nodes. Analysis of the patterns by failure revealed that in up to 90% of cases there is evidence of locoregional recurrence [2]. It has been suggested that a combined modality approach, including the delivery of radiation therapy to the tumor bed concomitant with chemotherapy as an adjuvant to surgery, may eradicate microscopic residual disease, reduce the local recurrence rate, and improve survival [3].

In our present study we describe our experience with patients who had locally advanced but resectable gastric carcinoma who were treated with combined 5-FU and radiation therapy as an adjuvant to surgery.

Materials and Methods

A prospective study of combined radiochemotherapy as an adjuvant to surgery for locally advanced gastric cancer was initiated in November 1976 and the data were updated in January 1985. Patients have been followed up for a median of 60.0 months from surgery (range 16 to 110 months).

The treatment program included the delivery of external irradiation with a 6-MeV linear accelerator machine to the tumor bed and its lymph node-bearing areas, given in two opposed, anterior/posterior fields to a total dose of 5000 rads, with daily fractions of 200–250 rads each. The spine was shielded posteriorly after 4000 rads. In planning the radiotherapy we used a UGI study to determine the stomach and its lymph node-bearing areas. Treatment was given over 7 weeks, with a 2-week interval following the initial 2500 rads. 5-FU was administered by intravenous push 3 h before the irradiation at a dose of 500 mg daily during the first 3 days of each 2.5-week treatment period. Following completion of the radiotherapy, 5-FU was continued at weekly doses of 500 mg for a minimum of 1 year. Patients' pretreatment evaluation included physical examination, complete blood count, blood biochemistry, serum carcinoembryonic antigen, chest roentgenogram

Recent Results in Cancer Research, Vol. 110
© Springer-Verlag Berlin · Heidelberg 1988

and liver and bone scans. During treatment, blood counts and biochemistry were evaluated every 4 weeks. Chest roentgenography and liver scan were repeated every 4 months and UGI and endoscopic studies and an abdominal CT-scan were performed at the completion of treatment to document absence of disease activity.

Patients' Characteristics (Table 1)

Between November 1976 and September 1984, 27 patients with locally advanced gastric carcinoma were entered into the study (Table 1). There were 21 men and six women with a median age of 62 years. The primary tumor was located in the gastric body in ten patients, in the antrum in ten, and in the cardia in four; in three patients the tumor was multifocal. Twenty-three patients underwent subtotal gastrectomy and four proximal esophagogastrectomy. Splenectomy was also carried out in three patients.

Twenty-four patients had histologic evidence of regional lymph node metastases. Of the remaining three patients, two had microscopic evidence of residual tumor in the surgical margin and in one the tumor was multifocal and penetrated through the gastric wall.

The median time from surgery to the onset of adjuvant radiochemotherapy was 55 days (range 19–141). All patients had a good performance status at the onset of treatment.

Table 1. Patients' characteristics

Number of patients	27
Sex: male/female	21/6
Age (in years): median (range)	62 (24–74)
Location of primary tumor	
Body	10
Antrum	10
Cardia	4
Multifocal	3
Type of surgery	
Subtotal resection	23
Proximal esophagogastrectomy	4
Regional lymph node status	
Positive	24
Negative	3
Surgical margins' status	
Negative	16
Positive	8
Unknown	3

Table 2. Survival (months) by patient and tumor characteristics

Characteristic	No. of cases	Survival in months Median (Range)	
Age			
<60 years	12	23.5	(9–98+)
≥60 years	15	27	(11–94+)
Sex			
Male	21	19	(9–98+)
Female	6	31	(11–86+)
Tumor histology			
Moderately to well differentiated	19	27	(9–98+)
Anaplastic	8	23.5	(12–86+)
Tumor location			
Body	10	23	(11–84+)
Antrum	10	17	(9–62)
Cardia	4	63.5	(29–98+)
Multifocal	3	19	(16+–32+)
Lymph node status			
Positive	24	27.5	(9–98+)
Negative	3	19	(19–42)
Surgical margins status			
Tumor-free	16	23.5	(11–98+)
Infiltrated	8	28	(9–43+)
Unknown	3	19	(12–42+)
Degree of leukopenia to 5-FU			
<3000/mm^3	7	42	(16+–86+)
≥3000/mm^3	20	19	(9–98+)

Results

Survival

Survival data are summarized in Table 2 and Fig. 1. The median survival after surgery for the whole group was 27 months (range 9–98). Nine patients remain alive; six disease-free for a median of 62 months and three with disease for 53 months. Seventeen patients died, one of myocardial infarction 27 months after surgery, without clinical evidence of tumor activity, and the remaining 16 patients of gastric carcionoma after a median survival of 19 months. One patient was lost to follow-up.

We correlated the patients' and tumor characteristics with survival. No significant difference has been observed in median survival by age, sex, tumor histology, and lymph-node involvement and surgical margins' status. However, there was a difference in survival by the location of the tumor in the stomach. The median survival of patients with a tumor located in the cardia was 63 months as compared with 23 and 17 months in patients with a tumor located in the gastric body and in

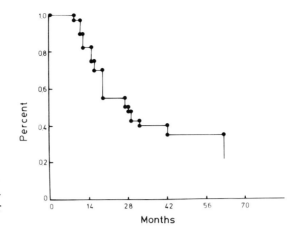

Fig. 1. Actuarial survival following "curative" resection and adjuvant radio- and chemotherapy for locally advanced gastric cancer

the antrum, respectively. There was a difference in survival by the degree of leukopenia induced by 5-FU treatment. The median survival for patients with WBC below $3000/mm^3$ was 42 months, as compared with 19 months for patients whose leukocyte count did not drop below $3000/mm^3$ during 5-FU treatment.

Nineteen patients relapsed at a median of 15 months from surgery (range 5–95). The sites of failure included the peritoneal cavity in ten patients, the liver in seven patients, the mediastinum in two patients, and the pleura and the skeleton in one patient each. In three patients there was local recurrence. The median survival of these 19 patients was 19 months (range 9–98) from surgery and 4 months from relapse.

Toxicity

The treatment was well tolerated. The main side effects occurred during the administration of radiotherapy and included weakness, anorexia, and nausea with vomiting.

The nadir of the leukocyte count ranged between 1900 and $5300/mm^3$ and of platelets between 40000 and $278000/mm^3$. There were no episodes of leukopenia with fever and no episodes of bleeding.

Discussion

A number of trials of adjuvant therapy following resection of gastric carcinoma have been published. In a randomized study the Veterans Administration Surgical Oncology Group found no significant difference in the 2-year survival between a group treated with 5-FU and methyl-CCNU and the control group following curative surgery for gastric carcinoma [4]. However, the Gastrointestinal Tumor Study Group used the same type of adjuvant chemotherapy following curative resection of gastric cancer and found an increase in survival for the treated group over controls [5]. In addition, the combination of chemotherapy with local irradiation (5000 rads) improved the survival of patients with locoregional gastric cancer which was not completely resected [4]. The Massachusetts General Hospital used a number of combination chemotherapy protocols with local irradiation as an adjuvant to curative surgery in gastric cancer; the median survival was 24 months, with 43% survival at 3 years [6].

Our patients represent a group at high risk for tumor recurrence, because regional lymph node involvement and surgical margin infiltration were found in 26 of 27 patients. Although this is a small group of patients and not a randomized study, the results of the local control and survival were encouraging.

In conclusion, the survival of our patients is similar to those in other studies using adjuvant radiochemotherapy following resection of locally advanced gastric cancer.

This combined modality may eradicate minimal residual disease. It may also improve survival and, finally, the morbidity is low.

References

1. Silverberg E (1984) Cancer statistics, 1984. CA 34: 7–23
2. MacDonald JS, Hunderson L, Cohn I (1982) Cancer of the stomach. In: DeVita VT, Hellman S, Rosenberg SA (eds) Cancer principles and practice of oncology. Lippincott, Philadelphia, pp 534–562
3. Douglass HO, Stablein DM (1982) Controlled trial of adjuvant chemotherapy following curative resection for gastric cancer. Cancer 49: 1116–1122
4. Higgins GA, Amadeo JH, Smith DE et al. (1983) Efficacy of prolonged intermittent therapy with combined 5-FU and methyl-CCNU following resection for gastric carcinoma: a Veterans Administration Surgical Oncology Group Report. Cancer 52: 1105–1112
5. Schein PS, Stablein DM, Novak JW, Bruckner HW, et al., for the GITSG (1982) A comparison of combination chemotherapy and combined modality therapy for locally advanced gastric carcinoma. Cancer 49: 1771–1777
6. Gunderson LL, Hoskin RB, Cohen AC, et al. (1983) Combined modality treatment of gastric cancer. Int J Radiat Oncol Biol Phys 9: 965–975

The Value of a Multidisciplinary Approach in the Management of Gastric Cancer

J. W. L. Fielding

Consultant Surgeon, Queen Elizabeth Hospital, Birmingham, Great Britain

Carcinoma of the stomach is the most common cause of death in Japan, Finland, Chile and the U.S.S.R. It was thought to be decreasing in incidence, but a recent necroscopy study from Norway has cast serious doubt on this, as the histologically proven incidence has been constant over a 15-year period [1]. In the United Kingdom carcinoma of the stomach remains a common condition, accounting for over 10000 deaths a year. In the West Midlands, a multidisciplinary approach to the management of this disease has been developed over a 20-year period. The basic data for this work have been collected by the Birmingham Cancer Registry. Between 1957 and 1976, 25255 patients with gastric cancer were registered and the 5-year survival is 5% (Fig. 1). An analysis of these patients by quinquennium and sex (Figs. 2 and 3) shows that there has been no change in the results of the management of this condition over this period.

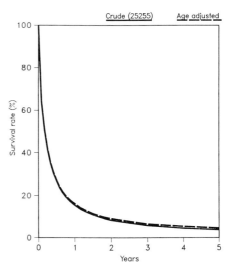

Fig. 1. Survival for gastric cancer cases in the West Midlands

Recent Results in Cancer Research, Vol. 110
© Springer-Verlag Berlin · Heidelberg 1988

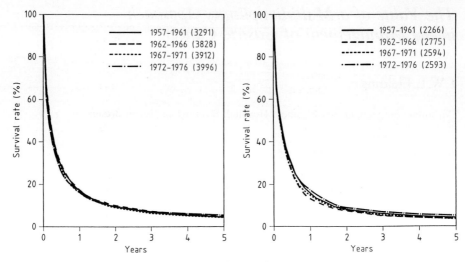

Fig. 2 *(left).* Survival of male patients by quinquennium

Fig. 2 *(right).* Survival of female patients by quinquennium

Current Treatment

The Registry data document the types of treatment that have been used during this period: these have been classified as "curative", "palliative" and "no treatment" (Table 1). It can be seen that 42.5% of patients receive no specific anti-cancer therapy, and in the remainder, the mainstay of treatment has been surgery, with a limited number receiving either chemotherapy or radiotherapy.

Surgery

There are no randomised studies of the benefits of surgery. The results for "curative" and "palliative" treatments can be seen in Figs. 4 and 5, and these can be compared with those for laparotomy alone or no treatment in Fig. 6. The survival is best among those undergoing curative resection. The difference between the partial and total gastrectomy groups can be accounted for by a 20% operative mortality for a curative total gastrectomy. There is no doubt that of the treatment options available, surgery appears to produce the best results. However, the results are stage dependent. The Birmingham staging system [2] is similar to that described by the TNM, and the results by stage are demonstrated in Fig. 7. Curative surgery has been undertaken (stages I–III) in 20% of Registry cases.

Table 1. Type of treatment: Distribution

	No. of patients	%
Curative		
Total gastrectomy	984	3.9
Total gastrectomy + adjuvant therapy	12	0.1
Partial gastrectomy	4006	15.9
Partial gastrectomy + adjuvant therapy	48	0.2
Palliative		
Total gastrectomy	356	1.4
Partial gastrectomy	1747	6.9
Bypass	1892	7.5
Tube with laparotomy	512	2.0
Tube only	249	1.0
Laparotomy + adjuvant therapy	261	1.0
Radiotherapy/chemotherapy	221	0.9
Other		
Laparotomy only	4106	16.2
Treatment not to primary tumor	131	0.5
No treatment	10744	42.5
Total	25269	100.0

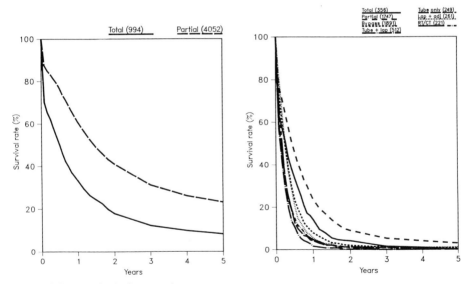

Fig. 4 *(left).* Survival after curative gastrectomy

Fig. 5 *(right).* Survival after palliative treatment

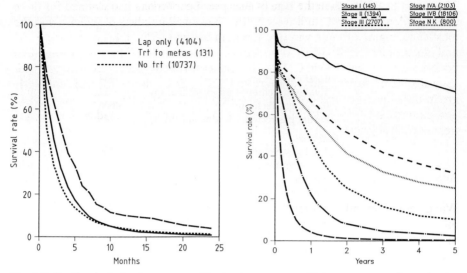

Fig. 6 *(left).* Survival after laparotomy *(Lap)* only, treatment *(Trt)* to metastases *(metas)* only, or no treatment

Fig. 7 *(right).* Overall survival by stage. *NK*, not known

Non-surgical Treatment

The advanced stage of disease at presentation has excluded many patients from the chance of having curative surgery, and the stage-dependant results of surgery are such that it has become imperative to explore other possible treatments for this malignancy. In the mid 1970s there were many reports suggesting that chemotherapy might have a useful part to play. Many trials were uncontrolled and were based on an inadequate evaluation of response prior to commencing the trial. Even the published randomised trials could be criticised as follows:

1. The numbers are too small in each group (to have 95% chance showing 20% difference requires over 100 patients in each group).
2. Response rate is used as an end point, rather than survival. The response rate is notoriously difficult to assess in gastric cancer and has rarely been related to a significant benefit in survival.

In the West Midlands chemotherapy has been evaluated in both advanced disease and as an adjuvant to curative surgery. The first trial [3] was based solely in the West Midlands and was a double-blind trial of 5-fluorouracil (20 mg/kg i.v. weekly) and methyl-CCNU (125 mg/m^2 every 6–10 weeks p.o.) versus a placebo. The groups were stratified for age and length of history but not for performance status. However, the two groups were found to be equivalent in this respect. There were 100 patients in each group and no survival advantage was found. A review of the major randomised studies of combination chemotherapy in advanced gastric cancer [4] showed that this was the only study which had 100 patients in each group.

This failed to substantiate the benefit that previous workers had claimed for these drugs [5, 6]. More recent studies have often had small numbers of patients and the most encouraging of these was that reported by the GITSG [7] comparising 5-FU and doxorubicin with 5-FU, doxorubicin and methyl-CCNU and with 5-FU, doxorubicin and mitomycin C. With 241 patients randomised, there was a statistically significant survival advantage for the 5-FU, doxorubicin and methyl-CCNU group over the 5-FU and doxorubicin group but not over the 5-FU, doxorubicin and mitomycin C group. Unfortunately, this, like many other studies, had no untreated control group.

Adjuvant Therapy

When most currently reported adjuvant studies were established in the 1970s, there was general optimism that drugs only partially effective in advanced disease might still be effective in an adjuvant setting. The West Midlands joined the British Stomach Cancer Group in a study of 411 patients randomised into a trial to receive either long-term (up to 2 years) mitomycin C and 5-FU with an induction course of 5-FU, cyclophosphamide, vincristine and methotrexate (group B), 5-FU and mitocycin C alone (group C) or a placebo (group A).

Stratification was for age, sex, length of history and stage, and the groups proved to be well matched. In the preliminary report of this study there was no benefit from received adjuvant chemotherapy [8]. The study also demonstrated 16 drug-related deaths, 11 of which were due to a haemolytic uraemic syndrome. An update of this study (Fig. 8) confirms the earlier results and demonstrates that no benefit accrued from chemotherapy over a longer period of follow-up.

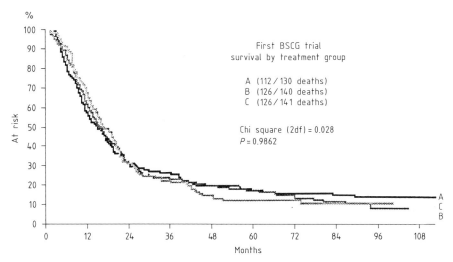

Fig. 8. Results of chemotherapy. *BSCG,* British Stomach Cancer Group; *A,* placebo group; *B,* 5-FU and mitomycin C plus cyclophosphamide, vincristine and methotrexate; *C,* 5-FU and mitomycin C alone

There have been many other studies of adjuvant chemotherapy in gastric cancer and these are extensively reviewed by Hockey and Fielding [4] and Jones [9]. Most of these studies are in agreement with the result demonstrated by the British Stomach Cancer Group, though the combinations of drugs that had been used were different. It is encouraging that most adjuvant studies have included a control group and that significant numbers of patients have been randomised. Perhaps the most important of these, which originated in Japan [4, 10–12], demonstrated an improvement in survival. Mitomycin C, FT207 and 5-FU seem to be the drugs most frequently associated with improvement in survival.

Radiotherapy

There are no randomised trials of radiotherapeutic regimes in advanced disease, but an excellent case has been made for adjuvant radiotherapy [13]. The British Stomach Cancer Group commenced its second adjuvant study in 1981. Patients were randomised into one of three groups: a control group, patients who were to receive mitomycin C, adriamycin and 5-FU, and a radiotherapy group. Entry into this study has now been closed after the randomisation of over 400 patients, and early results are awaited.

Screening for Gastric Cancer

At the same time that chemotherapeutic agents were being evaluated, there were major advances in diagnostic technology, particularly the development of the double-contrast barium meal and the fibro-optic endoscope. Clearly, the results of surgery were stage dependent and it was proposed that if the number of patients receiving treatment for stage-I gastric cancer could be increased, this would significantly improve the results of treatment. The Japanese have fostered this hypothesis and provided convincing evidence that this early-diagnosis approach is the most important development in the management of gastric cancer [14]. Early detection programmes for gastric cancer were started in 1960. In Japan about 3–4 million people have been screened annually by mass radiology, and the programme is thought to have screened 9% of the population between the ages of 14 and 69 and to have achieved a detection rate of 1:1000. Long-term results demonstrate that the 5- and 10-year survival is significantly higher for gastric cancer cases detected by mass screening than for cases detected in outpatient clinics. The follow-up results show a significantly lower cancer-adjusted death rate among screened compared with unscreened patients: in men this was 61.9 of 38 377,5 screened person years versus 137.2 of 20 653.0 screened years and in women 28.1 of 48 888.5 screened person years versus 53.8 of 21 579.5 unscreened person years. Hirayama [14] also reports on the gastric cancer death rate from 1969–1972 to 1973–1977 in 14 municipalities having an average screening rate of 17.7%. This was compared with that of 28 randomly selected comparable controlled municipalities having an average screening rate of 7.7%. The death rate from gastric cancer decreased by 25.5% in high-screening areas.

This suggests that surgery in the early stage of disease is able to influence natural history. However, a detection rate of 1:1000 in a country with a high incidence of gastric cancer is unlikely to be cost-effective when transferred to other countries with a lower incidence. For screening to be applicable in other areas it is necessary to define high-risk groups: particular attention should be given to symptomatic patients with predisposing conditions (pernicious anaemia and a previous gastrectomy for a benign condition) and precancerous lesions (chronic atrophic gastritis, intestinal metaplasia and dysplasia) [15]. Such a study has been initiated in the West Midlands [16]. Dyspepsia clinics have been established in a population of 60000, allowing the referral and diagnosis by endoscopy of patients to be made within 2 weeks of presentation to their family doctor. Endoscopy is repeated in patients with gastric ulcers, intestinal metaplasia, chronic atrophic gastritis or dysplasia. The results of the first 683 patients have been reported and the pick-up rate of gastric cancer is 1:50 patients screened. The incidence of stage-I disease is 14%, and 67% of the patients have disease suitable for curative surgery. This latter figure is to be compared with the 20% of patients undergoing curative surgery in the West Midlands (Table 1).

The Multidisciplinary Approach

The data presented have outlined the multidisciplinary approach to gastric cancer, particularly as seen in the West Midlands of Great Britain. Certain features become clear, particularly the importance of a regionally based cancer registry that provides data on a condition as managed in a population. This provides important baseline information against which all further therapies must be judged. These type of data can be collected only with the co-operation of epidemiologists, surgeons, physicians, pathologists and radiation oncologists. They also provide indicators of future therapeutic strategies. Also important are the stage-dependent survival curves and the need to diagnose the disease at an early stage.

The therapeutic mainstay in gastric cancer is surgery, and to date it seems that this is the only therapy capable of influencing survival. Chemotherapy has been extensively evaluated, and the only consistently reported positive results have been seen with chemotherapy as an adjuvant to surgery. Certainly, none of the modern therapeutic agents appear to influence advanced disease. Despite some conflicting results, it does appear that the agents mitomycin C, FT207 and 5-fluorouracil are worthy of further study as adjuvants to surgery. However, it is quite clear that there is no place for these cytotoxic agents outside of controlled prospective clinical trials.

References

1. Maartmann-Moe H, Martveit F (1985) On the reputed decline in gastric carcinoma; necroscopy study from Western Norway. Br Med 290: 103–105
2. Fielding JWL, Roginsk C, Ellis DJ, Jones BG, Powell J, Waterhouse JAH, Brookes VS (1984) Clinicopathological staging of gastric cancer. Br J Surg 71: 677–680

3. Kingston RD, Ellis DJ, Powell J, Brookes VS, Waterhouse JAH, Hurst MD, Smith JA (1978) The West Midlands gastric carcinoma chemotherapy trials: planning and results. Clin Oncol 4: 55–69
4. Hockey MJ, Fielding JWL (1986) In: Stevin ML, Staquet MJ (eds) Gastric cancer in randomised trials in cancer: a critical review by sites. Raven, New York, pp 221–240
5. Kovach J, Moertel C, Schutt A, Hahn P, Reitemeier R (1974) A controlled study of 1, 3,-B 15 (2 chloroethyl)-1-nitrosourea and 5-fluorouracil therapy for advanced gastric cancer and pancreatic cancer. Cancer 33: 563–567
6. Mortel CG, Mittelman JA, Bagemeier RF et al. (1976) Sequential and combination chemotherapy of advanced gastric cancer. Cancer 38: 678–682
7. Gastrointestinal Tumour Study Group (1982) A comparative clinical assessment of combination chemotherapy in the management of advanced gastric carcinoma. Cancer 49: 1362–1366
8. Fielding JWL, Fagg SL, Jones BG, Ellis D, Hockey MS, Minawa A, Brookes et al. (1983) An interim report of a prospective, randomised, controlled study of adjuvant chemotherapy in operable gastric cancer. British Stomach Cancer Group. World J Surg 7: 390–399
9. Jones BG (1986) In: Fielding JWL, Priestman TJ (eds) Therapeutic options: chemotherapy in gastrointestinal oncology. Castle House, Tunbridge Wells, pp 26–40
10. Imanaga H, Nakazoto H (1977) Results of surgery for gastric cancer and the effect of adjuvant mitomycin C on cancer recurrence. World J Surg 1: 213–227
11. Kondo T, Inokuchi K, Hattori T et al. (1982) Multihospital randomised study on adjuvant chemotherapy with mitomycin C and Futraful for gastric cancer v estimation of 5-year survival rate. Gan To Kagaku Ryoho 9: 2016–2024
12. Fujimoto S, Akao T et al. (1977) Protracted oral chemotherapy with fluorinated pyrimidines as an adjuvant to surgical treatment for stomach cancer. Ann Surg 1985: 462–466
13. Gunderson LL, Sosin H (1982) Adenocarcinoma of the stomach: areas of failure in a reoperation series (second or symptomatic look)-clinicopathological correlation and implications for adjuvant therapy. Int J Radiat Oncol Biol Phys 8: 1–11
14. Hirayama T (1984) Gastric carcinoma. In: Bouchier J, Allan R, Hodgson H, Keighley MRB (eds) Textbook of gastroenterology. Bailliere Tindall, Eastbourne, pp 219–224
15. Fielding JWL (1984) Non-radiological screening. Clin Oncol 3 (2): 259–271
16. Allum WH, Hallissey MT, Dorrell A, Low J, Fielding JWL (1986) Programme for early detection of gastric cancer. Br Med J 293: 541

The Approach to Hepatobiliary-Pancreatic Cancer

Approach to Primary Liver Cancer

R. Pichlmayr, B. Ringe, W. O. Bechstein, W. Lauchart, and P. Neuhaus

Klinik für Abdominal- und Transplantationschirurgie, Medizinische Hochschule Hannover, Konstanty-Gutschow-Straße 8, 3000 Hannover 61, FRG

Primary malignant liver tumor is the most frequent malignoma worldwide. This is due mainly to a high incidence in Asian and African countries. Particularly in these countries, but also in Europe and other continents, most hepatocellular carcinomas are associated with liver cirrhosis. In contrast to this high frequency, therapeutic experience with hepatocellular or cholangiocellular carcinomas has been very limited, at least in Europe. This is not only because of the relative infrequency of this tumor in our countries in comparison with other malignancies; such tumors were generally diagnosed very late and liver resection therapy was uncommon, particularly in cirrhotic but also in non-cirrhotic patients. Similarly, experience with non-surgical methods is limited. This situation has changed in part within the past few years: ultrasonography and CT scanning, as well as the determination of alpha-fetoprotein, have significantly increased the number of diagnosed tumors and have enabled diagnosis in earlier stages. More specific methods of liver surgery have been developed and, finally, liver grafting was added. Many other approaches for therapy were also instituted. Thus, therapeutic access to a primary liver malignoma became more frequent.

The general theme of this symposium is combined therapy. Thus, this paper should also give an overview of combination therapies, strategies for combination, etc., but this appears very difficult today: It seems that we have too few exact data on the success rate and indication for each individual therapy. This is particularly so in comparison with other cancers: For example, in gastric or colonic cancer we know how to resect the tumor, we know the 5-year survival rates according to stage, and we have good evidence for the response rate of chemotherapy. Thus, we can consider combinations of treatments for these tumors and calculate how effective these combinations are. With liver tumors, in contrast, it appears that we are just beginning to clarify the worth of individual therapies. There have been reports about combined efforts, but up to now these appear preliminary, and results will depend largely on the performance of each individual therapy, for example on how surgery is done, and not so much on the effect of the combinations used. Moreover, the fact that most liver tumors are associated with cirrhosis renders a combined approach difficult, and the final outcome may depend on the tumor as well as on the underlying disease.

Recent Results in Cancer Research, Vol. 110
© Springer-Verlag Berlin · Heidelberg 1988

Table 1. Natural course of primary hepatocellular carcinoma without therapy. (From Okuda [14])

Stage	n	Survival (%)				
		3	6	12	24	36 months
I	23	80	70	35	10	0
II	90	30	10	5	<5	<5
III	56	0	–	–	–	–

Staging	Factor	pos.	neg.
I mildly advanced (factors 1–4 neg.)	1 Ascites	+	–
II moderately advanced (factors 1–2 pos.)	2 Tumor size	>50%	<50%
	3 Albumin	<3 g/dl	>3 g/dl
III very advanced (factors 3–4 pos.)	4 Bilirubin	<3 mg/dl	>3 mg/dl

A further difficulty in judging results of the different modes of treatment lies in the fact that too little is known about the natural history and course of a malignant liver tumor. It is well known from several historical studies that the overall prognosis is very limited; however, the published data about survival times refer mainly to patients in whom the tumor has been diagnosed based on massive symptoms and who thus were already in a very late stage of the disease. Very short survival times of 3–6 months after diagnosis are true mainly for tumors diagnosed in such an advanced stage. Only recently there have been a few reports about survival time in patients with smaller tumors, particularly cirrhotic patients with subclinical hepatocellular carcinoma [15], but no comparative observations have been reported on non-cirrhotic patients.

A third difficulty concerns the missing staging and classification of malignant liver tumors[1]. There are some proposals for a classification according to tumor size, tumor extent, and clinical science [14] (Table 1), but these classifications are not in common use. Thus, all results of treatment of primary liver malignomas are preliminary. This is particularly true of non-surgical, chemotherapeutic, or immunotherapeutic methods; for surgery more experience has been accumulated and published within the past few years. The following is an overview of surgical therapy for malignant liver tumors.

Liver Malignancy in Cirrhotic Patients

On the whole, the therapeutic situation seems very unfavorable. It is well known that major liver surgery is highly complicated and dangerous in cirrhotic livers. This is due to intraoperative difficulties, mainly those of pronounced blood loss and of clotting problems, as well as to the danger of liver insufficiency through in-

---

[1] At the time of printing, a new edition of the "TNM classification of malignant tumors" (P. Hermanek and L. H. Sobin, eds.) was used, which now comprises for the first time TNM staging of liver tumors.

competence of the remaining liver tissue. While the former problem may be ameliorated by improvement of technique, at least in some cases, the latter problem is always existent. When planning a resection it is desirable to measure or calculate the functional capacity of the cirrhotic liver. The loss of functioning liver through surgery must of course be considered. Several proposals for such a calculation have been made – recently, for example, by Bismuth et al. [4]. Briefly, if liver function tests – particularly clotting factors and cholinesterase values – are normal, some typical method of liver resection may be applicable; if they are pathologic, larger resections are excluded. This means that any larger tumor in a cirrhotic liver in an advanced stage of disease will not be resectable. However, resection of a smaller tumor in a cirrhotic liver, if done as a typical lobectomy, is also highly dangerous. Thus, the concept of segmentectomy or subsegmentectomy has been elaborated, particularly in Asian countries. Further studies are necessary to determine whether these smaller resections are feasible for the majority of cirrhotic tumor patients and are sufficiently radical for a malignant tumor. Data available at present, particularly in Europe, are preliminary [4]. It must be stated that all types of resections in cirrhotic patients have been performed more frequently and with higher success rates in Asian countries than in Europe or the USA.

Other therapeutic modalities are also hindered by the cirrhotic state. Chemoembolization may offer some chance for palliation. Apparently, systemic chemotherapy is not particularly effective in these tumors, and the required dosage may be dangerous because of liver insufficiency.

Liver Malignancy in Non-cirrhotic Patients

The situation of hepatic malignancy in the absence of cirrhosis is better for all kinds of therapy, particularly for surgery. In non-cirrhotic livers typical large anatomical resections such as lobectomies, hemihepatectomies, or enlarged hemihepatectomies can be performed without significant danger of liver insufficiency. Because they are radical these typical resections are preferred. Technically, this means the primary isolation and ligation of the hilar vessels, followed by the dissection of hepatic veins and finally of liver tissue. When the tumor is located near another segment, an appropriately enlarged resection seems justified to obtain at least a 2–3 cm distance between the tumor and the resection line. During resection, clamping of the remaining hilar structures seems worth while to reduce blood loss; clamping can be done without severe damage to the liver for at least 45–60 min; in most cases the ischemic period is much shorter.

Results of liver resection in non-cirrhotic patients are much superior to those in cirrhotics (Table 2). The postoperative mortality has decreased in recent years. This and other results support the view that liver resection significantly prolongs the median survival time of these patients, is the most effective treatment, and can cure a small percentage of patients. This statement seems justified, although exact comparative figures are missing (see above). Thus, surgery is always the first choice of treatment, if at all possible. But the frequency of recurrence and metastases makes trials of a multimodality treatment necessary. So far, little has been contributed to this question.

Table 2. Results of hepatic resection for primary liver malignancies. Untreated ("natural course") (Asia, America, Europe) survival time is 2–6 months

Author, Year	No. of patients	Operative mortality (%)	Survival time – years (%)				
			1	2	3	4	5
Foster (1977) [4] Asian patients	365	21			23		7
Non-Asian patients	149	19			61		35
Foster (1974) cirrhotics	10	Excluding operative			25		0
"LTS" non-cirrhotics	77	mortality	83	72	60	42	34
Lin (1973/1976) [11]	118	11.8	35	24	20		19
Lee and Wong (1982) [10]	165	20.0	45	30	20		20
Wu (1980) [16]	181	8.8	56	37	39		16
Almersjö et al. (1976) [2]	46	30			31		
Bengmark et al. (1982) [3]	21	14.3	47.6	38			
Fortner et al. (1978/1981) [7]	42	16.7	85		50		37
Adson and Weiland (1981) [1]	60	6.7			65		36
Iwatsuki et al. (1983) [9]	43	9.3	78	60	56		46
Okamoto et al. (1984) [13]	90		65		26.7		13.3
Zirngibl and Gebhardt (1983) [17]	53	41.5	~20	~15	~10	7	7
Funovics and Fritsch (1983) [8]	25	24	20	9	9		
Own results (1.1.86)							
HCC overall	62	13	72	54	49	42	42
HCC + cirrh. excluded	54	6	79	63	58	49	49

Personal Experience

As many tumors in the liver are found today by routine ultrasonography, a differential diagnosis between benign and malignant tumors is essential. During the past few years we have found that with a combination of ultrasonography, angio-CT scanning, and scintiphotographic methods, a differentiation between focal nodular hyperplasia and hemangioma on the one side and all other tumors (adenoma and malignoma) on the other side is feasible, with a high degree of reliability [5].

Sixty-five hepatocellular carcinomas (45 male, 20 female patients) were resected at Medizinische Hochschule Hannover during the period from 1974 through 1985. Details on the operative technique used in these cases will be published elsewhere.

The results support the views mentioned above. There is a particularly high postoperative mortality among the few patients with hepatocellular carcinomas in

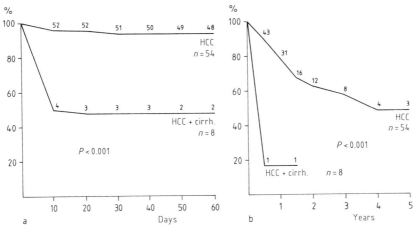

Fig. 1a, b. Survival after liver resection for hepatocellular carcinoma *(HCC)* for 62 patients with complete follow-up, 1974 through 1 January 1986, Medizinische Hochschule Hannover. **a** Operative; **b** long-term

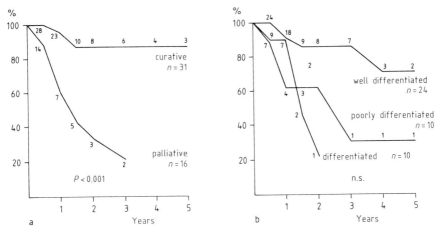

Fig. 2a, b. Long-term survival (>60 days) for 48 noncirrhotic patients. **a** Palliative vs. curative resections, $n=47$ (one classification missing); **b** according to histological grading of tumor, $n=44$ (four gradings missing)

cirrhotic liver; the resections in severely cirrhotic livers were done in the earlier years of our experience, and large anatomical resections in cirrhotic livers are no longer performed unless liver function tests are normal or nearly normal. In contrast, operative mortality in patients without cirrhosis is about 6%. The overall short- and long-term survival is presented in Fig. 1.

If only the tumors in non-cirrhotic livers are studied more closely and operative mortality is excluded, some differences in prognosis can be seen (Figs. 2, 3); there is some evidence that tumor size might be a relevant factor, although this differ-

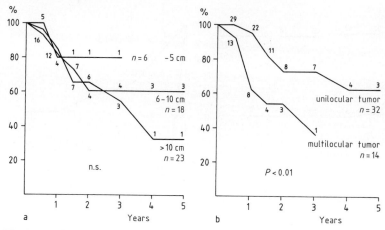

Fig. 3a, b. Survival after liver resection for hepatocellular carcinoma: $n = 47$, patients with cirrhosis and operative mortality excluded. **a** According to tumor size; **b** according to number of tumor nodes

ence has not reached statistical significance so far. The same is true for histological gradings of the tumor. There was a statistically significant difference in the outcome between unilocular and multilocular tumors and between curative and palliative resections. A resection has been classified as palliative if positive lymph nodes were found and were incompletely resected or not resected, and/or if the margin of tumor resection in liver parenchyma was not tumor free or was directly contiguous to tumor tissue.

Role of Liver Grafting in Primary Hepatic Malignancy

While liver grafting is not justified at the moment in liver tumors which can be resected – although multilocular tumor genesis or early intrahepatic recurrences of these tumors lead us to consider this possibility – it may be justified in non-resectable liver tumors, because, or as long as, any other effective mode of treatment is lacking. This indication for liver grafting has been used at most liver transplant centers, particularly in Pittsburgh, Denver, Cambridge, and Hannover. We have performed liver grafting in 31 patients; 16 of these had hepatocellular carcinoma with cirrhosis, and 15 had a noncirrhotic liver (Fig. 4). Not too surprisingly, overall results in our experience are very limited regarding long-term survival. The 2-year survival rate in our series is 34% in the group without cirrhosis and 6% in the group with cirrhosis. There are two main reasons for death: particularly in the cirrhotic group there is a high mortality, partly due to our lack of experience and partly due to the severe illness of these patients. But most deaths are due to early recurrence of the tumor. One should bear in mind that the tumor stage is nearly always very late, as the resectable tumors are excluded. The exception would be a smaller tumor in a cirrhotic liver which cannot be resected because of functional abnormalities of the liver.

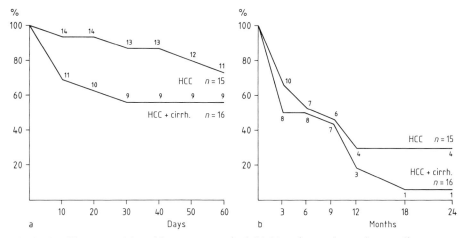

Fig. 4a, b. Short-term (**a**) and long-term survival (**b**) 31 patients who underwent liver transplantation for hepatocellular carcinoma *(HCC)*

While overall results are unsatisfactory, individual long-term survivors show the potential of this treatment under suitable conditions. An example is our patient with the longest survival after liver grafting, at present over 12 years; she suffered from a huge hepatocellular carcinoma. There will be differences between different kinds of tumors regarding the chance for cure or longer survival by liver grafting. Some preliminary scale for this chance may be given on the basis of worldwide and personal experience with hepatocellular carcinomas: those of the fibrolamellar type appear to be superior to all other kinds of tumors; liver grafting because of cholangiocellular-type tumors has always been followed by an early recurrence. So far, however, these prognostic scales are preliminary, as greater experience with individual tumors and tumor stages is needed. In particular, many of the transplant patients already had positive lymph nodes or other extrahepatic tumor manifestations which could not be diagnosed prior to operation or during operation. For the future we must work out a more precise characterization of liver tumors with regard to prognosis, particularly that for liver grafting. In addition to there being some hope for cure, it should be stressed that the palliative effect for patients who suffer from huge tumors may be excellent, at least for several months or perhaps for years. Of course, a liver transplantation is a major procedure for a palliative aim, but this may sometimes be justified.

Conclusions

Improved techniques in liver surgery have introduced liver resection procedures for primary and, even more, for secondary malignant tumors into many hospitals. The indications are steadily expanding. The most significant change from historical results is a reduction of mortality and morbidity after liver resection. Although some favorable results may be obtained by surgery in hepatocellular tumors, many patients will have recurrence. Thus, there is a need for an efficient multimodality treatment. What is the situation at present? We are just beginning to accumulate exact data from comparative and cooperative studies. More are urgently needed. A prerequisite would be a comparable staging and perhaps grading of tumors and patient situations.

In cirrhotics the roles of surgery and other methods seem very limited. If regular examinations of cirrhotic patients enabled the diagnosis of subclinical hepatocellular carcinomas in the west as it does in Asia, the performance of segmentectomies or subsegmentectomies might be one possibility. But preliminary experience indicates that these minor resections might also have significant dangers and perhaps only a small chance of curing the tumor.

Given the situation, more liberal indications for liver grafting for hepatocellular carcinoma in cirrhotic patients might be considered, even – or particularly – if these tumors are small and diagnosed early. If the condition of the patients is "elective" for liver grafting, mortality will not be too high, and cure or at least long-term survival might be possible. This approach would cover the possibility of multifocal tumor genesis and would cure the cirrhotic status of the patient. Further experience with such tumors is extremely important. It is most unfortunate that the country which could clarify this question in a short time and which has all technical and scientific prerequisites for liver grafting, namely Japan, is not yet able to perform it because brain death is not an accepted legal definition of death, and thus livers cannot be harvested from heart-beating donors.

In non-cirrhotic patients surgery plays the major role. Apparently, surgery is highly effective in smaller tumors, i.e., in those tumors which can be resected radically. In all other situations, particularly with combinations of multilocular tumors, large tumors or palliative resections, any type of combined approach should be investigated, because the prognosis with surgery alone is very poor.

Thus, finally, the present status – as also this paper – represents more the search for an appropriate approach by mutual discussion than a final concept.

References

1. Adson MA, Weiland LH (1981) Resection of primary solid hepatic tumors. Am J Surg 141: 18–21
2. Almersjö O, Bengmark S, Hafström L (1976) Liver resection for cancer. Acta Chir Scand 142: 139–144
3. Bengmark S, Hafström L, Jeppsson B, Sundquist K (1982) Primary carcinoma of the liver: improvement in sight? World J Surg 6: 54–60
4. Bismuth H, Houssin D, Ornowski J, Meriggi F (1986) Liver resections in cirrhotic patients: a Western experience. World J Surg 10: 311–317
5. Creutzig H, Brölsch C, Gratz K, Neuhaus P, Müller S, Schober O, Lang W, Hundeshagen H, Pichlmayr R (1984) Nuklearmedizinische Differentialdiagnostik intrahepatischer Raumforderungen. Dtsch Med Wochenschr 109: 861–863
6. Foster JH, Berman MM (1977) Solid liver tumors. In: Major problems in clinical surgery, vol 22, Saunders, Philadelphia, pp 62–104
7. Fortner JG, Kim DK, MacLean BJ, Barrett MK, Iwatsuki S, Turnbull AD, Howland WS, Beattie EI jr (1978) Major hepatic resection for neoplasia: personal experience in 108 patients. Ann Surg 188: 363–370

8. Funovics I, Fritsch A (1983) Leberresektionen bei primären Tumoren und Metastasen. In: Häring R (ed) Chirurgie der Leber. edition medizin, Weinheim, pp 237–245
9. Iwatsuki S, Shaw BW, Starzl TE (1983) Experience with 150 liver resections. Ann Surg 197: 247–253
10. Lee NW, Wong I, Ong GB (1982) The surgical management of primary carcinoma of the liver. World J Surg 6: 66–75
11. Lin TY (1973) Results in 107 hepatic lobectomies, with a preliminary report on the use of clamp to reduce blood loss. Ann Surg 177: 413–421
13. Okamoto E, Tanaka N, Yamanaka N, Toyosaka A (1984) Results of surgical treatments of primary hepatocellular carcinoma: some aspects to improve long-term survival. World J Surg 8: 360–366
14. Okuda K, Obata H, Nakajima Y, Ohtsuki T, Okazaki N, Onishi K (1984) Prognosis of primary hepatocellular carcinoma. Hepatology 4 [Suppl]: 3–6
15. Tang ZY (ed) (1985) Subclinical hepatocellular carcinoma. Springer, Berlin Heidelberg New York Tokyo
16. Wu MC (1978) Resection of primary hepatic carcinoma during a period of 18 years. Reprint from the First Affiliated Hospital of the Second Military Medical College, Shanghai, China
17. Zirngibl H, Gebhardt C (1983) Ergebnisse der operativen Therapie maligner Lebertumoren. In: Häring T (ed) Chirurgie der Leber. edition medizin, Weinheim, pp 229–235

Biliary Duct Cancer: Therapeutic Nihilism or Prospect

S. Bengmark

Institutionen för Kirurgi, Lunds Universitet, 22185 Lund, Sweden

Infection and Stasis Predispose for Cancer

Bile duct cancer is as frequent as cancer of the tongue. The number of cases detected each year is increasing. It is not clear whether this is a true reflection of increase in incidence or a consequence of better methods for imaging the biliary tree in obstructive jaundice. Benign tumors in the biliary tract do exist, but the overwhelming majority of tumors resulting in obstruction of the bile duct are malignant. In more than 90% of cases these tumors are cholangiocarcinomas and are often located at the confluence of the bile ducts. Its etiology is unknown, but the disease is frequently seen in patients with chronic suppurative cholangitis, in patients with biliary ductal parasites, in patients with sclerosing cholangitis, and in patients with chronic inflammatory changes and stasis for other reasons. In addition, a small percentage of patients with previous history of ulcerative colitis will sooner or later develop bile duct cancer. The disease is also said to be more frequent in patients with malformations of the bile ducts, especially with choledochal cysts. It is probably also worth mentioning that a large percentage of patients with bile duct cancer in the past have been employed in the rubber industry. The common denominators in the etiology thus seem to be infection, bile stasis, and bacterial degradation of bile salts.

Extensive Invasive Growth Locally

Most of the cases involve a rather scirrhous type of cancer. As a matter of fact the fibrous component is almost always dominant. Sometimes the dominance of fibrous components is so extensive that the epithelial tumor components might be difficult to find. The tumor grows diffusely locally, under the mucosa, along the nerves, venules, arteries, and lymphatics, and can extend far beyond macroscopic margins. It has also a tendency to affect the portal vein, especially at the confluence where the duct and the vein are very close. This is the reason why, despite the fact that distant metastases are rare and late, radical resection is often not possible. Even in cases where the surgeon has felt that his resection is macroscopically

Recent Results in Cancer Research, Vol. 110
© Springer-Verlag Berlin · Heidelberg 1988

radical, the subsequent microscopical examination has often shown residual cancer.

Tumors in the bile ducts differ considerably from cancers of the gallbladder, not only in macroscopic and microscopic appearance but also in relation to their growth speed and clinical course.

Patients with rapidly increasing bilirubin levels are very often suspected to have malignant obstruction. However, a slower, obstruction is often seen. The careful history will in such cases reveal prodromal complaints such as loss of appetite, loss of weight, abdominal discomfort, diarrhea, and pruritus.

Representative Biopsies Often Difficult to Get

Infectious manifestations are frequent. The experience of the group at the Royal Postgraduate Medical School in London and ours in Lund is that positive cultures of bile occur in approximately one third of the cases at initial percutaneous transhepatic intubation. The pattern of detection of these tumors has changed in the recent years. Not long ago, almost all such tumors were detected at exploratory laparotomy after – sometimes very difficult and time-consuming – attempts to make representative biopsies. Today, with the availability of ultrasonography, CT, percutaneous cholangiography, ERCP, etc. the tumors in most cases are diagnosed before laparotomy, although the problem of getting representative biopsies to confirm the diagnosis still exists.

Results of Stenting Are not very Encouraging

There is no doubt that the difficult preoperative diagnosis, the difficult histological confirmation, and the extreme difficulty – from a technical point of view – of resecting the tumors and constructing intrahepatic or subhepatic biliary-enteric anastomoses were the reasons for a very pessimistic attitude in the past. It is thus natural that when new developments such as PTC and ERCP brought new possibilities of treating these cases, such as percutaneous placement of catheters for external and/or internal drainage, percutaneous placement of stents, or endoscopic placement of endoprostheses, these techniques were widely used. It should, however, be emphasized that the results with these treatments have been far from good. Voegeli et al. [17] recently presented six cases treated with external percutaneous drainage. Five patients are dead and one is alive after 2 years. The median survival in this small group is 6 months. The results of endoscopic treatment with an endoprosthesis or percutaneously placed stents are not very encouraging; the 30-day mortality varies between 17% and 31% and the median survival between 2 and 5 months [8, 9, 12].

Parallel to the development of new diagnostic tools, the possibilities for extensive surgical intervention in the hepatopancretobiliary region have increased. Extensive liver resection has become a surgical routine. All these facts taken together lead us to believe that all patients with a tumor in the common duct, including those at the confluence, should be regarded as potential candidates for curative surgery. Extensive bilateral intrahepatic ductal spread or multifocal disease, involvement of the main trunk of the portal vein, or bilateral involvement of blood vessels and particularly the portal vein are usually associated with a preoperative judgement of nonresectability [4, 18].

Early Cases - Potential Candidates for Curative Surgery

There are essentially two objectives in the therapy of tumors of the biliary tract: Firstly, if possible, to eliminate the tumor and second, to restore bile flow to the bowel. The ideal is to combine these two objectives. There are four main options: local or hepatic resection, transtumoral drainage, or paratumoral bypass. Only the first two alternatives can achieve both objectives. However, results with a combination of transtumoral drainage and radiotherapy have been encouraging [11, 15].

Although high bile duct cholangiocarcinomas were described by Altemeier et al. in 1957 [1] and Klatskin in 1965 [13], the first local resection was described even earlier [6]. Boerma [5] reviewed the literature and found 75 patients in whom local resection had been performed during the almost 30 years since 1954. He calculated a postoperative mortality of 11% and 1-, 2-, and 3-year survivals of 70%, 33%, and 20% respectively. The mean survival was 19 months.

Most of the cases were reported by surgeons who had had experience with one or two operations. Very few reported on series of more than ten patients. Cameron et al. [7] reported on ten patients with local resections. They had no postoperative mortality and the mean survival was 21 months. It is obvious, however, that the mean survival is a poor measurement of the success with this type of treatment. A few radically resected long-living patients will contribute to the mean survival, hereby hiding the fact that quite a few of the patients - those not radically resected - die rather early. Instead, the use of median survival should be encouraged.

Liver Resection - A Logical Alternative

In his extensive review, Boerma [5] found another 77 cases in which a local resection had been combined with liver resection. Again, most of the cases were reported by surgeons who had performed less than five, in most cases only one or two liver resections. If a clinical series is taken to consist of ten or more patients, the first data published on liver resection in combination with a local resection of a high bile duct tumor were reported by our group in 1980 [10]. At that time we were able to report on 15 such operations, almost all done in the years when exploratory laparotomy was necessary for diagnosis, i.e., between 1969 and 1977. Tsuzuki et al. [16] reported 15 cases with a 50% actuarial survival of 24 months. Three years later Blumgart et al. [4] reported on 12 cases with a mean survival of 22 months. Among our early 15 patients, three are surviving after 10 years; this looks very promising. Approximately ten 5-year survivors, but no 10-year survivors have previously been reported in the literature.

Microscopical Free Margin - A Must for Success

The complication rate in our early series was approximately 50%, most of the complications being related to leaking hepatojejunostomies and infection. This almost led us to give up surgery on this indication. However, as time has passed and we have seen that three of the first 15 patients survived 10 years, we have regained our enthusiasm. Reexamination of the patients showed that microscopic free margins were seen in only four patients. Three of these four survived 10 years. This should encourage us to select more suitable patients for resection as well as to better resect those selected. Leakage is probably almost always a manifestation of residual tumor growth in the margins and poor healing. Blumgart in London and Launois in Rennes pooled their data with ours [3]. We totaled 26 major hepatic resections, almost half of them with extended hepatic lobectomy. At the time of publication one quarter of the liver-resected patients (eight) were surviving after an average of 65 months. However, 18 were dead after an average of 13 months. We concluded from the study that resection of bile duct cancer can be performed with a 10%-15% hospital mortality, that the quality of life is good, and that the 3-year survival is 30%, the 5-year survival 12%. As elsewhere in the gastrointestinal tract, resection of cancer and restoration of continuity seem to offer the best palliation.

We believe that with experience, the results can be greatly improved. For this reason all patients should be approached with assessment for resection in mind. We believe that interventional radiology and endoscopy should not be employed in an indiscriminate manner.

References

1. Altemeier WA, Gall EA, Zinninger MM, Hoxworth PJ (1959) Sclerosing carcinoma of the major intrahepatic ducts. Arch Surg 75: 450-460
2. Bengmark S, Ekberg H, Evander A, Klöfver-Ståhl B, Tranberg KG (1987) Major liver resection for hilar cholangiocarcinoma (to be published)
3. Bengmark S, Blumgart LH, Launois B (1986) Liver resection in high bile duct tumours. In: Bengmark S, Blumgart L (eds) Liver surgery. Churchill Livingstone, Edinburgh
4. Blumgart LH, Benjamin IS, Hadjis NS, Beazley R (1984) Surgical approaches to cholangiocarcinoma at confluence of hepatic ducts. Lancet 1: 66-70
5. Boerma EJ (1983) The surgical treatment of cancer of the hepatic duct confluence. A clinical, anatomical and experimental study and literature survey. Veenman, Wageningen
6. Brown G, Myers N (1954) The hepatic ducts. A surgical approach for resection of tumour. Aust NZ J Surg 23: 308-312
7. Cameron JL, Broe P, Zuidema GD (1982) Proximal bile duct tumours. Ann Surg 196: 412-419
8. Classen M, Hagemüller F (1983) Biliary drainage. Endoscopy 15: 221-229
9. Cotton PB (1982) Duodenoscopic placement of biliary prosthesis to relieve malignant obstructive jaundice. Br J Surg 69: 501-503
10. Evander A, Fredlund P, Hoevels J, Ihse I, Bengmark S (1980) Evaluation of aggressive surgery for carcinoma of the extrahepatic bile ducts. Ann Surg 191: 23-29
11. Fletscher MS, Brinkley D, Dawson JL, Nunnerley H, Wheeler PG, Williams R (1981) Treatment of high bile duct carcinoma by internal radiotherapy with iridium-192 wire. Lancet II: 172-174

12. Huibregtse K, Tytgat GNT (1984) Endoscopic placement of biliary prosthesis. In: Salmon P (ed) Advances in gastrointestinal endoscopy 1984, vol 1. Chapman and Hall, London
13. Klatskin G (1965) Adenocarcinoma of the hepatic duct and its bifurcation within the porta hepatis. Am J Surg 38: 241–256
14. Launois B, Campion JP, Brissot P, Gosselin M (1979) Carcinoma of the hepatic hilus. Surgical management and the case for resection. Ann Surg 190: 151–158
15. Terblanche J, Saunders SJ, Louw JH (1972) Prolonged palliation in carcinoma of the main hepatic duct junction. Surgery 71: 720–731
16. Tsuzuki T, Ogata Y, Hosoda Y (1981) Hepatic resection upon patients with jaundice. Surg Gynecol Obstet 153: 387–391
17. Voegeli DR, Crummy AB, Weese JL (1985) Percutaneous transhepatic chlangiography, drainage and biopsy in patients with malignant biliary obstruction. Am J Surg 150: 243–247
18. Voyles CR, Bowley NJ, Allison DJ, Benjamin IS, Blumgart LH (1983) Carcinoma of the proximal extrahepatic bile tree. Radiological assessment and therapeutic alternatives. Ann Surg 197: 188–194

The Problem of Radical Surgery in Pancreatic Cancer and Its Implications for a Combined-Treatment Approach

F. P. Gall and F. Köckerling

Chirurgische Klinik und Poliklinik, Universität Erlangen-Nürnberg, Maximiliansplatz, 8520 Erlangen, FRG

It is a well known fact that the prognosis of ductal adenocarcinoma of the pancreas is still very poor. Gudjonsson [10] found an overall 5-year survival of only 0.4% among 15000 histologically verified cases collected from the literature.

The pancreas is hidden in the retroperitoneal space. At first, tumor growth causes vague and uncharacteristic symptoms such as loss of appetite and weight, while alarming signs like jaundice or intractable back pain appear rather late. Another unfavorable feature is the very small anterior-posterior and superior-inferior diameter of the pancreas. Any tumor originating near the organ surface will penetrate through the capsule into the adjacent tissue at an early stage. In many instances, therefore, despite a small tumor diameter of only 2–3 cm, these lesions have automatically moved to a far advanced, almost incurable stage.

While for most gastrointestinal cancers the present resection rate is 70%–90%, for ductal cancer of the pancreas it is very low, around 15%–20%. By application of extended resection this rate was increased to 30% in some centers (Fig. 1), but the benefit of it has still not been documented. Partial duodenopancreatectomy

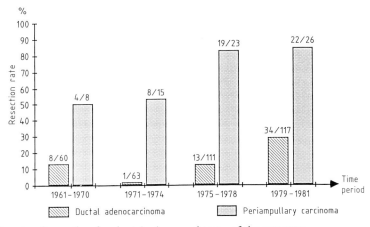

Fig. 1. Increase in rate of resection for ductal adenocarcinoma of the pancreas

Recent Results in Cancer Research, Vol. 110
© Springer-Verlag Berlin · Heidelberg 1988

Table 1. Mortality and survival with total duodenopancreatectomy as reported in the literature

Author	Year	*n*	Mortality (%)	Mean survival (months)	5-Year survival *n*	%
Brooks and Culebras [2]	1976	17	12.5	23.0	3	22.0
Coopermann et al. [3]	1981	43	28.0	15.0	2	5.0
Edis et al. [6]	1980	38	16.0	10.0	1	4.4
Forrest and Longmire [8]	1979	6	17.0	26.0	1	17.0
van Heerden et al. [26]	1981	51	14.0	13.0	1	2.3
Hicks and Brooks [12]	1971	11	9.1	15.4	0	
Hollender and Meyer [14]	1978	5	0.0	16.0	0	
Ihse et al. [16]	1977	58	23.0	20.0	2	4.6
Knight et al. [17]	1978	4	25.0	23.0	1	33.0
Matsui et al. [18]	1979	4	0.0	7.0	1	25.0
Moossa and Levin [19]	1981	45	8.9	33.0		
Pliam and ReMine [21]	1975	33	21.0		1	
ReMine et al. [22]	1970	23	21.7		2	
Trede et al. [24]	1977	5	0.0		0	
Tryka and Brooks [25]	1979	25	12.0	24.0	4	19.0
Total		368	17.4	18.8 ± 7.4	19	6.3

was the operation of choice in the 1940s and 1950s for cancer of the head of the pancreas. However, it soon became evident that this procedure was inadequate to avoid local recurrences at the resection line, which were seen in 25%–30% [5] of autopsied cases. Therefore, the radical operation was extended to a total pancreatectomy, avoiding spillage of tumor cells with the pancreatic juice and local recurrence, as well as dealing with multifocal cancer origin. Total duodenopancreatectomy, however, is combined with an increased operative mortality of 10%–30%, averaging 17%, and its mean survival time of 18 months is equal to that with partial duodenopancreatectomy (Table 1).

After total duodenopancreatectomy, 80% of tumors (24/28) were classified as pT4 because of local infiltration of the retroperitoneal tissue at the cephalic region. We therefore questioned the use of total duodenopancreatectomy, which cannot control local tumor invasion into the retroperitoneum any better than a more limited resection. To reduce the high frequency of local recurrence at the resection line as seen after partial duodenopancreatectomy, an extension of this operation to the left to a subtotal duodenopancreatectomy was initiated by us in 1982 (Fig. 2). This type of resection guarantees a much larger margin of safety (30–120 mm) than can be achieved by a regular partial duodenopancreatectomy. With this procedure our previous operative mortality of 20% was reduced to 2.3% in 36 consecutive cases. This reduction is especially beneficial for patients with early carcinomas. With this new operation the rate of diabetes is increased from 14% preoperatively to only 40% postoperatively. Due to preservation of the pancreatic tail, diabetic control is greatly facilitated by preserved glucagon production for the rest of our patients. The follow-up is still too short for evaluation of 5-year

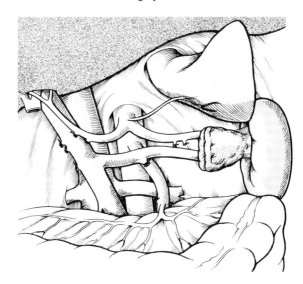

Fig. 2. Situs following subtotal duodenopancreatectomy

Table 2. Median survival for periampullary carcinoma with and without lymph node dissection

	n	Stage IVa	Stage IVb	Median survival (months)
Without lymph node dissection	20	2	3	42
With lymph node dissection	24	2	2	> 60

survival, but the mean survival of 12 months confirms that subtotal duodenopancreatectomy is as radical as a total pancreatectomy.

Another improvement in the effectiveness of radical operations was the introduction of extended regional lymph node dissection, which has been routinely performed since 1978. Positive lymph nodes were found in 85% of ductal carcinomas removed by a total pancreatectomy with extended regional lymph node dissection. While the benefit of extended lymph node dissection is clear in periampullary cancer, where we found an increase in median survival from 42 to 60 months (Table 2), the prognosis of pancreatic cancer remained unchanged for patients with positive lymph nodes, with a mean survival of 9 months after regional lymph node dissection. Patients without nodal involvement had a median survival of 60 months (Table 3).

Adherence of the tumor to the portal vein is still considered a sign of inoperability by many surgeons. However, it can be dealt with by partial resection of the portal vein and an end-to-end anastomosis without increasing the operative risk. In our series the median survival time was 12 months for patients with and 11 months for those without portal vein resection (Table 4). In total there were 35 cases of curative resected ductal adenocarcinoma of the pancreas without resection of the portal vein, 21 cases of stage IVa and 6 cases of stage IVb; the rest

Table 3. Median survival for ductal adenocarcinoma of the pancreas with and without lymph node involvement

	n	Stage IVa	Stage IVb	Median survival (months)
pN_0	12	7	2	>60
pN_1	13	11	2	9
pN_2	20	10	7	9

Table 4. Median survival for ductal adenocarcinoma of the pancreas with and without resection of portal vein

	n	Stage IVa	Stage IVb	Median survival (months)
Without resection of portal vein	35	21	6	11
With resection of portal vein	12	7	5	12

Fig. 3. Staging of exocrine carcinoma of the pancreas according to UICC, 1987

had tumors in lower stages. Despite all surgical efforts the 5-year survival rate for resected pancreatic cancer patients is very low at around 5%–10%. This fact promoted a rather nihilistic attitude on the part of some authors who question the advisability of radical resections in favor of only palliative procedures on the basis of equal mean survival time [4, 7, 11].

We, like many others, are opposed to this policy, because it deprives patients with an early resectable tumor of the only chance to date of a curative operation with longer survival.

The Union Internationale Contre le Cancer (UICC) has introduced a new stage grouping for exocrine carcinoma of the pancreas (Fig. 3). The T classification is divided into T1 for tumors limited to the pancreas, T1a for tumors smaller than 2 cm in diameter, T1b for those larger than 2 cm, T2 for tumors extending to the duodenum, bile duct or peripancreatic tissue, and T3 for extension to the stomach, the colon, the spleen, and large vessels (Table 5).

For lymph node involvement the staging distinguishes only N0 and N1, and no further subdivisions of positive nodal involvements are made.

According to Ichikawa [15] T1a has a 5-year survival of 86%, T1b of 25%, T2 of 6%, and T3 of 3% (Table 6). The calculated 4-year survival in stage I is 32%, stage II 24%, stage III (=N1 cases) 8%, and stage IV 0% (Table 7).

Table 5. UICC T-classification of exocrine carcinoma of the pancreas, 1987

T_1	Limited to pancreas
	T_{1a} 2 cm or less
	T_{1b} more than 2 cm
T_2	Extends directly to duodenum, bile duct, peripancreatic tissues
T_3	Extends directly to stomach, spleen, colon, adjacent large vessels

Table 6. Prognosis for exocrine carcinoma of the pancreas based on UICC T-classification ($n = 2194$) [15]

	n	(%)	5-year survival
T_{1a}	8	(0.4)	86%
T_{1b}	58	(2.6)	25%
T_2	507	(23.1)	6%
T_3	1621	(73.9)	3%

Table 7. Prognosis for exocrine carcinoma of the pancreas according to stage grouping ($n = 902$) [15]

Stage	n	(%)	4-year survival
I	143	(15.9)	32%
II	82	(9.1)	24%
III	367	(40.7)	8%
IV	310	(34.4)	0%

Table 8. Prognosis for exocrine carcinoma of the pancreas in 105 patients at the Department of Surgery, University of Erlangen (FRG), based on T-classification

	n	(%)	5-year survival
T_{1a}	5	(5)	/
T_{1b}	12	(11)	($52 \pm 32\%$)
T_2	77	(73)	$12 \pm 10\%$
T_3	11	(10)	0%

In our own series of 105 resected ductal carcinomas, early carcinoma (T1a) was found in 5% of cases, but none of these patients survived 5 years; for T1b tumors the 5-year survival was 52%, T2 tumors 12%, and in T3 lesions 0% (Table 8).

The prognosis of ductal carcinoma has remained unchanged by resective surgery alone during the past decade. Is there any indication that it can be improved by adjuvant therapy? The adjuvant treatment of resectable carcinoma of the pancreas is still in an experimental stage.

Radiation Therapy

Pilepich and Miller [20] used preoperative radiotherapy in 17 patients considered clinically to have localized cancers of the pancreas; the patients received up to 5000 rads in 5 weeks. In the irradiated group 11 patients underwent exploration and six had pancreatic resection. Only two patients remained free of disease for longer than 5 years.

Hiraoka et al. [13] used intraoperative irradiation combined with resection for cancer of the head of the pancreas to prevent local recurrence. Thirty gray of the electron beam from a linear accelerator were administered to the operative field, including the celiac axis and mesenteric artery, following pancreaticoduodenectomy. Results of the combined therapy in 12 patients were compared with the results in 12 patients who had undergone pancreaticoduodenectomy alone. The combined-therapy group showed improvement in the 1-year survival rate but not in the 2-year survival rate.

There is only a small amount of evidence currently available suggesting that adjuvant radiation therapy may play a role in the treatment of resectable pancreatic cancer. The National Institute of Health in the United States is currently conducting a randomized trial evaluating adjuvant conventional and intraoperative radiotherapy combined with resection of localized pancreatic carcinoma.

Chemotherapy

Chemotherapy as an adjuvant to surgical resection has not been used extensively in pancreatic carcinoma. Some institutions have occasionally given chemotherapy after pancreatic resection, with some claims of benefit by longer survival than would be expected with surgical resection alone.

Combined-Modality Therapy

Adjuvant combined-modality therapy in resectable pancreatic cancer has been suggested to be of benefit in prolonging survival, although the available experience is small. Appelqvist et al. [1] treated eight patients with pancreatic carcinomas by resection, postoperative radiotherapy of 4500 rads, and 5-FU chemotherapy. The 1-year survival was 75%, the 2-year survival 25%, and the 3-year survival 12.5%. None of the 11 patients treated by resection alone survived up to 3 years.

The Gastrointestinal Tumor Study Group has conducted a prospective randomized trial evaluating combined-modality treatment in resectable pancreatic cancer [23]. Patients with localized carcinomas of the pancreas who underwent pancreatectomy and removal of all gross disease were prospectively randomized to surgical resection alone and resection with adjuvant combined-modality therapy consisting of 4000 rads of external beam radiotherapy and 5-FU chemotherapy. Indicative of the rarity of surgical resection, only 59 patients were entered into the multi-institutional study during an 8-year period, and 43 patients are available for current analysis. After an average follow-up of more than 5 years, the median survival for the group of patients treated with adjuvant radiation and chemotherapy after resection was 20 months, significantly longer than the median survival of 11 months for the resection-alone control group. The probability of survival after 2 years favored the adjuvant combined-modality treatment group with 42% over the surgery-alone control group with 15%. The majority of all patients, however, experienced local or disseminated disease recurrence, with 71% of the adjuvant therapy group and 86% of the control group failing treatment. Only 14% (three of 22) of the patients receiving adjuvant radiotherapy and chemotherapy and only 5% (one of 21) of the surgery-alone control patients were projected to be alive 5 years after pancreatic resection.

Conclusions

At present radical resection is the only chance for cure or long survival. Therefore, no patient should be denied exploration, unless inoperability is verified histologically by fine-needle biopsy of liver or other metastases.

Prospectively randomized trials are needed to compare surgery alone with surgery in combination with various chemotherapy regimens and methods of radiation therapy. The demonstrated benefit of combined therapy over surgery alone in carefully performed trials will be needed before adjuvant combined-modality treatments can be justified for routine use.

Early diagnosis of pancreatic cancer must be improved. In patients with unspecific symptoms, a careful evaluation must also include a complete examination of the pancreas to detect an early pancreatic cancer.

References

1. Appelqvist P, Viren M, Minkkinen J, Kajanti M, Kostiainen S, Rissanen P (1983) Operative finding, treatment, and prognosis of carcinoma of the pancreas: an analysis of 267 cases. J Surg Oncol 23: 143
2. Brooks JR, Culebras JM (1976) Cancer of the pancreas: palliative operation, Whipple procedure or total pancreatectomy. Am J Surg 131: 516
3. Coopermann AM, Herter FP, Morboe CA, Helmreich ZV, Persin KH (1981) Pancreatoduodenal resection and total pancreatectomy: an institutional review. Surgery 90: 707
4. Crile G (1970) The advantages of bypass operations over radical pancreaticoduodenectomy in the treatment of pancreatic carcinoma. Surg Gynecol Obstet 130: 1049
5. Diamond D, Fisher B (1975) Pancreatic cancer. Surg Clin North Am 55: 363
6. Edis AJ, Kiernan PD, Taylor WF (1980) Attempted curative resection of ductal carcinoma of the pancreas. Review of Mayo Clinic Experience 1951-1975. Mayo Clin Proc 55: 531
7. Feduska NJ, Dent TL, Lindenauer SM (1971) Results of palliative operations for carcinoma of the pancreas. Arch Surg 103: 330
8. Forrest JF, Longmire WP (1979) Carcinoma of the pancreas and periampullary region. Ann Surg 189: 129
9. Fuchsjäger N (1973) Ergebnisse nach partieller Duodenopankreatektomie. Wien Klin Wochenschr 85: 147
10. Gudjonsson B, Livstone EM, Spiro HM (1978) Cancer of the pancreas. Diagnostic accuracy and survival statistics. Cancer 42: 2494

11. Hertzberg J (1974) Pancreatico-duodenal resection and bypass operation in patients with carcinoma of the head of the pancreas, ampulla and distal end of the common duct. Acta Chir Scand 140: 523
12. Hicks RE, Brooks JR (1971) Total pancreatectomy for ductal carcinoma. Surg Gynecol Obstet 133: 16
13. Hiraoka T, Watanabe E, Mochinaga M, Tashiro S, Miyanchi Y, Nakamura I, Yokoyama I (1984) Intraoperative irradiation combined with radical resection for cancer of the head of the pancreas. World J Surg 8: 766
14. Hollender LF, Meyer C (1978) Operative Behandlung des Pankreaskarzinoms. Zentralbl Chir 103: 1256
15. Ichikawa H (1986) Report of the Japanese Joint Committee to the UICC, Geneva, May 6
16. Ihse J, Lilja P, Arnesjö B, Bengmark S (1977) Total pancreatectomy for cancer. Ann Surg 186: 675
17. Knight RW, Scarborough JP, Goss JC (1978) Adenocarcinoma of the pancreas. A 10-year experience. Arch Surg 113: 1401
18. Matsui Y, Aoki Y, Ishikawa O, Iwanaga T, Wada A, Tateishi R, Kosaki G (1979) Ductal carcinoma of the pancreas. Rationales for total pancreatectomy. Arch Surg 114: 722
19. Moossa AR, Levin B (1981) The diagnostic of "early" pancreatic cancer: the University of Chicago experience. Cancer 47: 1688
20. Pilepich MV, Miller HH (1980) Preoperative irradiation in carcinoma of the pancreas. Cancer 46: 1945
21. Pliam MB, ReMine WH (1975) Further evaluation of total pancreatectomy. Arch Surg 110: 506
22. ReMine WH, Priestley JT (1970) Total pancreatectomy. Ann Surg 172: 595
23. Sindelar WF, Kinsella TJ, Mayer RJ (1985) Cancer of the pancreas. In: De Vita VT, Hellmann S, Rosenberg SA (eds) Cancer, Principles and practise of oncology. Lippincott, Philadelphia, pp 691–739
24. Trede M, Kersting K-H, Hoffmeister A (1977) Das Pankreaskopfkarzinom. Diagnostik, chirurgische Indikation und Ergebnisse. mmw 119: 617
25. Tryka AF, Brooks JR (1979) Histopathology in the evaluation of total pancreatectomy for ductal carcinoma. Ann Surg 190: 373
26. van Heerden JA, ReMine WH, Weiland CH, McIlrath OC, Ilstrup OM (1981) Total pancreatectomy for ductal adenocarcinoma of the pancreas. Am J Surg 142: 308

Treatment of Pancreatic Carcinoma: Therapeutic Nihilism?

J. A. Wils

Department of Internal Medicine, Laurentius Hospital,
6043 CV Roermond, The Netherlands

Introduction

The incidence of pancreatic carcinoma is rising in Western countries and it now ranks fourth in causes of cancer deaths. The disease is highly lethal and the vast majority of patients die within 1 year of diagnosis. Overall survival at 3 years is practically zero [1]. The diagnosis of adenocarcinoma of the pancreas is most often made when the disease is already far advanced. It tends to spread rapidly intra-abdominally and can be called the silent killer of the upper abdomen as opposed to ovarian carcinoma, the silent killer of the lower abdomen. Theoretically, surgery offers the best hope for cure, but only a very small minority of patients are resectable for cure, and the survival of these patients after 3 years drops to about 15%. Nevertheless, this survival is better than that with any other method of treatment. It is clear that all patients must be carefully evaluated as candidates for curative surgery. Although only a small minority of the patients will be resectable for cure, these patients are the only ones with a potential for long-term survival. During the past 10 years new diagnostic facilities such as echography, computerized tomography (CT) and endoscopic retrograde studies (ERCP) have been developed, but to date this enhanced ability to detect earlier disease has not changed the dismal outlook. The outcome for a patient for whom no therapeutic attempts are made is death within a very short time. To accept this outcome does not follow the best concepts of medicine. Palliation and improvement of survival for patients with advanced disease with other treatment modalities (i.e., irradiation, chemotherapy) must be continuously pursued.

Radiotherapy

Conventional photon irradiation with 4000–6000 rads may offer some palliation for locally advanced disease, but its impact on survival is questionable. The Gastrointestinal Tumor Study Group (GITSG) study has shown some evidence that combination of irradiation and 5-fluorouracil (5-FU) is superior to radiotherapy alone for locally advanced disease [2]. In this study patients were randomized to receive either 4000 rads + 5-FU or 6000 rads ± 5-FU. The radiotherapy-alone group was discontinued with 25 patients because early analysis had shown a statistically inferior survival for this group. Median survival in patients treated with 6000 rads + 5-FU was slightly but not significantly better than that for patients receiving the lower dose of irradiation, but this early benefit was not sustained much beyond 1 year. At 60 weeks both survival curves intercepted, and at 2 years all curves approached zero. A subsequent study has evaluated doxorubicin and radiation versus the superior 5-FU radiation combination. Among 143 evaluable patients median survival in the doxorubicin group was 32.5 weeks and in the 5-FU group 38 weeks [3]. A beneficial role for combined radiation-chemotherapy is further suggested by the results of a prospective trial comparing adjuvant radiation (4000 rads) + 5-FU with no adjuvant treatment in 43 patients following potentially curative surgery. The median survival of 20 months for the treated group was significantly better than the 11 months for the control group [4]. Because of the relatively small number of patients, these results cannot be considered definitive. In a study conducted by the Eastern Cooperative Oncology Group (ECOG), 91 evaluable patients with locally advanced disease were randomized to receive either 5-FU alone or 5-FU combined with 4000 rads. The median survival time was 8 months for both treatment programs, but serious toxicities were significantly increased in the combined-modality group [5], thus making questionable the relative merit of conventional irradiation.

Newer radiation techniques for locally advanced disease, such as implantation of radioactive materials, intraoperative radiotherapy [6], and the use of specialized beams (neutrons, protons, mesons, etc.) are of interest and may benefit some patients. Impact on survival, however, can be expected to be relevant only if these techniques are combined with some form of systemic treatment. Irradiation with high-energy neutrons resulted in a median survival of 6 months in 77 patients; 26 of these patients experienced severe late side effects or complications, and there were two treatment-related deaths [7]. The combination of external radiation, implantation of iodine 125, and chemotherapy resulted in a median survival of 11 months in 20 patients with locally advanced disease. The survival of patients treated with chemotherapy in addition to external radiation or external radiation plus iodine 125 implant was significantly better than that of the patients who received no additional chemotherapy. Patients in this study, however, were not randomized [8]. The sequential use of 5-FU, adriamycin, mitomycin C, and radiotherapy was reported to yield an overall median survival of 12 + months in 26 patients [9]. In another study, six cycles of 5-FU, adriamycin, and cisplatin followed by radiation (40 Gy) + 5-FU resulted in four partial responses in ten patients and a median overall survival of 13 + months [10]. These studies encourage exploration of new radiation techniques combined with new drugs, including analogs of existing drugs such as doxorubicin and cisplatin with attenuated toxicity.

Chemotherapy

The development of chemotherapy in pancreatic carcinoma has proceeded relatively slowly. One of the problems is the fact that response to chemotherapy can often be measured only by techniques such as echography and CT. These techniques can be accepted as reliable parameters only if they are interpreted by experienced investigators. It is questionable whether measurements of vaguely defined abdominal lumps are more accurate. Furthermore, patients with pancreatic carcinoma frequently present with a low performance status, a bad prognostic factor in many malignant diseases, which makes the evaluation and tolerance of chemotherapy particularly difficult. Another reason why phase-II chemotherapy studies in pancreatic cancer have lagged behind those of other common malignancies is the nihilism which still prevails in approaching this disease.

Survival time in chemotherapy trials also has to be viewed in light of the patient population studied. Whereas radiation therapy studies investigate patients with locally inoperable disease, chemotherapy studies are based on patients with metastatic disease (most often liver metastases), and their survival tends to be lower. Furthermore, studies conducted by different institutions or by different cooperative groups may produce vastly different response rates. Part of this variability is explained by patient selection difference and part by a stricter definition of measurable disease.

Only a few single agents have been adequately tested in more than 20 patients, and four drugs appear to have a response rate of over 20% (Table 1). 5-FU is the most extensively evaluated drug, with a response rate of 28% in collected series [1, 11], which is probably an overestimation because this result is obtained from 15 series with response rates ranging between 0% and 67%. All these studies were performed between 1960 and 1971 using nonstandardized response criteria, the greater part of which would be unacceptable today. Response rates for mitomycin C and streptozotocin as shown in Table 1 are also compilations from collected series [1, 12]. Ifosfamide was recently reported to yield a response rate of 22% [14]. Adriamycin has been tested by the GITSG and yielded a response in two (13%) of 15 patients [13]. All other drugs tested so far were reported to have an activity of less than 20%. These drugs include melphalan [15], the nitrosoureas [16], methotrexate [13], actinomycin [13], and vindesine [17].

Despite the relatively few active drugs there has been continued interest in combination chemotherapy. Table 2 gives an overview of phase-II pilot studies

Table 1. Activity of single agents in pancreatic cancer

Drug	Number of responses/patients	Response rate (%)	Reference
5-FU	60/212	28	[1, 11]
Mitomycin C	12/44	27	[1, 12]
Streptozotocin	8/22	36	[1, 12]
Ifosfamide	6/27	22	[14]
Adriamycin	2/15	13	[13]
Melphalan	2/15	13	[15]
Methyl-CCNU	3/34	9	[16]
Vindesine	1/15		[17]
Methotrexate	1/25		[13]
Actinomycin C	1/28		[13]
BCNU	0/20		[18]

Table 2. Combination chemotherapy in advanced pancreatic carcinoma (excludes comparative studies – see text)

Regimen	No. of patients	No. of responders	Median survival, responders (months)	Median survival, all patients (months)	Survivors > 1 year	Reference
SMF	23	10	10	6	4	[19]
SMF	22	7	9	6		[20]
FAM	27	10	12	6	4	[21]
FAM	15	6	13+	4	1	[22]
FAM-S	25	12	10	7	7	[23]
FAP	15	3	10+			[24]
FAP	21	5		4		[25]
HEXA-FAM	30	5		4		[26]
HEXA-FM	21	2		10		[27]
	199	60 (30%)	10	6	16 (8%)	

S, Streptozotocin; *M*, mitomycin; *F*, 5-fluorouracil; *A*, adriamycin; *P*, *cis*platinum; *HEXA*, hexamethylmelamine.

in advanced pancreatic carcinoma. FAM and SMF are the regimens most employed.

The response rate is about 30%; the median survival of responders is about 10 months, but the overall median survival does not exceed 6 months. About 10% of patients seem to survive over 1 year. A randomized study comparing FAM with SMF in 184 patients, however, showed response rates of only 14% and 4% and median overall survival of 26 and 18 weeks respectively [28]. In another randomized study of 116 patients with measurable disease conducted by the South West Oncology Group (SWOG), SMF was compared with MF. Response rates were 34% and 8% respectively, but median survivals were similar, 18 versus 17 weeks [29]. Despite these disappointing results, one must discard cynicism in the treatment of this disease. There should be a continuous search for new drugs of greater efficacy through phase-II studies which include new evaluation procedures such as CT scan in previously untreated patients.

Epirubicin and Epirubicin Combined with 5-FU in Advanced Pancreatic Carcinoma (EORTC trials 40821 and 40841)

Epirubicin (4′-epi-adriamycin, 4′-epi-doxorubicin, EPI) is a new anthracycline antibiotic. If differs from doxorubicin (DOXO) by the epimerization of the hydroxyl group in position 4′ of the aminosugar side chain and was synthesized in an effort to find agents with a therapeutic index superior to that of the parent compound doxorubicin. The pharmacokinetics of the two drugs are different, and the acute and chronic toxicity of epirubicin are less than those of doxorubicin in equimolar doses [30]. Two preliminary communications suggested that epirubicin might be active in pancreatic carcinoma [31, 32], and this was confirmed in another pilot study [33]. This prompted the EORTC Gastrointestinal Group to conduct a phase-II study with this drug, and results have been reported [34]. CT and ultrasound were accepted as methods of measuring lesions. Epirubicin was given in a dose of 90 mg/m^2, i.v., every 4 weeks, with dose escalation in the absence of major toxicity. Definition of response was according to WHO criteria. The median number of courses was 4 (range 2–11) and the mean dose per course 96 mg/m^2 (range 90–120 mg/m^2). Including only the eligible and adequately treated (at least two full cycles of chemotherapy) patients, the response rate was 27% (8/30), but keeping all eligible patients in the denominator the response rate was 20% (8/40) and the median survival time 5 months. The median duration of response was 7 months. The two complete remissions were documented by CT scanning and the duration of remission was 8 and 17 months. One patient had locally advanced disease plus liver metastases, the other only locally advanced disease. Their survival was 9 and 24 months respectively. Four responses were observed at the first evaluation, i.e., after the second cycle. There were four patients who developed a remission after at least four cycles and in three of them the dose of epirubicin had been escalated up to 110 mg/m^2. Toxicity of epirubicin was relatively mild. Major toxicity consisted of alopecia, median grade 2 (WHO), and nausea/vomiting, median grade 1. The median white cell count on day 14 was 2.7×10^9/l (range 0.6–11.5). Thrombocytopenia was not observed and there were no toxic deaths.

The EORTC Gastrointestinal Group has subsequently conducted a trial evaluating the activity of the combination of EPI with 5-FU. In this new study EPI was given in a dose of 90 mg/m^2, day 1, i.v., and 5-FU in a dose of 500 mg/m^2, days 1–4, i.v. in a 2-h infusion. Courses were repeated every 4 weeks. Eligibility criteria were the same as in the previous trial. A total of 47 patients were registered, three of whom were not eligible and one not evaluable. From ten patients the data are too early. There were seven early deaths, six due to tumor progression and one due to a cerebrovascular insult. There were six partial responses, giving response rates of 23% excluding and 18% including the early deaths. The median duration of response was 7 months and the median survival for all patients 4 months. The toxicity in this trial was low, with a median white cell nadir of 2.4×10^9/l and only 3% of the patients experiencing grade-3 or -4 nausea/vomiting.

These were two subsequent studies with different patient selection (lower performance status and fewer patients with locally advanced disease only in the second trial). Moreover, the dose of EPI was different in both trials. Nevertheless, these results would suggest that the addition of 5-FU to EPI offers no advantage over EPI alone.

Endocrine Therapy

There are some preliminary data suggesting that pancreatic cancer might be sensitive to endocrine therapy. Pancreatic tumor cytosols can bind estradiol at high levels, and pancreatic adenocarcinoma cell lines have shown steroid sensitivity in vitro [35]. Recently, tamoxifen was reported to yield a median survival of 8.5 months in 14 patients; three male patients with locally advanced disease survived 22 months [36]. In another study, however, none of 13 patients responded to endocrine treatment; nine of these patients were treated with tamoxifen [37].

Discussion

There is still considerable skepticism in the treatment of advanced pancreatic carcinoma because of the disappointing results obtained so far. To ameliorate the outlook for patients with pancreatic adenocarcinoma, all treatment modalities must be improved and must be integrated in an optimal way. We need earlier diagnosis, which may raise the incidence of curative resections. It is possible that in the future, perioperative chemotherapy may have an impact on the survival of resectable cases [4]. For locally advanced disease we need better radiotherapeutic options, probably in combination with chemotherapy, and for metastatic disease we need better drugs and new combinations.

The results of the EORTC Gastrointestinal Group study 40821 have shown that EPI is an active drug in pancreatic cancer and can be administered with low toxicity. These results have been confirmed by others [38]. Several studies with other solid tumors have demonstrated that EPI administered in equimolar doses is as effective as DOXO but less myelosuppressive and less cardiotoxic [39–42]. The diminished cardiotoxicity has been clearly demonstrated in the study by the Memorial Sloan-Kettering Institute showing that the median cumulative dose of EPI to the development of laboratory cardiotoxicity was definitely higher than that of DOXO, even when the data analysis took into consideration the difference in myelosuppressive potency between the two drugs [39]. The therapeutic effectiveness of EPI in pancreatic cancer might be due to the fact that this drug can be administered in a higher dose than DOXO. Another possibility may be that EPI has different biologic properties despite its chemical similarity with DOXO, as it has been shown that the pharmacokinetics of EPI are different from those of DOXO [43]. Unfortunately, the addition of 5-FU to EPI did not seem to enhance the results as has been suggested by the EORTC study 40841. Further studies with EPI in pancreatic cancer are currently being planned by the EORTC Gastrointestinal Group in the hope of improving the dismal outlook for these patients. To date, however, all treatment of advanced pancreatic cancer remains experimental, there is no impact on survival, and patients should be treated only within controlled clinical trials.

References

1. Macdonald JS, Gunderson LL, Cohn I (1982) Cancer of the pancreas. In: De Vita V, Hellman S, Rosenberg SA (eds) Cancer, Principles and Practise of Oncology. Lippincott, Philadelphia, pp 563–589
2. Moertel CG, Frytak S, Hahn RG, et al. (1981) Therapy of locally unresectable pancreatic carcinoma: a randomised comparison of high-dose (6000 rads) radiation alone, moderate dose radiation (4000 rads + 5-fluorouracil) and high-dose radiation + 5-fluorouracil. Cancer 48: 1705

3. Douglas HO, Stablein D, Thomas P, Schein P (1984) Treatment of locally unresectable pancreatic cancer with radiation (RT) combined with adriamycin (A) or 5-fluorouracil (FU) (abstract). Proc American Society of Clinical Oncology, no 3, p 137
4. Kalser MH, Ellenberg SS (1985) Pancreatic cancer. Adjuvant combined radiation and chemotherapy following curative resection. Arch Surg 120: 899
5. Klaassen DJ, MacIntyre JM, Catton GE, et al. (1985) Treatment of locally unresectable cancer of the stomach and pancreas: a randomized comparizion of 5-fluorouracil alone with radiation plus concurrent and maintenance 5-fluorouracil – an Eastern Cooperative Oncology Group study. J Clin Oncol 3: 373
6. Nishimura A, Nakano M, Otsu H, et al (1984) Intraoperative radiotherapy for advanced carcinoma of the pancreas. Cancer 54: 2375
7. Cohen L, Woodruff KH, Hendrickson FR, et al. (1985) Response of pancreatic cancer to local irradiation with high-energy neutrons. Cancer 56: 1235
8. Whittington R, Solin L, Mohiuddin M, et al. (1984) Multimodality therapy of localized unresectable pancreatic adenocarcinoma. Cancer 54: 1991
9. Schein PS, Smith FP, Dritschillo A, et al. (1983) Phase-I to -II trial of combined-modality FAM (5-fluourouracil, adriamycin and mitomycin C) plus split-course radiation (FAM-RT-FAM) for locally advanced gastric (LAG) and pancreatic (LAP) cancer: a mid-Atlantic oncology program study (abstract). Proc American Society of Clinical Oncology, no 2, p 126
10. Wagener DJT, Hoogenraad WJ, Kruiselbrink H, et al. (1985) Chemotherapy (5-fluorouracil, adriamycin and cisplatin) preceding irradiation in locally advanced unresectable carcinoma of the pancreas: a phase-II study. In: Wagener D, Blijham G, Smeets J, Wils J (eds) Primary chemotherapy in cancer medicine. Liss, New York, pp 301–315
11. Smith FP, Schein PS (1979) Chemotherapy of pancreatic cancer. Semin Oncol 6: 368
12. Carter SK, Comis RL (1975) Adenocarcinoma of the pancreas: current therapeutic approaches, prognostic variables, and criteria of response. In: Staquet MJ (ed) Cancer therapy: prognostic factors and criteria of response. Raven, New York, pp 237–253
13. Schein PS, Lavin PT, Moertel CG (1978) Randomized phase-II clinical trial of adriamycin in advanced measurable pancreatic carcinoma: a GITSG report. Cancer 42: 19
14. Loehrer PJ, Williams SD, Einhorn LH, Ansari R (1985) Ifosfamide: an active drug in the treatment of adenocarcinoma of the pancreas. J Clin Oncol 3: 367
15. Smith DB, Kenny JB, Scarffe JH, Maley WV (1985) Phase-II evaluation of melphalan in adenocarcinoma of the pancreas. Cancer Treat Rep 69: 917
16. Douglass HO, Lavin PT, Moertel CG (1976) Nitrosoureas: useful agents for treatment of advanced gastrointestinal cancer. Cancer Treat Rep 60: 769
17. Magill GB, Cheng EW, Currie VE (1981) Chemotherapy of pancreatic carcinoma with vindesine (DVA) (abstract). Proc American Society of Clinical Oncology, no 22, p 458
18. Kovach JS, Moertel CG, Schutt AJ, et al. (1974) A controlled study of combined 1,3-bis (2-chloroethyl)-1 nitrosourea and 5-fluorouracil therapy for advanced gastric and pancreatic cancer. Cancer 33: 563
19. Wiggans G, Woolley PV, MacDonald JS, et al. (1978) Phase-II trial of streptozotocin, mitomycin C and 5-fluorouracil (SMF) in the treatment of advanced pancreatic cancer. Cancer 41: 387
20. Bukowski RM, Abderhalten RT, Hewlett JS, et al. (1980) Phase-II trial of streptozotocin, mitomycin C and 5-fluorouracil in adenocarcinoma of the pancreas. Cancer Clin Trials 3: 321
21. Smith FP, Hoth DF, Levin BL, et al. (1980) 5-Fluorouracil, adriamycin and mitomycin C (FAM) chemotherapy for advanced adenocarcinoma of the pancreas. Cancer 46: 2014
22. Bitran JD, Desser RK, Kozloff MF, et al. (1979) Treatment of metastatic pancreatic and gastric adenocarcinoma with 5-fluorouracil, adriamycin and mitomycin C (FAM). Cancer Treat Rep 63: 2049
23. Bukowski RM, Schacter LP, Groppe CW, et al. (1982) Phase-II trial of 5-fluorouracil, adriamycin, mitomycin C, and streptozotocin (FAM-S) in pancreatic carcinoma. Cancer 50: 197

24. Gisselbrecht C, Smith FP, Woolley PV, et al. (1981) Phase-II trial of FAP (5-fluorouracil, adriamycin and cisdiammine dichloroplatinum) chemotherapy for advanced measurable pancreatic cancer (PC) and adenocarcinoma of unknown origen (AUO) (abstract). Proc American Society of Clinical Oncology, no 22, p 454
25. Moertel C, Fleming T, O'Connell M, et al. (1984) A phase-II trial of combined intensive course 5-FU, adriamycin and cis-platinum in advanced gastric and pancreatic carcinoma (abstract). Proc American Society of Clinical Oncology, no 3, p 137
26. Smith FP, Priego V, Lohey L, et al. (1983) Phase-II evaluation of hexamethylmelamine + FAM (HEXA-FAM) in advanced measurable pancreatic cancer (PC) (abstract). Proc American Society of Clinical Oncology, no 2, p 126
27. Bruckner HW, Storck JA, Brown JC, et al. (1983) Phase-II trial of combination chemotherapy for pancreatic cancer with 5-fluorouracil, mitomycin C and hexamethylmelamine. Oncology 40: 165
28. Oster MW, Gray R, Panasci L, Perry MC, et al. (1986) Chemotherapy for advanced pancreatic cancer: a comparison of 5-fluorouracil, adriamycin and mitomycin (FAM) with 5-fluorouracil, streptozotocin and mitomycin (FSM). Cancer 57: 29
29. Bukowski RM, Balcerzak SP, O'Bryan RM, et al. (1983) Randomized trial of 5-fluorouracil and mitomycin C with or without streptozotocin for advanced pancreatic cancer. Cancer 52: 1577
30. Ganzina F (1983) 4'-Epi-doxorubicin, a new analogue of doxorubicin: a preliminary overview of preclinical and clinical data. Cancer Treat Rep 10: 1
31. Ferrazzi E, Nicoletto O, Vinante O, et al. (1982) Preliminary clinical experience with 4'-epi-doxorubicin. In: Muggia FM, Young CW, Carter SK (eds) Anthracycline antibiotics in cancer therapy. Martinus Nijhoff, The Hague, pp 562-567
32. Green MD, Speyer JL, Muggia FM (1982) A phase-I/II study of 4'-epidoxorubicin administered as a 6-hour continuous infusion (abstract). Proc American Society of Clinical Oncology, no 1, p 20
33. Wils J, Thung P (1984) Treatment of pancreatic carcinoma. How do we proceed? In: Klein H (ed) Advances in the chemotherapy of gastrointestinal cancer. perimed, Erlangen, pp 143-149
34. Wils J, Bleiberg H, Blijham G, et al. (1985) Phase-II study of epirubicin in advanced adenocarcinoma of the pancreas. Eur J Cancer Clin Oncol 21: 191
35. Benz C, Wiznitzer I, Benz C (1983) Steroid binding and cytotoxicity in cultured human pancreatic carcinomas (abstract). J Steroid Bioch [Suppl] 19: 125S
36. Theve NO, Pousette A, Carlström K (1983) Adenocarcinoma of the pancreas - a hormone-sensitive tumour? A preliminary report on Nolvadex treatment. Clin Onc 9: 193
37. Miller B, Benz C (1985) Endocrine treatment of pancreatic carcinoma (abstract). Proc American Society of Clinical Oncology, no 4, p 90
38. Hochster H, Green MD, Speyer JL, Wernz JC, Blum RH, Muggia FM (1986) Activity of epirubicin in pancreatic carcinoma. Cancer Treat Rep 70: 299
39. Jain KK, Caspar ES, Geller NL, et al. (1985) A prospective randomized comparison of epirubicin and doxorubicin in patients with advanced breast cancer. J Clin Oncol 3: 818
40. Bonadonna G, Brambilla C, Rossi A, et al. (1985) Epirubicin in advanced breast cancer. The experience of the Milan Cancer Institute. In: Bonadonna G (ed) Advances in anthracycline chemotherapy: epirubicin. Masson, Milan, pp 63-70
41. Armand JP (1985) Phase II and phase III studies with epirubicin in breast cancer in France. In: Bonadonna G (ed) Advances in anthracycline chemotherapy: epirubicin, Masson, Milan, pp 75-82
42. Mouridsen HT, Somers R, Santoro A, et al. (1985) Doxorubicin vs epirubicin in advanced soft tissue sarcomas. An EORTC randomized phase-II study. In: Bonadonna G (ed) Advances in anthracycline chemotherapy: epirubicin. Masson, Milan, pp 95-103
43. Weenen H, Lankelma JP, Penders PGM, et al. (1983) Pharmacokinetics of 4'-epidoxorubicin in man. Invest New Drugs 1: 59

Adjuvant Portal Infusion Chemotherapy in Colorectal Cancer

U. Metzger

Department für Chirurgie, Universitätsspital, Rämistraße 100, 8091 Zürich, Switzerland

Introduction

Liver metastases are present on initial diagnosis of large-bowel cancer in 25%–30% of patients [2]. After curative resection of colorectal primary tumors, the liver again is the most frequent site of relapse in 40%–50% [4, 18]. Once liver metastases have developed, the prognosis is poor, with an expected median survival of 6–9 months [2, 14], the extent of the tumor being the most important prognostic factor [22]. A great deal of work has been done to determine the factors that influence development of liver metastases. There is evidence that tumor cells embolize into the portal venous system via the mesenteric veins and enter the liver. In 1957, Dukes [6] found evidence of venous spread in 17% of operative rectal cancer specimens. Fisher and Turnbull [7] discovered tumor cells in the mesenteric venous blood of 32% of colorectal carcinoma patients at surgery. They suggested that manipulation of the tumor may force malignant cells into the circulation, and they initiated the so-called no-touch isolation technique [21]. However, not all circulating cancer cells give rise to metastases. Several reports have shown that patients with malignant cells in the portal venous blood fare no worse than those without [15, 17].

Metachronous liver metastases may originate from microscopic deposits not visible at surgery for the primary tumor. These micrometastases are the most important target for adjuvant systemic therapy [5, 16]. Since adjuvant systemic chemotherapy has mostly failed in several well-designed prospective, randomized trials [8–10, 12], numerous studies have approached the issue of hepatic artery or portal venous infusion of fluorinated pyrimidines. Almersjö et al. [1] have shown the safety of portal venous infusion in man. It is generally accepted that adjuvant therapy should be started as soon as possible after surgery, when the tumor burden is minimal [3, 16]. In addition, surgical stress, anesthetics and other drugs, hypercoagulability, blood transfusion, and decrease of the immunological function due to surgery possibly render the perioperative period a vulnerable phase of tumor promotion.

In 1957, Morales et al. [13] advocated intraportal injection of cytotoxic agents at the time of surgery for colorectal cancer in an attempt to prevent liver metastases.

Recent Results in Cancer Research, Vol. 110
© Springer-Verlag Berlin · Heidelberg 1988

Renewed interest in adjuvant portal liver infusion is based on an early report of Taylor et al. [19], who reported in 1979 on a randomized study evaluating adjuvant cytotoxic liver infusion for colorectal cancer. After a follow-up of 26-28 months, 23 patients died in the control group and seven in the infusion group. In the control group, five had multiple liver metastases alone, eight had only local recurrences. One patient in the infusion group had liver metastases alone, one had liver metastases as well as metastases elsewhere, and four had local recurrences. The incidence of liver metastases in the two groups (13 control, two infusion) was significantly different statistically [19].

Overview of Randomized Trials with Adjuvant Portal Infusion

At the moment, there are at least seven prospective controlled adjuvant studies in progress using portal infusion chemotherapy following radical surgery for colorectal cancer. An overview of these trials is given in Table 1. Only randomized trials with a „no-treatment" control group were considered, and with the exception of Taylor's study in Liverpool, all trials are multicentric; some do not include rectal cancer. All studies require radical en bloc resection of the primary without residual disease; portal venous catheterization is done at laparotomy through various routes according to the protocol or the surgeon's preference. Adjuvant treatment is given immediately following surgery as continuous infusion for 7 days. In three protocols the effect of anticoagulants is tested by using heparin or urokinase alone in a three-arm trial design.

In a more recent analysis, Taylor et al. [20] reported on 127 control patients and 117 patients who received adjuvant infusion. Thirteen patients were excluded following randomization because of cirrhosis in one, liver metastases at laparotomy in three, and technical problems with catheter cannulation in nine. After a median follow-up of 4 years, 53 patients died with recurrent disease in the control group and 25 in the infusion group. In the control group, 22 patients developed liver metastases, and in the infusion group five developed liver deposits as the predominant site of recurrence. The patients in the infusion group appeared to have an improved overall survival. However, when individual groups are analyzed, only patients with Dukes B colon tumors show a significant improvement in overall survival. Postoperative morbidity was increased by the adjuvant treatment, more patients suffering from nausea and diarrhea. Overall postoperative mortality was 2.6%, five patients in each group. One patient receiving infusion died in the postoperative period and it was felt that cytotoxicity had contributed to her death. In this case, there was evidence of perirectal sepsis at the time of surgery and the patient died with gram-negative septicemia and leukopenia. Since this occurrence, patients with any evidence of intra-abdominal sepsis have been excluded from the study [20]. At St. Mary's and surrounding hospitals in the U.K. 451 patients have been entered in a three-arm study. No published data are available on this trial, but it is known that 145 of 160 control patients, 110 of 142 heparin-treated patients, and 106 of 149 heparin + 5-fluorouracil-treated patients completed the treatment according to the protocol. Postoperative mortality was 3% and there was one toxic death due to protocol violation.

Table 1. Prospective randomized trials with adjuvant portal infusion at May 1986

Institution	No. patients	Entry	Primaries	Treatment (vs. control)	Results
Liverpool	257	1976–1980	C + R	1 g 5-FU + heparin/d × 7	Survival (4 yrs) (Colon Dukes-B) 70% vs. 50% 92% vs. 60%)
St. Mary's	451	1978–1983	C + R	1 g 5-FU + heparin/d × 7 or 10000 U heparin/d × 7	Liver metas. 6.5% vs. 8.8% vs. 15.3% (control)
Rotterdam	303	1981–1984	C + R	1 g 5-Fu + heparin/d × 7 or 240 000 U urokinase/24 h	Liver metas. 7% vs. 12% vs. 15% (control) At 24 months
Mayo/NCCTG	?	1980–	C	1 g 5-Fu + heparin/d × 7	No data
NSABP	500	1984–	C	600 mg/M² 5-Fu + heparin/d × 7	No data
EORTC	150	1983–	C	500 mg/M² 5-Fu + heparin/d × 7 or 5000 U heparin/d × 7 alone	No data
SAKK	450	1981–1986	C + R	500 mg/m² 5-Fu + heparin/d × 7 + 10 mg/m² mitomycin C d 1	Relapses 19% vs. 24% (control) Liver metas. 6% vs. 10%

C, colon; R, rectum.

Liver metastases occurred in 15.3% (controls), in 8.8% (heparin alone), and in 6.5% (heparin + 5-FU) respectively at a median follow-up of more than 2 years (J. P. Fielding 1986, personal communication). A similar three-arm study has been conducted in Rotterdam with cooperating Dutch Hospitals using urokinase in the anticoagulation-alone arm. Again, in this study, preliminary findings at 24 months indicate a decrease in the incidence of liver metastases, by 15% in the control group, 12% in the urokinase group, and 7% in the 5-FU + heparin group respectively (J. Wereldsma 1986, personal communication).

No data are available so far from the American cooperative group trials. Excellent patient entry is known for the NSABP study (over 500 patients entered within 20 months by more than 40 participating institutions). Results of the Mayo clinical trial are awaited with interest, because this protocol has been active since 1980.

The EORTC Gastrointestinal Tract Cancer Cooperative Group study 40812 is evaluating portal vein infusion of 5-FU + heparin versus heparin alone versus no adjuvant therapy; 182 patients have been entered so far by 11 participating hospitals. Major complications have occurred in seven patients (five septic, one pneumonia, one myocardial infarction) and minor complications in 16 patients, with no differences among the three groups. Heparin infusion had to be stopped in two patients due to postoperative hemorrhage; in the 5-FU-treated patients no dose reductions were necessary, with a mean total dose of 6.3 g 5-FU (4.3–8 g). A strong correlation was found between disease-free survival and local tumor extent and lymphatic invasion. Further data are not available at this moment.

The Swiss group study SAKK 40/81 [11] will be closed in the near future; 450 patients have been entered by seven participating institutions. For various reasons (21 liver metastases, ten other distant metastases detected at laparotomy, 11 incomplete resections, 23 other histology and five protocol violations), 70 patients are not evaluable for the study, and 25 patients are too early for evaluation, leaving 355 fully evaluable patients for interim analysis (179 controls, 176 infusions). Hospital mortality was 2.25% (8/355), duration of hospitalization was 17.9 days for the control group versus 21.2 days for the infusion group ($P < 0.01$). Overall morbidity was slightly increased in the infusion group.

At a median follow-up of 24 months, 30 patients died in the control group and 20 patients in the infusion group. In the control group 18 patients developed liver metastases and 25 patients had recurrent disease outside the liver; in the infusion group 14 patients developed liver metastases and 20 patients had disease progression outside the liver. For various reasons (intraoperative surgical problems in 11, anesthesiological problems in four, technical catheter problems in five, postoperative hemorrhage in three, refusal by three patients, etc.), 29 patients did not receive catheter and/or infusion according to the protocol outline. Analysis according to treatment revealed a 24% relapse rate and a 2-year survival of 83.2% for the control group and a 17.7% relapse rate and a 90.5% survival at 2 years for the patients who had had prophylactic liver infusion. Additional follow-up of 2–3 years is needed in this study for definitive conclusions.

Discussion

Access to the portal vein is possible through various routes. The actual method employed in the Swiss and the EORTC trials using any side branch of the mesenteric vein according to the surgeon's preference was easy to perform; cannulation proved to be technically impossible in less than 2% of patients only, which seems to be superior to a 7% failure rate in cannulating the umbilical vein [20]. Using the transabdominal route there have been no direct catheter-related complications with therapeutic consequences.

Despite a large cumulative dose of 5-FU given during the immediate postoperative period, the systemic side effects were minimal and morbidity of large-bowel surgery was only slightly increased, as was the hospital stay in at least one study. There is a tendency to slightly increased postoperative hemorrhage in the infusion patients, but this was not recorded in all studies.

Toxic deaths have been recorded in at least three trials. One was in Taylor's study, due to perirectal sepsis [20], and one was in the St. Mary's trial in a patient over 80 years old (JP Fielding 1986, personal communication). Another unfortunate course was reported in the Swiss group trial: A 72-year-old insulin-dependent diabetic man had a persistent purulent secretion following right hemicolectomy. On the 11th postoperative day he developed necrotizing fasciitis of the abdominal wall with bronchopneumonia and irreversible gram-negative septicemia. At this time he had marked leukopenia of $2200/mm^3$. For future studies of adjuvant portal infusion, exclusion is recommended for patients over 75 years of age, for insulin-dependent diabetics, and for patients with any evidence of intra-abdominal sepsis at laparotomy or during the early postoperative period.

Interestingly, the overall operative mortality in all the trials cited above is in the range of 2%, considerably lower than that reported by previous multicenter trials and in the surgical literature. This indicates a possible advance in surgical technique and pre-/postoperative patient management in this type of elective cancer surgery.

Preliminary analysis of three different trials at 2 years appears encouraging and tends to support the data of Taylor [20]. Reduction of liver metastases, reduced overall incidence of relapses, and a tendency toward better survival for infusion patients were consistently recorded in these trials. They also confirmed the feasibility of locoregional adjuvant portal chemotherapy in the immediate postoperative period following colorectal cancer surgery. The role of anticoagulation in portal vein infusion has not yet been clearly defined, but there are at least three studies in progress (St. Mary's, the Dutch, and the EORTC trial) evaluating this topic. Within another 2–3 years, definitive conclusions can be made on the usefulness of adjuvant portal infusion. Detailed analysis of all the studies is awaited with interest; subgroup analysis may reveal the candidates most suitable for this type of adjuvant treatment. Until these data are available, adjuvant portal infusion should be restricted to well-designed protocols, and its use is not recommended outside a clinical trial setting.

References

1. Almersjö O, Brandberg A, Gustavsson B (1975) Concentration of biologically active 5-fluorouracil in general circulation during continuous portal infusion in man. Cancer Lett 1: 113–118
2. Bengmark S, Hafström L (1969) The natural history of primary and secondary malignant tumors of the liver. 1. The prognosis for patients with hepatic metastases from colonic and rectal carcinoma by laparotomy. Cancer 23: 198–202
3. Burchenal JH (1976) Adjuvant therapy – theory, practice, and potential. The James Ewing Lecture. Cancer 37: 46–57
4. Cedermark BJ, Schultz SS, Bakshi S, Parthasarathy KL, Mittelman A, Evans TJ (1977) Value of liver scan in the follow-up study of patients with adenocarcinoma of the colon and rectum. Surg Gynecol Obstet 144: 745–748
5. De Vita VT (1983) The relationship between tumor mass and resistance to chemotherapy. Imlications for surgical adjuvant treatment of cancer. The James Ewing Lecture. Cancer 51: 1209–1220
6. Dukes CE (1957) Discussion on major surgery in carcinoma of the rectum, with or without colostomy, excluding the anal canal and including the rectosigmoid. Proc R Soc Med 50: 1031–1052
7. Fisher ER, Turnbull RB (1955) The cytological demonstration and significance of tumor cells in the mesenteric venous blood in patients with colorectal cancer. Surg Gynecol Obstet 100: 102–106
8. Gastrointestinal Tumor Study Group (1984) Adjuvant therapy of colon cancer – results of a prospectively randomized trial. N Engl J Med 310: 737–743
9. Higgins GA, Amadeo JH, McElhinney J, McCaughan JJ, Keehn RJ (1984) Efficacy of prolonged intermittent therapy with combined 5-fluorouracil and methyl-CCNU following resection for carcinoma of the large bowel. Cancer 53: 1–8
10. Lawrence W, Terz JJ, Horsley S, Donaldson M, Lovett WL, Brown PW, Ruffner BW, Regelson W (1975) Chemotherapy as an adjuvant to surgery for colorectal cancer. Ann Surg 81: 616–623
11. Metzger U, Aeberhard P, Egeli R, Harder F, Largiadèr F, Muller W, Pettavel J, Weber W, Cavalli F (1982) Adjuvante portale Leberperfusion beim kolorektalen Karzinom. Helv Chir Acta 49: 175–178
12. Metzger U, Schneider K, Largiadèr F (1982) Adjuvant therapy of colorectal cancer, an overview. Oncology 5: 228–236
13. Morales F, Bell M, McDonald GD, Cole WH (1957) The prophylactic treatment of cancer at the time of operation. Ann Surg 146: 588–595
14. Pestana C, Reitemeier RJ, Moertel CG, Judd ES, Dockerty MB (1964) The natural history of carcinoma of the colon and rectum. Am J Surg 108: 826–829
15. Roberts S, Jonasson O, Long L, McGrath R, McGrew EA, Cole WH (1961) Clinical significance of cancer cells in the circulating blood: 2- to 5-year survivals. Ann Surg 154: 362–371
16. Schabel FM (1975) Concepts for systemic treatment of micrometastases. Cancer 35: 15–24
17. Sellwood RA, Kuper SW, Burn JI, Wallace EN (1965) Circulating cancer cells: the influence of surgical operations. Br J Surg 52: 69–72
18. Swinton NW, Legg MA, Lewis FG (1964) Metastases of cancer of the rectum and sigmoid flexure. Dis Colon Rectum 7: 273–277
19. Taylor I, Rowling JT, West C (1979) Adjuvant cytotoxic liver perfusion for colorectal cancer. Br J Surg 66: 833–837
20. Taylor I, Machin D, Mullee M, Trotter G, Cocke T, West C (1985) A randomized controlled trial of adjuvant portal vein cytotoxic perfusion in colorectal cancer. Br J Surg 72: 359–363
21. Turnbull RB (1970) Cancer of the colon: 5- to 10-year survival rates following resection utilizing the isolation technique. Ann R Coll Surg Engl 46: 243–250
22. Wanebo H (1984) A staging system for liver metastases from colorectal cancer. Proc American Society of Clinical Oncology, no 3, 143 C-560

Interim Analysis of a Double-Blind Phase-III Clinical Trial of Adjuvant Levamisole Versus Control in Resectable Dukes-C Colon Cancer: A Study of the EORTC Gastrointestinal Tract Cancer Cooperative Group

J. P. Arnaud, M. Buyse, M. Adloff, B. Nordlinger, J. C. Pector, and N. Duez

CMCO Schiltigheim, Straßburg, France

The 5-year survival of patients with Dukes-C colon cancer is about 35%. Adjuvant therapy after surgical resection is therefore warranted, but since no therapy has proven effective so far, a control group receiving no further treatment is ethically justified and scientifically required. Results that had been obtained with immunotherapies (BCG, MER-BCG, Corynebacterium Parvum and Levamisole) in colorectal cancer were either ambiguous or based on uncontrolled trials when this trial was initiated by the EORTC in 1978.

The aim of this study is to compare, in a two-arm prospective double-blind randomized trial which includes a placebo control, the efficacy of an adjuvant treatment with Levamisole with respect to (a) overall survival and (b) tumor-free interval. Patients eligible for the trial are those who have had an excision for cure of a large bowel cancer and in whom a Dukes-C grade of tumor spread is found by the pathologist.

Patients and Methods

Criteria for Admission into and Exclusion from the Clinical Trials

The criteria of local disease for this protocol are as follows:

- Adenocarcinoma of the colon, from the cecum to the sacral promontory
- Curative surgical resection, without any macroscopic or histologic residual tumor tissue, local or metastatic
- Involvement of one or more lymph nodes observed by the histologist

Patients with ulcerative or graulomatous colitis and familial polyposis are excluded from the study.

Patient criteria for eligibility into this protocol are no age limit and no previous treatment, radio- or chemotherapy, for any other malignant disease or for the present lesions. Patient criteria of non-eligibility are as follows:

- Presence of another cancer
- Previous history of agranulocytosis or allergy to one or more drugs

Recent Results in Cancer Research, Vol. 110
© Springer-Verlag Berlin · Heidelberg 1988

- Leukopenia (white blound count $<2000/mm^3$)
- Thrombopenia (platelet count $<150000/mm^3$)
- Renal insufficiency (creatinine clearance <60 ml/mm)

Adjuvant Treatment with Placebo or Levamisole

The double-blind adjuvant treatment should begin as soon after surgery as possible within 7 days. Patients are randomized to receive, in double-blind fashion, either 100-250 mg (depending on body weight) of Levamisole on two consecutive days every week for 1 year or a placebo at the same schedule. Treatment is stopped before the end of 1 year if there is morphological evidence of relapse or if symptoms related to toxicity are observed.

Patients

From 1978 to January 1985, 297 patients were accrued in the trial by 14 European institutions. The distribution of the patients to the two groups (placebo or Levamisole) was similar if different subgroups according to the main characteristics are considered (sex, median age, extent of direct tumor spread, presence of lymphatic or venous invasion, proximal or distal involvement of lymph nodes).

Results

Toxicity

The toxicities are given for evaluable patients in the two groups according to the World Health Organization classification. For each patient, toxicities are reported at their highest degree. Mild and moderate side effects (grades 1-3) of therapy were reported equally frequently in the placebo and in the Levamisole groupe (Table 1).

Table 1. Comparison of most frequent side effects (grades 1-3)

	Placebo 132 patients		Levamisole 125 patients	
	n	(%)	n	(%)
Depression	15	11	18	14
Insomnia	19	14	18	14
Anorexia	20	15	15	12
Nausea/vomiting	10	8	20	16
Tiredness	27	20	28	22
	91	69	99	80

Severe toxicities (grades 3 or 4), observed only in the Levamisole group, were reported in 19 of 125 patients (15%): fever in eight patients, agranulocytosis in four, flush-like syndrome in four and skin rash in three. The reaction was reversible in all cases after treatment was stopped.

Survival Data

Patient status by treatment group at February 1986 is summarized in Table 2. There was no difference between Levamisole and placebo in terms of frequency, timing, and site of first disease recurrence: 34% of the recurrences were only local, 8% were only distant, and 58% were both.

There was no difference between placebo and Levamisole in terms of time of death: median survival was 3 years and median disease-free survival 2 years in both groups. There was no advantage of Levamisole in any of the sub-groups examined.

Table 2. Patient status by treatment group

	Placebo	Levamisole
No follow-up information	16	8
Alive without recurrence	62	70
Alive with recurrence	17	18
Dead without recurrence	8	3
Dead with recurrence	48	47
Total	151	146

Conclusion

Unless a long-term benefit of Levamisole appears when more follow-up is available on the patients still alive, we conclude that non-specific immunotherapy with Levamisole is useless in the management of Dukes-C colon cancer.

The Northwest of England Rectal Cancer Trial

R. D. James*

The Christie Hospital and Holt Radium Institute, Withington,
Manchester M20 9BX, Great Britain

Introduction

In 1979 and 1980 more than 4000 cases of large-bowel cancer were treated annually in the Northwest region of England. Of these, 35.5% were within 13 cm of the anal verge. The prognosis following surgery in operable rectal cancer is 30% surviving at 5 years. A large proportion of patients die with evidence of recurrent rectal cancer in the pelvis. Local recurrence appears to be associated with invasion of tumor into surrounding structures which are not removed by conventional surgery [2, 3]. Of 48 patients with locally recurrent tumour investigated by computerised axial tomography (CAT) scanning at the Christie Hospital, 38 had disease limited to structure which were in contact with the original tumour before surgery [10]. In a recent MRC study [5] 765 cases of rectal cancer were assessed before surgery. When tumour appeared to have penetrated into surrounding structures, causing some loss of mobility, it was found that local recurrence following surgery was twice as common (70% versus 37% at 5 years). Furthermore, in over 60% of the cases with tumour penetration it was felt that a complete surgical resection could not be performed. Residual tumour in surrounding structures can regrow to give recurrence.

The prognosis following surgery for rectal cancer may be improved by the addition of radiotherapy at the time of surgery. The aim is to eradicate tumour cells in organs which are not routinely removed by the radical anterior or abdominoperineal excision of the rectum. When radiotherapy is given before surgery its effect can be seen as a reduction in tumour size in irradiated patients compared with non-irradiated controls [5]. Small rectal cancers can be completely eradicated with

* On behalf of the North West of England Rectal Cancer Group: Doctors Baillie, Bancewicz, Bell, Buckler, Cade, Clegg, Cooper-Wilson, Crumplin, Done, Duari, Duthie, Eddleston, England, Forrest, Fussell, Haboubi, Hancock, Hartley, Hoare, Howat, Humphrey, Ingram, James, Johnson, Irving, Kingston, MacLennan, Main, Matheson, Moore, Neill, O'Brien, Ostick, Paley, Pearsonn, Salem, Schofield, Shafiq, Todd, Tweedle, Wilkinson, and Williams.
Acknowledgements to Mr. R. Swindell, Mrs. R. Hannom and Mrs. D. Driver for statistical Analysis.

excellent long-term survival when the dose of radiation is taken to higher levels [6, 9]. Postmortem examinations carried out in one controlled study of preoperative radiotherapy showed a significant reduction in local recurrence for irradiated patients compared with controls [8]. The results are awaited of randomised trials using higher doses conducted by the MRC in Great Britain and by the Veterans' Administration and other groups in the U.S.A. None of these trials have evidenced an increase in surgical morbidity following moderate doses of radiotherapy.

When radiotherapy is given before rather than after surgery there appears to be less risk of severe radiation damage to the small bowel [7]. Radiation fields can be more accurately located around the tumour bed and the small bowel is less likely to adhere to the pelvis postoperatively.

Patients and Methods

Surgeons participating in the Northwest of England Cancer Trial are invited to refer patients with carcinoma of the true rectum (below 12 cm) suitable for a radical resection in whom there is a reasonable risk of local recurrence following surgery. This decision will depend on the personal experience of individual surgeons. They are asked, however, to give an estimate of those factors known to influence local recurrence, the height of the tumour above the anal verge and its apparent fixity in the pelvis, in order to correct any apparent bias in selection of cases. Surgeons are also asked to register patients with rectal cancer unsuitable for the trial.

Patients in the study group are randomly allocated to no treatment or to a 4-day course of preoperative radiotherapy. The tumours of patients in the latter group are marked by the insertion of a radio-opaque clip into the lower border. Radiotherapy (2000 cGy in 4 days to the posterior pelvis), based on this marker and a computerised axial tomograph, is designed to allow anterior *or* abdominoperineal resection. The radiotherapy field is a cylinder 10 cm in diameter and 10 cm long, centred on the tumour. Radiation is delivered with the patient prone using a wedge rotation technique and a 4 MeV linear accelerator. Patients are returned to the referring surgeon for definitive operation unless a specific request is made that surgery be carried out at the Christie Hospital, in which case this is arranged. Participating surgeons are asked to supply operative and postoperative details as well as a copy of the pathology report on irradiated and non-irradiated patients. A 10-ml specimen of clotted blood is set aside preoperatively for the measurements of CEA.

Follow-up is conducted as usual by the referring surgeon. Events which are of particular interest in this study are (a) the definition of local recurrence, (b) the detection of distant metastases, and (c) death. In a recent analysis of 142 cases of recurrent rectal cancer treated at the Christie Hospital, it was found that the accurate determination of time of recurrence was extremely difficult and depended largely on the subjective impressions of surgeon and patient [4]. This subjective variation can be largely eliminated by the measurement of CEA in the serum and by CAT scanning of the pelvis and abdomen.

In this study 10 ml clotted blood is collected at each visit and transferred by the local biochemistry laboratory to the Referral Service in South Manchester. Serial results are available to the referring surgeon and are monitored for each patient by the Trial Secretariat. It is suggested that when a significant rise in CEA occurs, patients should be recalled for a repeat measurement 1 month later. If the rise is sustained surgeons are invited to refer patients for CAT scanning at the Christie Hospital. If local or distant recurrence is confirmed, the patient is no longer in the trial and appropriate treatment will be instituted by consultation with the referring surgeon. Local recurrence can occur without previous rises in CEA, and surgeons are invited to refer patients for CAT scanning if there is reasonable suspicion following AP or anterior resection.

The trial aims to enter 300 patients, assuming a proportion may prove to be inoperable, 150 in each arm. This will give a 90% chance of detecting an increase of 20% in the 3-year local recurrence-free survival rate. It is hoped that recruitment will be complete in 4 years.

Results

To date, 125 patients have been randomised to surgery alone (control) and 128 patients to radiotherapy followed by surgery. The median age of these patients is 67 years, with 98 aged 70 or more, the oldest being 87 years. Data on surgical resections are available on 235 patients and are presented in Tables 1-4. Abdominoperineal resection has been performed on 149 patients, anterior resection on 59, and a Hartman's procedure on eight (Table 1). Eighteen patients have proved to have unresectable tumours. Table 2 shows that the proportion of patients stated to have had a curative procedure is identical in both arms of the trial, suggesting that any differences in local recurrence-free survival times are likely to be the result of radiotherapy. Table 3 shows that the most common site which was felt by the surgeon to contain residual disease was the pelvic side wall. This trial is not designed to irradiate the pelvic side wall but to include the sacrum and bladder, which were felt to be the site of residual disease in 57 patients. Table 4 shows that postopera-

Table 1. Randomisation of patients according to type of surgery

Operation	No. randomised to:	
	XRT	Control
AP	75	74
AR + col.	14	8
AR, no col.	16	21
Hartman's	5	3
Lap. with col.	5	7
Lap., no col.	1	1
Cryosurgery		1
Local excision	1	0
No surgery	2	1

AP, abdominoperineal resection; *AR,* anterior resection; *col,* colostomy.

tive complications in this trial are identical to date in both arms, with no increase in the anastomotic leak rate in patients having low anterior resections following radiotherapy. Tables 5 and 6 record pathological data on histological grade (Table 5) and Dukes' stage (Table 6), indicating that there are equal proportions of each prognostic category in both groups.

Follow-up times have been tabulated in Table 7 for the 221 patients for whom we have accurate information, median follow-up being approximately 11 months. Data are available on survival and local recurrence-free survival in this trial, but they are of necessity tentative and publication at this stage is likely to be misleading. A total of 21 patients have died with no evidence of recurrence, 12 in the control group and nine in the radiotherapy group. To date, there have been a total of 78 deaths, 37 in the radiotherapy group and 41 in the control group. Nineteen deaths have occurred in the postoperative period, within 30 days of surgery, eight in the radiotherapy group and 11 in the control group.

Table 2. Randomisation of patients according to estimation of surgery

Operation considered to be:	No. randomised to:	
	XRT	Control
Curative	62	62
Palliative	40	40
Indeterminate	14	13
Not known	3	1

Table 3. Residual disease at operation

Site	No	Yes	N/K
Side wall	171	61	3
Sacrum	206	25	4
Bladder	200	32	3

N/K, "not known" means not recorded on data form by surgeon.

Table 4. Postoperative complications according to randomisation

Postoperative complications	No. Randomised to:	
	XRT	Control
Abdominal wound sepsis	15	18
Pelvic sepsis	18	11
Urinary obstruction	9	10
Intestinal obstruction needing surgery	5	3
Anastomotic leak	5	6
Haemorrhage	5	9
Other	28	13

Table 5. Histological grade of disease

Pathology	XRT	Control
Well diff.	28	41
Mod. diff.	59	60
Poorly diff.	19	5
N/K	10	8

Table 6. Classification of disease according to Dukes' stage

Dukes classification	XRT	Control
A	21	21
B	37	42
C	51	46
N/K	6	5

Table 7. Length of follow-up according to randomisation

Follow-up time in Months	No. randomised to:	
	XRT	Control
0– 6	29	33
7–12	23	21
13–18	17	21
19–24	15	16
25–30	20	10
31+	7	9

Discussion

Accrual to this trial has been satisfactory, and since all radiotherapy has been given in one centre, quality control of treatment in the combined arm has been easy to assess. Computerised axial tomography has been performed preoperatively in all patients receiving radiotherapy, the field being easily identifiable relative to the tumour. It should therefore be simple to determine whether pelvic recurrence occurs within or outside the radiotherapy field, provided each with local recurrence is rescanned in the same Institute. To date this has been possible in many but not all patients with local recurrence. A second feature of this trial is the provision for preoperative and serial postoperative CEA estimation, allowing an investigation of sites of recurrence as determined by CAT scanning, based on serial rises in CEA. A pathology review is in progress, incorporating staining of tumour sections for CEA, and this should give much-needed information on the usefulness of this histopathologic criterion for determining sites and times of recurrence of rectal carcinoma following combined surgery and radiotherapy.

It is unlikely that preoperative pelvic radiotherapy will alter overall survival rates following surgery for rectal cancer. Benefits may, however, be seen in local recurrence-free survival times, provided local recurrence is defined as recurrence within an irradiated field, which, for the purpose of each trial, should be considered a test-bed for the assessment of the biological activity of radiotherapy in this disease. The exact date of pelvic recurrence is notoriously difficult to determine following abdominoperineal resection, particularly in the male, whilst extraluminal recurrence in the pelvis is common following anterior resection and may remain silent until it ulcerates the bowel at the anastomotic site. These variables may, in themselves, be sufficient to explain the conflicting results of the benefits of radiotherapy in this condition. However, at least two other variables are likely to be involved, namely the extent of the radiotherapy field and the dose of radiation given. It has already been indicated that the radiotherapy field in this trial was limited to the presacral space, and the dose, although low in numerical terms, is probably equivalent to approximately 4000 cGy in 20 fractions over 4 weeks with respect to its effect on normal tissues. This has obviously not increased surgical morbidity, but it remains to be seen whether it will have a significant effect on microscopic disease left following resection in the presacral space. It is important to recognise that the effective radiotherapy dose for such disease is not known and is impossible to predict from radiobiological data which relate normal tissue damage to time-dose effects. A further, largely unconsidered variable in trials of preoperative radiotherapy, intimately related to the two already considered, is the timing of surgical intervention relative to the rate of repair and expression of radiation damage in tumour cells, which itself is an expression of the characteristic cell-kinetic parameters of each tumour. Radiation repair by tumour cells is more likely to be complete when a delay of 4-6 weeks is imposed on the surgeon, as has been the case with moderate and high-dose preoperative studies published to data [1]. Surgery immediately following irradiation, as recommended for this trial, may cause an expression of potentially lethal radiation damage in resting tumour cells stimulated to divide by surgical insult.

The relationship between these variables is likely to be too complex for simple predictions to be made, and the only reliable method for determining the effectiveness of preoperative radiotherapy will be to increase doses, field sizes and surgical extent as much as possible without increasing morbidity. In a recent review, Cummings recognised the importance of carefully controlled trials to assess the value of radiotherapy in rectal cancer [1]. It is the belief of the present author that, wherever possible, such trials should include an estimate of sites of recurrence relative to radiotherapy fields, preferably with the assistance of computerised axial tomography.

References

1. Cummings BJ (1986) A critical review of adjuvant pre-operative radiation therapy for adenocarcinoma of the rectum. Br J Surg 73: 332-338
2. Dixon AK, Kelsey Fry J, Morson BC, Nicholls RJ, Mason A (1981) Pre-operative computed tomography in carcinoma of the rectum. Br J Radiol 54: 655-659

3. Gunderson LL, Sosin K (1974) Areas of failure found at reoperation following "curative surgery" for adenocarcinoma of the rectum. Cancer 34: 1278–1292
4. James RD, Eddleston BE, Johnson RJ, Zheng G, Jones M (19833) Prognostic factors in locally recurrent rectal cancer treatment by radiotherapy. Br J Surg 70: 469
5. Medical Research Council, Rectal Cancer Working Party (1981) Newsletter No 10
6. Papillon J (1975) Intracavitary irradiation of early rectal cancer for cure. A series of 186 cases. Cancer 36: 696–671
7. Romsdahl MM, Withers HR (1978) Radiotherapy combined with curative surgery. Its uses as therapy for carcinoma of the sigmoid colon and rectum. Ann Surg 113: 446–453
8. Roswit B, Higgins GAJ, Geeha RJ (1975) Preoperative irradiation for carcinoma of the rectum and rectosigmoid colon – report of the National V.A. randomized study. Cancer 35: 1597–1602
9. Sischy B (1975) Treatment of carcinoma of the rectum by intracavitary irradiation. Surg Gynecol Obstet 141: 562–566
10. Zheng G, Johnson RJ, Eddleston BE, James RD, Schofield PF (1984) Computed tomography scanning in rectal carcinoma. JR Soc Med 77: 915

Five-Year Results of a Prospective and Randomized Study: Experience with Combined Radiotherapy and Surgery of Primary Rectal Carcinoma

W. Niebel, U. Schulz, M. Ried, J. Erhard, F. Beersiek,
G. Blöcher, H. Nier, H. Halama, E. Scherer, G. Zeller, F. W. Eigler,
with technical assistance of J. Tacken

Abteilung für Allgemeinchirurgie, Gesamthochschule Essen, Medizinische Einrichtungen der Universität, Universitätsklinikum Essen, Hufelandstraße 55, 4300 Essen, FRG

Introduction

In the past three decades there have been many reports dealing with different radio-therapeutic approaches, in combination with surgery, intended to improve the survival rates of patients with potentially curable rectal carcinoma. However, no clear-cut data have yet been presented in this field of clinical investigation, especially with respect to whether pre- or postoperative radiation should be applied and which kind of fractionation or dosage should be given.

Therefore, the University of Essen, the "Lutherhaus" Hospital Essen-Steele, and the City Hospital of Offenbach started a three-clinic study, first to evaluate the effect of low-dose preoperative radiotherapy with 25 Gy within 2.5 weeks; second, to see whether histological examination of the resected specimen revealed a pT3 or pT4 stage and if so, the effect of a postoperative 25-Gy boost; third, to evaluate postoperative radiotherapy with a 50-Gy dose within 6 weeks.

Material and Methods

The projected therapeutic schedule was originally set up so that the randomization between preoperative radiotherapy plus surgery and surgery alone took place after assessment of tumor growth by histological examination of the biopsy. No evidence was found that the randomization step was faulty. Unfortunately, the therapeutic schedule performed was different from the one projected, because many patients with pT3/pT4-stage disease postoperatively refused the intended radiation therapy in spite of having given informed consent or were not radiated for various reasons which reflect the doctor's or the patient's bias.

On the other hand, this provided us with two highly selected therapeutic groups, i.e., "preoperative radiotherapy plus surgery" and "surgery alone (controls)", which we then could compare. The other two groups which deal with postoperative radiation plus surgery can only be described.

From January 1978 to September 1981 a total of 142 patients with potentially curable rectal carcinoma were entered into the study. There were 71 male and

71 female patients with a mean age of 63.5 ± 9.0 years ($\bar{x} \pm SD$). No differences between the groups were found in relation to age, sex, Karnofsky index, CEA plasma levels, the clinical extent, and the distance of the tumor from the anal verge (data not shown). The ratio of sphincter-saving resections and abdominoperineal excisions was 1:1, the mortality was 2.2% the resectability rate 98% and the rate of curative resections 89%. The median follow-up time was 58 months as of April 1986.

Results

In five of 64 patients (8%) with preoperative radiotherapy the pathological assessment of excised tumors showed no further evidence of malignant tissue.

A comparison of the tumor sizes recorded by the pathologists, who measured the greatest diameters of length and breadth, reveals a significant difference: after preoperative radiotherapy plus surgery the tumors were significantly smaller than after surgery alone (9.7 ± 1.1 cm^2 versus 20.1 ± 2.0 cm^2; $\bar{x} \pm SEM$).

The distribution of pT-classification (according to the Heidelberg system) is as follows: the numbers of pT1 and pT2 cases are significantly higher and those of pT3 and pT4 cases lower after preoperative radiation plus surgery than after surgery alone.

There was no difference seen between the groups in the proportion of patients with positive lymph nodes.

After a median follow-up time of 58 months the rates of local recurrences, distant metastases, and deaths in 126 curatively resected patients were 10%, 20%, and 30% respectively. There were no differences between the two therapeutic groups.

Looking at tumor recurrence as a function of pT classification, there seems to be an advantage for pT1 and pT2 cases regarding local recurrence, but this advantage is diminished as regards distant metastases; therefore, there is no statistical difference.

The trends found before continue: After a median follow-up to 58 months the cumulative proportion of surviving patients with curative resection is $75\% \pm 7\%$ in the "surgery-alone" group and $73\% \pm 7\%$ in the "preoperative radiotherapy plus surgery" group. This is quite a high level in both groups, and preoperative irradiation does not influence it.

At 58 months after postoperative radiotherapy plus curative surgery we found a survival rate of $70\% \pm 10\%$. This is also a very high figure, considering that this group consists only of patients with pT3/pT4-stage disease.

Patients receiving pre- and postoperative radiotherapy and curative surgery show the poorest survival rate, i.e., $48\% \pm 14\%$ after 58 months. It is impossible to give a clear explanation for this finding. It must be said again that only pT3 and pT4 cases are in this group and that the total number of cases (15) is very small. In any case, the analysis of the data does not reveal any evidence that the combination of pre- and postoperative irradiation influences the morbidity or the mortality.

Discussion

After preoperative radiotherapy real biological effects can be found in the excised specimen of a rectal carcinoma. This can be demonstrated in cases in which the tumor can no longer be found pathologically and in the significant reduction of the tumor size. Another point is the imputed "down-staging". But regarding the most important parameter, i.e., the 5-year survival rate, there is no advantage of preoperative radiotherapy with 25 Gy within 2.5 weeks plus surgery compared with surgery alone. This conclusion can be drawn on the basis of the randomization in the study.

Surprisingly, another, more important result of the study is that after surgery and postoperative radiotherapy of high-risk patients with pT3/pT4-stage disease the 5-year survival rate was $70\% \pm 10\%$, a remarkable high figure. Unfortunately, our study did not contain a control for this group.

Conclusion

Regarding preoperative radiotherapy as part of the strategy for control of rectal carcinoma, this study has failed to obtain significant results, probably because of the good results obtained with surgery alone. Therefore, preoperative radiotherapy can not be recommended generally, but should be used only in selected cases or in prospective studies. On the other hand, postoperative radiotherapy in pT3/pT4 cases appears to improve the survival rate appreciatively, and this should be investigated in a more detailed study.

Acknowledgments. The authors wish to thank Prof. Dr. L. D. Leder, Pathological Institute of the University of Essen, and Dr. P. Müller, Pathological Institute of the City Hospital of Offenbach, for their kind cooperation, and L. Caron for his help with translation. This study was supported by a grant from the *Bundesministerium für Jugend, Familie und Gesundheit.*

The True Role of External-Beam Irradiation in the Initial Treatment of Cancer of the Rectum

J. Papillon

Department of Radiotherapy, Centre Léon Berard, 69008 Lyon, France

Among the several trials devoted to preoperative irradiation of rectal cancer, the second EORTC trial conducted by A. Gerard [1] between 1976 and 1981, which includes 318 cases, is one of the first to demonstrate decisively a significant gain in the 5-year survival rate – 70% vs 60%. For the radiation oncologists the trials are invaluable to show that irradiation is capable of improving the prognosis of cancer of the rectum after surgery. However, in almost all these trials the irradiation does not alter the surgical procedure, and the majority of cured patients have a permanent colostomy. In the EORTC trial more than 85% of the patients underwent a mutilating operation.

Optimal treatment of rectal cancer aims to give patients the highest chance of cure and the possibility of retaining normal anal function. The efficacy of external-beam irradiation may be improved by using appropriate protocols. Most methods of irradiation give homogeneous dose – 4500 rads in 5 weeks – to a large target area including most if not all of the pelvic cavity, and surgery is performed very soon after completion of the irradiation.

The dose/time relationship is the key factor of effectiveness of irradiation. The shorter the irradiaton protraction, the greater the effect of a delivered dose.

The second point concerns the time of surgery. Many radiobiological studies tend to indicate that the benefit of preoperative irradiation is the same irrespective of the interval between irradiation and surgery, since the proportions of cells killed and alive are identical in all cases. Moreover, radiobiologists fear a regrowth of the tumor if surgery is delayed.

The clinical experience is in contradiction with this rule [2]. Since 1977 we have used a protocol based on two principles: (a) nonhomogeneous dose of irradiation given to more a limited target area within a short period of time, (b) an interval of 2 months between the last application of radiotherapy and surgery.

The irradiation is performed as cobalt 60 120° arc rotation through a sacral field, the patient being in the prone position (Fig. 1). A dose of 3000 rads is delivered in ten fractions within 12 days. The dose is calculated at the isocenter situated at 10 cm depth. The target volume includes the tumor and a surrounding area with a substantial margin upwards, downwards, and laterally. Isodose distribution shows that the tumor area receives a higher dose of up to 3500 rads. The patient is

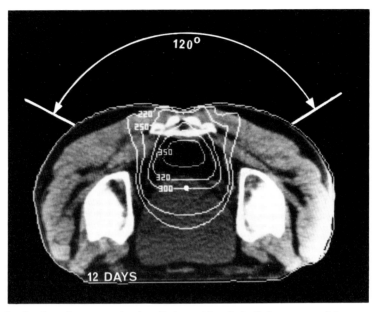

Fig. 1. Isodose distribution of preoperative irradiation with cobalt 60 for cancer of the rectum. Irradiation is performed by 120° arc rotation through a 9 × 12-cm sacral field. The patient is in the prone position with a full bladder. A dose of 30 Gy calculated at isocenter, which is at 10 cm depth, is delivered in ten fractions within 12 days. Note that a hot spot at 35–39 Gy is centered to the tumor area and that the target volume includes most of the posterior pelvic area with satisfactory protection of the small bowel, the urinary bladder, and bone structures

asked to have a full bladder at the time of irradiation, since bladder distension is the most efficient way to protect the small bowel which is then displaced superiorly and anteriorly. A roentgenogram of the small bowel is systematically taken to adapt the target volume to the location of the small bowel. One of the advantages of this method is that the isodose distribution may be adapted to the site and size of the tumor. The isocenter may be displaced laterally or situated at 8 cm instead of 10 cm according to the location of the tumor. The overall treatment time may be extended from 12 to 16 days for patients in poor general condition.

Such a dose given in a short period of time is well tolerated, the main complication being proctitis, which does not last more than 3 weeks and is easily relieved medically. There is no cystitis since most of the bladder is protected, and there is no risk of radiation enteritis.

The free interval of 2 month between irradiation and the second stage of treatment represents a decisive point of this protocol, which differs markedly from the usual methods of preoperative irradiation. Regrowth of the tumor has never been observed during the 2-month rest.

This protocol has been applied in 134 cases since 1977. Seventy patients underwent surgery and 64 patients were treated conservatively. This protocol has several advantages:

The 2-month rest following irradiation allows one to profit from the tumor regression and enlightens the selection process. It becomes easy to distinguish between deeply infiltrating tumors, tethered mobile, invading perirectal fat and surrounding structures on the one hand and the moderately infiltrating mobile lesions which have little or no extrarectal spread on the other.

The efficacy of the method may be assessed by the study of operative specimens, which shows a down-staging of the irradiated tumors. Table I reports the highest rate of tumor-free operative specimens ever published. Theoretically, these patients could have been spared major surgery. However, in spite of the tumor regression, surgery was considered to be absolutely necessary, both because of the size of the tumor at the time of presentation (4-7 cm) and because of the potential lymphatic involvement. Dukes A lesions were found in 18 cases (25%). One may assume that some initially Dukes B tumors have shrunk in such a manner that the residual lesion became confined to the bowel wall.

In this series the overall rate of tumor-free and Dukes-A surgical specimens is 42%. This figure may be seriously taken into consideration in the choice of the most appropriate terminal approach.

Timing of the operation 8 weeks after completion of the short-term irradiation makes the surgery easier and safer, and sometimes allows it to be less mutilating. Fifty-five patients underwent an abdominoperineal resection and 15 a low-anterior resection. No technical difficulties with defining fascial planes, no fibrosis, and no excessive bleeding related to the irradiation were noted during surgery. In many cases the surgeon stated that the excision was especially easy and quick.

The effectiveness of this protocol may be assessed by the study of pelvic failures. Among 47 patients followed up for more than 3 years, four developed local failures (8.5%), it should be kept in mind that most local failures occur during the first 3 years. Two patients died postoperatively. In the group of 15 patients who underwent a low-anterior resection, 13 had tumors located in or extended to the lower third of the rectum, which would have been treated by abdominoperineal resection if they had not been irradiated before. In such cases irradiation allowed an extension of the field of sphincter-saving procedures. No failures were observed in this group. Among these patients three developed anastomotic leakage which required temporary colostomy, closed after 3 months.

Table 1. Dukes' classification of 70 operative specimens following irradiation with cobalt 60 and delayed surgery[a] for rectal carcinoma

Classification	Percentage of cases
Tumor free	17.1
Dukes A	25.7
Dukes B	27.1
Dukes C	30

[a] AP resection ($n=55$) and LA resection ($n=15$; 13 tumors extended to lower one third of the rectum).

Particular cases are elderly, poor-risk patients with moderately infiltrating tumors of the lower rectum, too large (more than 4 cm) or too close to the sphincter area to be treated by traditional methods of conservation. Usually, all such patients undergo an abdominoperineal resection. But it is well known that a permanent colostomy in elderly patients, especially those in poor socioeconomic conditions or those living alone may give rise to profound depression, beside the non-negligible mortality and morbidity following major surgery. In such cases it may be rational to try to extend the field of conservation when the residual disease after a 2-month rest is limited and apparently suitable for intracavitary irradiation. This protocol was applied to 64 patients. Their median age is 77 years. The second stage of treatment consists in an iridium-192 implant, often associated with an application of contact radiotherapy.

Among the 47 patients followed up for more than 3 years, six developed pelvic failures, two of whom have been saved by AP resection, and six died of cancer, due either to distant metastasis (two) or to local failures (four). One 84-year-old patient died postoperatively; 28 patients are alive and well, 26 with normal anal function, two after salvage AP resection; 12 have died from intercurrent disease. The actuarial 5-year survival rate is 83% (Fig. 2). The average age of these patients at the time of death is 83 years. In the whole series, 94 patients have been followed up for more than 3 years. The results are reported in Table 2.

This experience shows that external-beam irradiation as the initial treatment is advisable in most cases of non-obstructive cancers of the lower rectum, but the technique of radiotherapy should be adapted to the intended purpose. Irradiation is able not only to improve the prognosis after radical surgery but also to extend the field of sphincter-saving and conservative procedure. To achieve such an ambitious task four conditions must be met: (a) Accurate pretreatment evaluation is necessary, with digital rectal examination and a systematic search for pelvic metas-

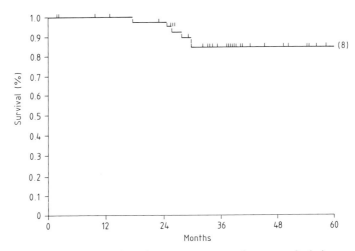

Fig. 2. Survival of patients with T_2 tumor of the lower rectum treated conservatively by external-beam irradiation (3000 rads in 12 days), followed by intracavitary irradiation 2 months later

Table 2. Results at 3 years with external-beam irradiation given as initial treatment (3000 rads, 12 days) for cancer of the lower rectum in 94 patients[a]

Result	No.	Percent
Alive and well	62	66
Dead of intercurrent disease	14	15
Dead of cancer ⎫ Post-op. deaths ⎭	18	19
Functioning w/o colostomy	47/76	61

[a] Radiotherapy + surgery: 47 patients (40 AP resection, 7 LA resection); radiotherapy + iridium: 47 patients.

tatic nodes by palpation and CT scan, proctosigmoidoscopy and biopsy, colonoscopy or double-contrast barium enema, and a general examination. These investigations allow a clinical staging which distinguishes the early rectal adenocarcinomas smaller than 4 cm suitable for intracavitary irradiation and larger tumors suitable for external-beam irradiation as initial treatment. (b) Short-term irradiation must be concentrated on a limited but sufficient target volume. (c) The second stage of treatment, surgical or radiotherapeutic, should be delayed for 2 months after completion of the first irradiation. (d) Careful follow-up is mandatory in order to detect as early as possible any abnormalities or recurrences. This strategy can spare a large number of patients with cancer of the lower rectum a permanent colostomy without jeopardizing their chance of cure.

References

1. Gerard A, Berrod JL, Pene F, Loygue J, Laugier A, Bruckner R, Camelot G, Arnaud JP, Metzger U, Buyse M, Dalesio O, Duez N (1985) Interim analysis of a phase-III study on preoperative radiation therapy in resectable rectal carcinoma. Trial of Gastrointestinal Tract Cancer cooperative group of the European organization for research on treatment of cancer. Cancer 55: 2373–2379
2. Papillon J (1982) Rectal and anal cancers. Conservative treatment by irradiation: an alternative to radical surgery. Springer, Berlin Heidelberg New York

Combined-Treatment Approaches in the Management of Rectal Cancer

L. L. Gunderson*

Mayo Medical School, Consultant in Radiation Oncology Mayo Clinic, 200 SW First Street, Rochester, MN, USA

Introduction

Irradiation (XRT) is being used in combination with surgery in the initial treatment of rectal cancer with increasing frequency. Incidence and areas of failure after operation alone will be outlined by site and stage, with implications for adjuvant therapy. Results of series utilizing radiation will be presented with an emphasis on North American studies. The potential for the future will be discussed.

Staging Systems

A comparison of common staging systems [1–4] is shown in Table 1. While the Dukes' staging system [1] is useful in predicting the outcome of survival after surgery, it is less functional in distinguishing subpopulations of patients at greatest risk for local failure who may benefit from adjuvant radiation. A modification of the Astler-Coller rectal staging system [2] by Gunderson and Sosin [3] differentiates by degree of extrarectal involvement in the B_2 and C_2 group, be it microscopic (m), gross (g) or macroscopic extension confirmed at microscopy, or adherence to or invasion of surrounding organs or structures (B_3 or C_3). This system has been used to analyze survival and patterns of recurrence after potentially curative surgery and indicates that within Dukes' stages B and C there are subgroups of patients with significantly different risks for both survival [2, 5] and local failure [3, 5–7]. For lesions that extend beyond the bowel wall in anatomically immobile sites, the amount of uninvolved tissue (circumferential or radial margins) may be as or more important than the degree of extrarectal extension.

* The author appreciates the efforts of Julie Boland and the Mayo Typing Service for assistance in the preparation of the manuscript.

Table 1. Staging systems for colorectal carcinoma – comparison of Dukes' scheme with TNM and a modification of the Astler-Coller system by Gunderson and Sosin. (Modified from Gunderson [42])

Staging system			
Dukes'	Modified Astler-Coller	TNM^a	
[1]	[3]	[4]	
A	A	T1N0	Nodes negative; lesion limited to mucosa
	B_1	T2N0	Nodes negative; extension of lesion through mucosa but still within bowel wall
B	$B_2{}^b$	T3N0	Nodes negative; extension beyond the bowel wall
C	C_1	T2N1	Nodes positive; lesion limited to bowel wall
	$C_2{}^b$	T3N1	Nodes positive; extension of lesion beyond the bowel wall

[a] By definition M_0 or no evidence of metastases.
[b] Separate notation is made regarding degree of extension beyond the bowel wall: microscopic only (m); gross extension confirmed by microscopy (g); surgical or pathologic adherence to or invasion of surrounding organs or structures ($B_3 + C_3$; TNM system – T_5).

Table 2. Rectal cancer – pelvic failure by Astler-Coller stage

Modified* A–C stage	Clinical series								Re-Op'n	
	U Florida [11]^a		Portland, ME [7]		Mallinkrodt [6]		MGH [5]		U Minn [3]	
	(n)	*(%)*	*(n)*	*(%)*	*(n)*	*(%)*	*(n)*	*(%)*	*(n)*	*(%)*
Within wall										
A	0/14	0	0/1	–	2/12	17	0/3	–	–	–
B_1	5/23	22	6/42	14	0/21	0	3/36	8	–	–
C_1	9/24	38	1/5	–	2/7	29	2/4	–	4/17	24
Through wall										
$B_2 (+B_3)^b$	10/45	22	13/37	35	7/43	16	18/59	31	–	–
$C_2 (+C_3)$	11/29	38	24/37	65	15/40	38	20/40	50	28/40	70
Totals	35/135	26	44/122	36	26/123	21	43/142	30	–	–

[a] Modified from Mendenhall et al. [11] on basis of personal communication from WM Mendenhall, September, 1985.
[b] See Table 1 regarding definition of stage (Astler-Coller B_2 and C_2 include modified Astler-Coller stages B_3 and C_3 respectively).

Patterns of Failure After "Curative Resection"

The risk of local recurrence after "curative resection" is related to both disease extension beyond the bowel wall and nodal involvement [3, 5–11]. The incidence of local recurrence for lesions with nodal involvement but tumor confined to the wall (i.e., C_1) varies from 20% to 40%, which is approximately the same as in the group

Table 3. Rectal cancer – pelvic failure by modified Astler-Coller stage

Extent of disease (MD Anderson)	Clinical series						Modified Astler-Coller stage[a]
	MD Anderson [10] At risk		Mallinkrodt [6]		MGH [5]		
	(n)	(%)	(n)	(%)	(n)	(%)	
A	–	–	2/12	17	0/3	–	A
B_1	149	3	0/21	0	3/36	8	B_1
B_2			6/38	16			B_2
a) No unusual problems	146	12			2/12	17	a) $B_2(m)$
b) Adherence or difficult dissection(s)	52	22			8/32	25	b) $B_2(g)$
B_3 – Adjacent structure (p)	11	31	1/5	–	8/15	53	B_3
C_1	12	32	2/7	29	2/4	–	C_1
C_2			14/38	37			C_2
a) No unusual problem	92	28			2/7	29	a) C_{2m}
b) Adherence or difficult dissection(s)	23	70			14/27	52	b) C_{2g}
C_3 – Adjacent structure (p)	11	45	1/2	–	4/6	67	C_3

s, surgical; p, pathological.
[a] For B_2 and C_2 stages in the MGH series, the degree of extension beyond the muscularis propia was analyzed – microscopic (m) or gross (g).

with nodes negative but extending beyond the wall (i.e., $B_2 + B_3$) where the risk is 20%–35% (Table 2). The lesions that have both bad prognostic factors, nodal involvement and extension beyond the wall (i.e., $C_2 + C_3$), have nearly an additive risk of local recurrence, varying from 40% to 65% in the clinical series [5–11] and amounting to 70% in the preoperative series [3]. In an MGH series, the incidence of both total and local failure in the node-negative group increased with each degree of extension beyond the wall [5] (Table 3). In that series and in a separate one from M. D. Anderson [10], the degree of extrarectal extension appeared to be an independent factor, influencing the risk of local recurrence even in node-positive patients.

Adjuvant Irradiation

When both surgery and radiation may be indicated, differences of opinion exist regarding the preferred sequence. A theoretical advantage of preoperative XRT is the potential damaging effect on cells that may be spread locally or distantly at the time of resection. The major advantage of postoperative treatment is the ability to exclude patients with advanced but undiagnosed metastatic disease prior to exploration or those at low risk for local recurrence. Only those patients at high risk for local recurrence on the basis of operative and pathologic findings are irradiated.

Rectal Cancer

The potential value of XRT for large bowel cancer has been identified more clearly with rectal cancer than with colon cancer. When used as an adjuvant to "curative resection," both preoperative and postoperative radiation have decreased local recurrence and improved survival in selected subgroups in both randomized and nonrandomized studies.

Preoperative Irradiation. Preoperative series using a variety of dose and portal arrangements have demonstrated evidence of tumor response by virtue of partial or total regression of the primary lesion [12, 13]. Although survival was improved in selected subgroups of patients in two prospective randomized low-dose series (Princess Margaret Hospital, 500 rad × 1 [14]; VA Hospital, 2000–2500 rad in 2–2½ weeks [15], these results were not duplicated in a recently published Medical Research Council trial which compared these two treatment arms with a surgery-alone control arm [16]. Results from a second VA trial using higher doses of preoperative irradiation (3500 rad/4 weeks) do not reveal an advantage to the irradiated group [17], and an EORTC trial with similar doses also does not show a survival advantage [18]. In a high-dose nonrandomized Oregon series (5000–6000 rad/6–7 weeks), only one of 45 patients (2.3%) with subsequent "curative resection" was proven to have later pelvic recurrence [13] as compared with an incidence of 29% in an autopsy subset of irradiated patients in the initial low-dose VA trial [15].

Following moderate-dose preoperative irradiation (4500–5000 rad), only abdominoperineal resections used to be recommended, due to a possible increase in anastomotic leaks. Published data from Stevens et al. [19] and Roberson et al. [20] have shown that such doses do not preclude anterior resection and primary anastomosis. Unirradiated large bowel should be utilized for the proximal limb of the anastomosis, with temporary diverting colostomies done only on the basis of surgical indications.

Postoperative Irradiation ± Chemotherapy. In prospective but non-randomized postoperative series utilizing dose levels of 4500–5500 rad in 5–6½ weeks for high-risk patients (B_{2-3}; C_{1-3}), local recurrence has decreased from an expected 35%–50% with operation alone to 10%–20% in the XRT series [11–13, 28]. Distant failures continue to be a problem in 25%–30% of patients in spite of the improvement in local control.

In a published MGH analysis by Hoskins et al. [21], local recurrence was compared at the 3-year interval from resection in non-randomized but sequential series for operation alone (103 patients) versus operation and postoperative irradiation (95 patients; Table 4). A statistically significant reduction in local recurrence was found for most stages in patients who received irradiation ($B_2[g]$, B_3, $C_1 + C_2[g]$). In a recent update of that series by Tepper et al. [22], the irradiated patients continued to have a significantly lower incidence of local recurrence by stage and the 5-year NED survival had improved (Table 5). The incidence of local recurrence in irradiated B_2 and B_3 patients was quite low at 8% (5/60). In node-positive patients, however, the incidence was $\geq 20\%$ (C_1-2/10, 20%; C_2-16/77, 21%; C_3-8/15,

Table 4.   Rectal cancer – pelvic failure at 3 years, MGH. (Modified from Hoskins et al. [21])

Modified A–C stage	Surgery		Postoperative XRT	
	At risk	LF	At risk	LF
	(n)	*(%)*	*(n)*	*(%)*
B_2 (m)	12	8	6	18
B_2(g)	32	25	23	0*
B_3	15	58	7	0*
C_1 C_2(m)	11	43	15	7*
C_2(g)	27	53	34	9*
C_3	6	100	10	31
Total	103		95	

LF, local failure.
* Significant at $P \le 0.05$.

Table 5.   Rectal cancer, MGH: 5-year NED survival – operation $\pm$ XRT. (Modified from Tepper et al. [22])

Stage	Surgery (%)	Surgery + XRT (%)
B_2	47	76
B_3	27	69
C_1	25	69
C_2	27	34
C_3	0	13

53%) suggesting either the need for higher doses of irradiation or the need to combine irradiation with chemotherapy or a radiation dose modifier. The figures for C_2 and C_3 may be falsely high, as three and five patients respectively had diffuse peritoneal seeding with a pelvic component; minimum pelvic failure rates with those patients excluded would be C_2–13/74 (18%), C_3–3/10 (30%).

A Gastrointestinal Tumor Study Group trial [23] randomized patients with Dukes' B or C lesions to a surgery-alone control arm versus adjuvant treatment arms of postoperative irradiation (4000 or 4800 rad), postoperative chemotherapy (5-FU + methyl-CCNU), or a combination thereof (4000 or 4400 rad). The disease-free survival of all three treated groups was higher than that for the surgery-alone group, but only the observed difference between the combined adjuvant arm versus surgery alone is statistically significant ($P < 0.009$). When patterns of initial failure were analyzed, however, the combined treatment resulted not in a decrease in the incidence of distant metastases but rather in a decrease in local recurrence. In spite of improvements in disease-free survival in both groups with irradiation, the local recurrence rates were too high in the irradiation-only group, with a $\ge$

20% incidence versus ≥ 11% with radiation plus chemotherapy (this may be higher, as only initial patterns of failure have been published).

Since radiation doses were low and local recurrence rates were high in the radiation-only group in the GITSG study, there was still uncertainty regarding radiation plus chemotherapy versus radiation alone as the preferred postoperative adjuvant treatment. A recently completed randomized trial by the Mayo Clinic and the North Central Cancer Treatment Group may clarify this uncertainty, since the minimum XRT dose within the boost field in both the XRT and XRT+CT arms was 5000 rads. Preliminary results were presented at the 1986 ASCO meeting [24] and demonstrated a statistically significant improvement in disease-free survival with the combined adjuvant treatment versus irradiation alone ($P<0.02$). The incidence of both local recurrence and systemic failure was lower in the combined group.

Preoperative± Postoperative Irradiation. Low-dose preoperative irradiation (500 rad × 1 or 5 × 200 rad) has been combined with selective postoperative irradiation (4500–5000 rad/25–28 fractions) in view of some theoretical advantages over either high-dose preoperative or postoperative irradiation [25–27]. In pilot studies from Thomas Jefferson University Hospital (TJUH) [26, 27] and MGH [25], indications for delivering the postoperative component were as follows: (a) extension beyond the wall, nodes negative (MGH excluded some patients with only focal microscopic extension and good circumferential margins - preferably ≥ 1.5–2 cm; (b) confined to the bowel wall, nodes positive (patients with only 1–2 adjacent nodes were excluded at MGH if 15–20 were examined); or (c) nodes positive and extension beyond the wall. The recent analyses of both series [25, 27] suggest that one can safely exclude patients who do not require the postoperative component of irradiation (Stages A and B_1 ± select early B_2[m] and C_1 lesions) and yet achieve excellent local control in Dukes' B and C patients and good survival rates. In the TJUH series, the addition of the postoperative component significantly reduced both total and local failure when compared with low-dose preoperative alone (total failure, 52% versus 19%; local failure, 34% versus 6%). While such an approach may be preferable to either high-dose preoperative or postoperative irradiation for mobile lesions, it would be difficult to develop a meaningful comparison with high-dose preoperative XRT since clinical staging at present is so inaccurate. A randomized comparison with postoperative XRT is in progress in a combined RTOG-ECOG trial, in which 50% of patients with clinically resectable rectal cancer receive 500 rad × 1 preoperatively. After resection, all patients with disease extension beyond the rectal wall (B_2, B_3), nodes involved (C_1), or both in conjunction (C_2, C_3) receive 4500–5000 rad in 180-rad fractions.

Complications and Therapeutic Ratio

A suitable therapeutic ratio between local control and complications is achieved only with close interaction between the surgeon and the radiotherapist and with the use of sophisticated radiation techniques [28]. In the postoperative MGH series with shaped multiple-field techniques, use of bladder distention, etc., the incidence of small-bowel obstruction requiring operative intervention is essentially equal in the group receiving irradiation and that with operation alone, at 6% versus 5% respectively [21, 22]. In the GITSG trial [23], severe or worse non-hematologic toxicity occurred in 35% of patients in the combined-adjuvant group arm versus 16% of those with radiation alone – two patients in the combined-treatment group died of complications of enteritis, free of disease. In the Mayo/NCCTG trial using multiple-field techniques, the incidence of small-bowel problems has been ≤5% with either XRT alone or in combination with chemotherapy [24].

Residual, Unresectable, Medically Inoperable, or Recurrent Disease

External-Beam Irradiation

Although results with radiation seem to be better in most series in those patients with inoperable (surgical or medical) and/or residual carcinoma as opposed to those with recurrence, there is need for improvement. Wang and Schulz [29] obtained cures in 12.5% (two of 16) of the inoperable group and 22% (two of nine) of the group with partial resection.

In a Princess Margaret Hospital series, 123 patients were treated with radical external-beam irradiation (usual dose of 4500–5000 rad delivered in 250-rad fractions, 5 days per week) [30]. Of 67 patients who presented with tumor fixation, local control was achieved in only six (9%), and the 5-year actuarial survival was 2%. Of 56 patients who presented with mobile lesions, local control was achieved in 21 (38%), and the 5-year actuarial survival was 40% (relative 5-year survival, 55%). While primary radiation produces superb palliation and an occasional cure with fixed lesions and decent local control and cure with mobile lesions (40%), the results do not compare favorably with those of combined surgery and irradiation [8]. Primary irradiation should be reserved for the patient who is a poor medical candidate for resection or refuses the procedure.

External Radiation ± Systemic Therapy or Surgical Resection

When external-beam radiation is combined with surgery for residual disease after resection [31–33] or for disease that is unresectable for cure due to fixation [12, 13, 34, 35], although local control and survival can be obtained in some patients, the risk of local progression is too high. In the residual disease subgroups from MGH [33] and Albert Einstein [32], the incidence of local recurrence after external-beam irradiation varied according to the amount of residual disease, being 50%–54% if there was gross residual (AE – 9/18; MGH – 13/24) versus 15%–26% if there was only microscopic residual (AE – 2/13; MGH – 8/31). In the MGH analysis, a possible dose-response correlation was seen in the group with microscopic residual, with an 11% LF risk (1/9) if the boost was ≥6000 rad and 33% (7/21) if the boost dose was ≤5500 rad. In the patients with gross residual, a dose-response correlation could not be discerned. With initially unresectable lesions, the resectability rate after preoperative doses of 4500–5000 rad has varied from 50% to 75%

by series (13, 34, 35). Even in those patients who were resected, the incidence of local recurrence has been excessive at 36%–45%. In the MGH series [34], long-term survival was seen only in patients who were resected (30% ≥ 5-year survival versus 0% 3-year survival for non-resected patients).

Intraoperative (IORT) and External-Beam Irradiation ± Resection

In an attempt to decrease local recurrence and improve survival, both MGH and Mayo have initiated pilot studies which add an intraoperative electron boost to the previous combinations of external-beam irradiation and resection [36–41]. In the initial published MGH trial of 32 patients, local control appeared to be improved in both the residual disease and initially unresectable patients, and survival was better in the latter group when compared with historical controls treated only with preoperative irradiation and resection [37]. In their ongoing trials, survival in the group of patients who present with recurrence is stable at ≥ 30% between 3 and 4 years in contrast to an expected long-term survival of 5%–10% when treated with standard techniques [38]. The incidence of moderate or severe soft-tissue complications has not appeared to increase as a result of the aggressive combinations [39]. In a series of 35 patients treated at the Mayo Clinic (recurrent – 24, primary – 11), results parallel those achieved at MGH but the follow-up is not as long [40, 41]. Disease progression has occurred in only two of eight (25%) when resection was preceded by the external-beam component of irradiation (5000 rad/28 fractions) versus 11 of 27 (40%) when resection was performed before external irradiation. Similar improvements in disease control were found in the MGH series when irradiation preceded the resection [37].

Radiation Dose Aims

Although temporary palliation of unresectable primary or recurrent lesions can be achieved with radiation dose levels as low as 2000 rad in 2 weeks, prolongation of palliation requires dose levels of 4000–5000 rad in 4–5 weeks or higher, and doses of 6000–7000 rad may be indicated. At such levels, however, the incidence of radiation-induced small-bowel damage will be prohibitive unless information is available regarding the relative position of tumor and small bowel and is used to modify XRT doses and portals.

Doses above 4500–5000 rad should not be used unless there is good small-bowel mobility or minimal volumes of small bowel, and above 5500 rad only if the small bowel is completely outside the XRT portal. Operative techniques including clip placement and reconstruction procedures [28] can help the radiation oncologist to use appropriate field reduction after an initial 4500–5000 rad (i.e., make the field smaller for an additional 1500–2000 rad yet include tumor and miss the small bowel with the aid of lateral fields and bladder distension). A unique combination of the two utilizes an intraoperative electron-beam boost to areas of high risk while dose-limiting tissues are retracted out of the field.

Conclusions and Future Possibilities

Adjuvant Irradiation ± Chemotherapy

In an adjuvant setting, doses of 5000 rad in 5½–6 weeks given either preoperatively (XRT alone) or postoperatively (XRT ± 5-FU) in conjunction with resection of all known disease produces good local control in most patients with rectal and rectosigmoid carcinoma. Complications appear to be satisfactory, provided multified techniques, bladder distention, etc., are utilized. In those patients with both node involvement and extension through the wall, although the incidence of local recurrence appears to have been reduced from 45%–65% down to 15%–20%, one may ultimately have to routinely add 5-FU to irradiation and/or increase the radiation dose to 5500–6000 rad whenever the volume of small bowel within the boost field is minimal to non-existent. The recently completed Mayo/NCCTG study suggests that combined treatment with XRT plus chemotherapy can reduce the risk of systemic as well as local failure. Future studies should address the sequencing of XRT and chemotherapy, whether methyl-CCNU is necessary, and the method of chemotherapy delivery (bolus versus continuous infusion). Distant failures via either the hematogenous or peritoneal route are too high at a level of 25%–30%.

Unresectable, Residual, Recurrent Disease

When unresectable or residual disease is treated with a combination of conventional irradiation and resection, local control and long-term survival can be achieved in 30%–50% of patients. The presence of dose-limiting normal tissues, however, prevents delivery of adequate levels of external-beam irradiation in the majority of patients. In early colorectal pilot studies from MGH and Mayo, the addition of intraoperative electron boosts appears to improve both local control and survival. Randomized trials comparing standard treatment ± IORT electron boosts are indicated.

For locally advanced or recurrent colorectal lesions in which operative resection is not feasible, a combination of external-beam irradiation and chemotherapy can achieve useful palliation in 75%–80% of patients and an occasional cure. If lesion size and location are such that intraoperative boosts with electrons, implantation techniques, or orthovoltage can be safely used to supplement external beam doses, further gains may be possible.

References

1. Gabriel WB, Dukes C, Bussey HJR (1935) Lymphatic spread in cancer of the rectum. Br J Surg 23: 395–413
2. Astler VB, Coller FA (1954) The prognostic significance of direct extension of carcinoma of the colon and rectum. Ann Surg 139: 846–851
3. Gunderson LL, Sosin H (1974) Areas of failure found at reoperation (second or sympto-

matic look) following "curative surgery" for adenocarcinoma of the rectum: clinicopathologic correlation and implications for adjuvant therapy. Cancer 34: 1278–1292

4. Wood DA (1971) Clinical staging and end-results classification. TNM system of clinical classification as applicable to carcinoma of the colon and rectum. Cancer 28: 109–113

5. Rich T, Gunderson LL, Galdabini J, et al. (1983) Clinical and pathologic factors influencing local failure after curative resection of carcinoma of the rectum and rectosigmoid. Cancer 52: 1317–1329

6. Walz BJ, Green MR, Lindstrom ER, Butcher HR (1981) Anatomic prognostic factors after abdominoperineal resection. Int J Radiat Oncol Biol Phys 7: 477–484

7. Gilbert SB (1978) The significance of symptomatic local tumor failure following abdomino-perineal resection. Int J Radiat Oncol Biol Phys 4: 801–807

8. Gunderson LL, Tepper JE, Dosoretz DE, et al. (1983) Patterns of failure after treatment of gastrointestinal cancer. In: Cox J (ed) Proceedings of CROS-NCI conference on patterns of failure after treatment of cancer. Cancer Treatment Symp, vol 2, pp 181–197

9. Romsdahl M, Withers HR (1978) Radiotherapy combined with curative surgery. Arch Surg 113: 446–453

10. Withers HR, Cuasay L, Mason KA, et al. (1981) Elective radiation therapy in the curative treatment of cancer of the rectum and rectosigmoid colon. In: Strocklein JR, Romsdahl MM (eds) Gastrointestinal cancer. Raven, New York pp 351–362

11. Mendenhall WM, Million RR, Pfaff WW (1983) Patterns of recurrence in adenocarcinoma of the rectum and rectosigmoid treated with surgery alone: implications in treatment planning with adjuvant radiation therapy. Int J Radiat Oncol Biol Phys 9: 977–985

12. Kligerman MM, Urdanetta N, Knowlton A, et al. (1972) Preoperative irradiation of rectosigmoid carcinoma including its regional lymph nodes. Am J Roentgenol 114: 498–503

13. Stevens KR, Allen CV, Fletcher WS (1976) Preoperative radiotherapy for adenocarcinoma of the rectosigmoid. Cancer 37: 2866–2874

14. Rider WD (1975) Is the Miles operation really necessary for the treatment of rectal cancer? J Can Assoc Radiol 26: 167–175

15. Roswit B, Higgins GA, Keehn RJ (1975) Preoperative irradiation for carcinoma of the rectum and rectosigmoid colon: report of a National Veteran's Administration randomized study. Cancer 35: 1597–1602

16. MRC Working Party (1984) The evaluation of low-dose preoperative X-ray therapy in the management of operable rectal cancer: results of a randomly controlled trial. Br J Surg 71: 21–25

17. Higgins GA, Humphrey EW, Dwight RW, et al. (1987) Preoperative radiation and surgery for cancer of the rectum: Veterans Administration Surgical Oncology Group Trial II. Cancer (in press)

18. Laugier A, Pene F (1984) Adjuvant radiotherapy in the management of rectal carcinoma. Proceedings of 3rd Annual Meeting, European Society for Therapeutic Radiology and Oncology, Jerusalem

19. Stevens KR, Fletcher WS, Allen CV (1978) Anterior resection and primary anastomosis following high-dose preoperative irradiation for adenocarcinoma of the rectosigmoid. Cancer 41: 2065–2071

20. Roberson SH, Kerman HD, Heron HC, Bloom TS (1985) Is anterior resection of the rectosigmoid safe after preoperative radiation? Dis Colon Rectum 28: 254–259

21. Hoskins B, Gunderson LL, Dosoretz D, Galdabini J (1985) Adjuvant postoperative radiotherapy in carcinoma of the rectum and rectosigmoid. Cancer 55: 61–71

22. Tepper JE, Cohen AM, Wood WC, Orlow EL, Hedberg SE (1987) Postoperative radiation therapy of rectal cancer. Int J Radiat Oncol Biol Phys 13: 5–10

23. Gastrointestinal Tumor Study Group (1985) Prolongation of the disease-free interval in surgically resected rectal cancer. N Engl J Med 312: 1465

24. Krooks J, Moertel C, Wieand H, et al. (1986) Radiation vs sequential chemotherapy-radiation-chemotherapy. A study of the North Central Cancer Treatment Group and the Mayo Clinic. Proc American Society of Clinical Oncology

25. Gunderson LL, Dosoretz DE, Hedberg SE, et al. (1983) Low-dose preoperative irradiation, surgery, and elective postoperative radiation therapy for resectable rectum and rectosigmoid carcinoma. Cancer 52: 446–451

26. Mohüidden M, Kramer S, Marks G, Dobelbower RR (1982) Combined pre- and postoperative radiation for carcinoma of the rectum. Int J Radiat Oncol Biol Phys 8: 133–136

27. Mohüidden M, Derdel J, Marks G, Kramer S (1985) Results of adjuvant therapy in cancer of the rectum. Cancer 55: 350

28. Gunderson LL, Russell AH, Llewellyn HJ, et al. (1985) Treatment planning for colorectal cancer: radiation and surgical techniques and value of small bowel films. Int J Radiat Oncol Biol Phys 11: 1379–1393

29. Wang CC, Schulz MD (1962) The role of radiation therapy in the management of carcinoma of the sigmoid, rectosigmoid, and rectum. Radiology 79: 1–5

30. Cummings BJ, Rider WD, Harwood AR, et al. (1983) External-beam radiation therapy for adenocarcinoma of the rectum. Dis Colon Rectum 26: 30–36

31. Turner SS, Vieira EF, Agar PT, et al. (1977) Elective postoperative radiotherapy for locally advanced colorectal cancer. Cancer 40: 105–108

32. Ghossein NA, Samala EC, Alpert S, et al. (1981) Elective postoperative radiotherapy after incomplete resection of a colorectal cancer. Dis Colon Rectum 24: 252–256

33. Allee PE, Gunderson LL, Munzenrider JE (1981) Postoperative radiation therapy for residual colorectal carcinoma. ASTR Proceedings. Int J Radiat Oncol Biol Phys 7: 1208

34. Dosoretz DE, Gunderson LL, Hoskins B, et al. (1983) Preoperative irradiation for localized carcinoma of the rectum and rectosigmoid: patterns of failure, survival, and future treatment strategies. Cancer 52: 814–818

35. Emami B, Pilepich M, Willett C, et al. (1982) Management of unresectable colorectal carcinoma (preoperative radiotherapy and surgery). Int J Radiat Oncol Biol Phys 8: 1295–1299

36. Gunderson LL, Shipley WU, Suit HD, et al. (1982) Intraoperative irradiation: a pilot study combining external-beam irradiation with "boost"-dose intraoperative electrons. Cancer 49: 2259–2266

37. Gunderson LL, Cohen AM, Dosoretz D, et al. (1983) Residual, unresectable or recurrent colorectal cancer: external-beam irradiation and intraoperative electron-beam boost ± resection. Int J Radiat Oncol Biol Phys 9: 1597–1606

38. Gunderson LL, Tepper JE, Biggs PJ, et al. (1983) Intraoperative ± external-beam irradiation. Current Probl Cancer 7: 1–69

39. Tepper JE, Gunderson LL, Orlow E, et al. (1984) Complications of intraoperative radiation therapy. Int J Radiat Oncol Biol Phys 10: 1831–1839

40. Gunderson LL, Martin JK, Earle JD, et al. (1984) Intraoperative and external-beam irradiation ± resection. Mayo pilot experience. Mayo Clin Proc 59: 691–699

41. Gunderson LL, Martin JK, Beart RW, Fieck J (1987) Intraoperative radiation for colorectal cancer. In: Abe Am, Dobelbower R (eds) Intraoperative radiation therapy. CRC Press, Boca Raton (in press)

42. Gunderson LL (1976) Staging systems for colorectal carcinoma. Current Probl Cancer 1: 40

Preoperative Radiotherapy and Radical Surgery as Combined Treatment in Rectal Cancer

A. Gerard, J. L. Berrod, F. Pene, J. Loygue, A. Laugier, R. Bruckner,
G. Camelot, J. P. Arnaud, U. Metzger, M. Buyse, O. Dalesio,
and N. Duez*, **

Institut Jules Bordet, Rue Héger Bordet 1, 1000 Brussels, Belgium

In 1976, the Gastrointestinal Group of the EORTC activated a clinical trial on rectal cancer with the aim of studying the efficacy of high-dose preoperative irradiation therapy (34.5 Gy) as an adjuvant before radical surgery. This was a multicentric prospective phase-III clinical trial.

Patients and Methods

Patients with histologicaly proven localized adenocarcinoma of the rectum within 15 cm from the anal margin, no clinical evidence of distant metastases (T2, T3, T4 NXMO), and a resectable tumor were registered. A previous clinical trial, activated as a first-generation trial by the same group [1, 2], had shown the necessity of not including patients older than 75 years.

Patients were randomized into two groups: Patients in the first group were treated by radical surgery. The second group of patients were treated by radiotherapy at a dose of 34.5 Gy, delivered in 15 fractions of 2.3 Gy daily over period of 19 days. Radical surgery took place within 2 weeks after the last fraction of irradiation therapy. Based on experience, the surgeon chose the shortest period after irradiation therapy to perform a radical resection.

Radiotherapy was given by megavoltage machines (preferably betatron or linear accelerator) in two parallel opposing anterior and posterior fields, covering the pelvic area and extending upward to the upper border of the second lumbar vertebra. Both fields covered the true pelvis and the para-aortic chain of lymph nodes.

The duration of the clinical trial was 5 years. The 466 patients registered were in a male/female ratio of 1.5; the median age was 60 years.

Sixteen patients were ineligible: two patients had rectal tumors classified as T1; five patients had a tumor which was not a rectal carcinoma; one patient had a synchronous tumor of the colon; three patients had a tumor located more than 15 cm

---

* Trial of the Gastrointestinal Tract Cancer Cooperative Group of the European Organization for Research and Treatment of Cancer (EORTC).
** The authors thank Mrs. S. Devaux for her secretarial help.

from the anal margin; and five patients had other cancers associated with rectal carcinoma. No follow-up data were available for 40 patients.

Ninety-two patients were unevaluable. The assigned treatment was not performed as described in the protocol by treatment group for eight patients. The irradiation therapy was stopped during administration because patients refused further treatment or for medical reasons in six cases. On the other hand, one patient refused a surgical procedure after registration. Three patients were lost to follow-up before treatment; one patient received chemotherapy. Twenty-six patients had a residual local tumor after the surgical procedure, 15 in the group treated by surgery alone and 12 in the group treated by preoperative radiotherapy. Fifty-three patients had distant liver metastases discovered during surgery, 25 in the group treated by surgery alone and 28 in the group treated by preoperative irradiation therapy.

Surgical Procedures

Three hundred eighteen patients underwent radical resection with a curative aim; 257 of the surgical procedures were rectal excision by an abdominoperineal resection, 126 in the control group and 131 in the group treated preoperatively by irradiation. 41 patients were treated by a sphincter-saving procedure including an anterior resection, 24 patients in the control group and 17 in the group treated preoperatively by irradiation therapy. Seventeen patients had a pull-through technique, 13 in the control group and four in the group treated preoperatively, and three patients registered in the control group had a Hartmann procedure.

Most of the tumors were located within the last 10 cm of the rectum, 132 within the last 5 cm and 152 between 6 and 10 cm from the anal margin. The distribution between the two groups of the clinical trial was well balanced. The distribution of the T categories showed that 170 of the 318 evaluable patients were staged as having a T3 or T_4 tumor, which means a locally extended adenocarcinoma.

Histologic Examination

Histologic examination showed an absence of any tumor in four cases at the time of surgery in the group treated preoperatively by irradiation therapy. On the other hand, there was no down-staging effect on Dukes C. There were 33.7% of patients classed as Dukes C, with 33.1% in the control group and 34.2% in the combined-modality therapy group.

Postoperative Mortality and Morbidity

Thirteen postoperative deaths during hospitalization were reported among these patients, which is an overall mortality of 4%; six patients were in the control group and seven in the group treated by preoperative radiotherapy. The causes of the postoperative deaths are well balanced in the two groups: cardiac failure, cerebrovascular disease, pulmonary embolism, sepsis, and colon necrosis. Postoperative morbidity was reported slightly more frequently and at a higher degree of severity after preoperative irradiation therapy, but the differences were not statistically significant. The most frequently reported complications were infections of the perineal wound, affecting 29% in the control group and 48% of the preoperatively irradiated patients. Persistence of the perineal sinus occurred in 21% and 26%, infection of the abdominal wound in 15% and 16%, and cystitis in 20% and 26% of the control group and the combined-modality therapy group respectively. Perineal wound healing took significantly longer in patients receiving preoperative radiotherapy, with a median healing time of 60 days versus 40 days in the control group. The median duration of hospitalization likewise tended to be longer in irradiated patients, at 27 days versus 21 days.

Results

It is obvious that there is a reduced incidence of local recurrence after preoperative irradiation therapy: 85% of the patients were free of local recurrence at 5 years after radiotherapy; only 65% of the control group were free of local recurrence. The difference between the two groups is highly significant ($P = 0.002$). This statistically significant difference was observed with respect to all the patients for whom data were available as well as for the group of patients treated according to the protocol with a curative aim.

After a mean follow-up of 5 years, the survival of all the patients registered in this clinical trial including the palliative resection shows a slight advantage for the patients treated by preoperative irradiation therapy but without a statistically significant difference. On the other hand, after the same mean follow-up of 5 years, the survival of eligible patients treated with a curative resection, those patients for whom the protocol was strictly followed, shows an advantage for the group treated by preoperative irradiation therapy with a improvement of 10%. The five years survival rate reaches 70%. The difference with the control group is statistically significant ($P = 0.032$).

Discussion

The large number of abdominoperineal resections could be explained by the location of the tumors. Most of them were located in the last centimeters of the rectum. The distribution of the surgical procedures is nearly the same in both groups. Therefore, it is not possible to conclude that preoperative irradiation therapy influences the selection of the surgical procedure.

There was no obvious down-staging effect on the Dukes-C classification, but the efficacy of irradiation therapy in rectal cancer was illustrated by the sterilization of the tumor in four patients.

Adjuvant preoperative irradiation therapy in rectal cancer has a few disadvantages. It means a delay of surgery. It slightly increases the postoperative morbidity, and it may not be useful for patients with a Dukes-C tumor.

Nevertheless, adjuvant preoperative irradiation therapy at the dose of 34.5 Gy administered in 15 fractions is effective in terms of controlling local recurrence. Local disease will be prevented or delayed for 20% of the patients. Pelvic recurrence is painful and a decrease in local recurrence represents an improvement in the quality of life of these patients.

Finally, for the patients treated by a radical surgical procedure after irradiation therapy, the 5-year survival rate increased by 10% and reached a very satisfactory level of 70% in this clinical trial, considering that only patients with a locally extended tumor were registered.

References

1. Boulis-Wassif S, Gerard A (1978) EORTC clinical trial with rectal cancer (preliminary report). In: Gerard A (ed) Gastrointestinal tumors. A clinical and experimental approach. Pergamon, Oxford
2. Boulis-Wassif S, Gerard A, Loygue J, Camelot D, Buyse M, Duez N (1984) Final results of a randomized trial on the treatment of rectal cancer with preoperative radiotherapy alone or in combination with 5-fluorouracil, followed by radical surgery. Trial of the European Organization on Research and Treatment of Cancer, Gastrointestinal Tract Cancer Cooperative Group. Cancer 53: 1811–1818

Combined Therapy in Anal Carcinoma

Preoperative Radio-Chemotherapy in Anal Carcinoma

H. Denecke and R. Roloff

Klinik und Poliklinik für Chirurgie und Radiologie, Klinikum Großhadern,
Universität München, Marchioninistraße 15, 8000 München 70, FRG

Squamous carcinomas of the anus are relatively radiosensitive. Therefore, the combination of radical surgical treatment with radiotherapy seems reasonable. Nigro et al. [4] added chemotherapy to this two-modality treatment. The rationale of adding cytotoxic medication was to potentiate the radiosensitivity of the tumor cells. After their first extraordinarily satisfying results sphincter-sacrificing operations could be postponed for most of their patients [5]. Meanwhile, several publications have reported excellent remission rates [1–3, 6, 7].

Patients and Method

At the Departments of Surgery and of Radiology, Grosshadern-Hospital, University of Munich, 30 patients were treated by preoperative radio-chemotherapy between 1982 and March 31, 1985. There were 22 (73%) squamous and eight (27%) basaloid anal carcinomas. Five patients were male, 25 were female: the patients' ages ranged from 54 to 79 years. Treatment was for primary cancer in 25 patients, for recurrence in seven.

Chemotherapy was started with mitomycin C, 10 mg/m^2 on day 1, and was continued by 5-FU infusion, 1000 mg/m^2 days 2 through 5 (Fig. 1).

Mitomycin C
10 mg/m^2

5-FU infusion
1000 mg/m^2/24 h

	Radiation 4 × 250 cGy		5 × 200 cGy	each week up to	4000 cGy
Day	1 2	5	14	21	28

Fig. 1. Protocol for administration of chemotherapy combined with radiotherapy

Recent Results in Cancer Research, Vol. 110

Radiation therapy was started with 4×250 cGy between days 2 and 5 and was continued by single doses of 200 cGy until a dose of 40 Gy was reached at the end of the fourth week. The radiation field extended over 14×20 cm, covering both the anorectal region and the inguinal lymph nodes. After a radiation-free interval of 4-6 weeks to let the patient recover from acute radiation stress, the tumor was restaged, and radical or local surgery was performed.

Results

Not all patients underwent this protocol. Within the group of primary tumors, we had to stop the planned therapy because of severe granulocytopenia in one patient. Another patient suffered from radiation symptoms and refused further radiotherapy.

Twenty-one patients finished radio-chemotherapy (Fig. 2). In three only local excision of the tumor scar was performed. Ten were treated by radical abdominoperineal excision. In one patient, unresectable intrapelvic disease was found at laparotomy and palliative end-colostomy was performed. Seven patients had no surgery on the tumor locally, one because of distant spread, two because of intercurrent disease (bronchial carcinoma, gastric cancer), and four because they refused the surgery to which they had earlier agreed.

The results of preoperative radio-chemotherapy in 13 patients could be proved by histologic examination (Table 1). The specimen were negative in three patients

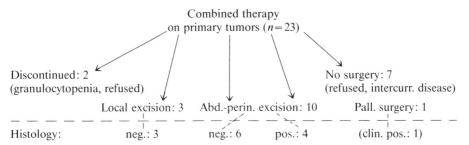

Fig. 2. Results of combined therapy for primary tumors in 23 patients

Table 1. Local success after radio-chemotherapy of primary tumors

Criterion	n	Locally	
		Free of disease	Not free of disease
Histol. examiantion after abd.-perin. excision	10	6	4[a]
Histol. examination after local scar excision	3	3	–
Clinical course (3-36 months)	8	2	6
	21	11	10

[a] One with severe atypia but not invasive carcinoma.

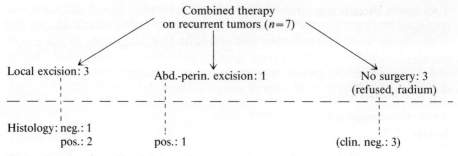

Fig. 3. Results of combined therapy for recurrent tumors in seven patients

Table 2. Local success after radio-chemotherapy of recurrent tumors

Criterion	n	Locally	
		Free of disease	Not free of disease
Histol. examination after abd.-perin. excision	1	–	1
Histol. examination after local scar excision	3	1	2
Clinical course (3–36 months)	3	2	1
	7	3	4

after local excision and in six patients after abdominoperineal excision. However, the tumor was still present in four patients. One specimen showed only severe atypia, but persistent invasive tumor was seen in the other three. Locally, radio-chemotherapy alone was successful in 11 of 21 patients. In two of them radiation had been completed up to a dose of 60 Gy. Preoperative therapy was not sufficient in four patients, and apparently radical surgery had been necessary. In addition, the clinical course revealed incomplete tumor regression in another six patients although the initial radio-chemotherapy had been followed by an additional radiation dose of 20 Gy or by radium therapy.

Figure 3 shows the results within the group of patients treated for recurrent cancer. In three patients a local excision was performed, with histologically negative results in one and tumor still present in two. In one patient, a T_3 tumor had disappeared locally, but a lymph node metastasis had remained and was removed by abdominoperineal excision. Three patients had no surgery. Histologically as well as clinically three patients were free of tumor after radio-chemotherapy and four were not (Table 2).

Twenty-four patients were evaluated after a follow-up of at least 6 months (Table 3). We excluded six patients for whom therapy was discontinued (three) or had been palliative (three). In the group in which treatment was completed by radical surgery, eight of ten patients are free of disease. After local surgery, which means excision of the tumor scar, three of five patients showed no evidence of disease. After additional radiation or radium therapy five of nine are free of disease. The mean follow-up time is comparable for all three groups.

Table 3. Combined treatment: late results (6–48 months)

Procedure	n	Mean follow-up (months)	Dead of disease	Alive with disease	Free of disease
Radio-chemotherapy and abdominoperineal excision	10	27.3	1	1	8
Radio-chemotherapy and local excision, with/without radiation	5	24.2	1	1	3
Radiochemotherapy and additional radiation/radium	9	22.7	1	3	5
Total	24	25.1	3	5	16

Table 4. Review of the literature on results of combined treatment of anal carcinoma

Authors		n	Operation		Histology neg.
			Abd.-perin. excision	Local excision	
Nigro et al.	1972–1982	104	31	62	83 (80%)
Sischy et al.	1980	10	4	6	10
Cummings et al.	1980	6	–	–	–
Wanebo	1981	4	4	–	1
Flam et al.	1983	12	–	12	12
Michaelson et al.	1983	37	5	32	22
Veidenheimer	1984	15	1	14	15
This series		28	11	6	10
		216	56	132	153

Table 4 shows a review of the results reported in the literature. In 153 patients who had surgery after radio-chemotherapy the specimens were free of tumor. This means 82% of all patients who were examined histologically.

Discussion

The best results were achieved after combined preoperative radio-chemotherapy and abdominoperineal excision. However, in six of the ten patients who underwent this extended operation, no tumor cells could be found within the specimens. In general, we were impressed by the quick response of the tumor to the radiochemotherapy. This was accompanied by a good effect on tumor pain. These facts often led the patients to refuse the initially planned abdominoperineal excision, so we had to complete the therapy by radiation or by radium. We did perform local excisions in a few patients in order to gain more information on tumor response and on further therapy. But we feel that this procedure is questionable, as it is

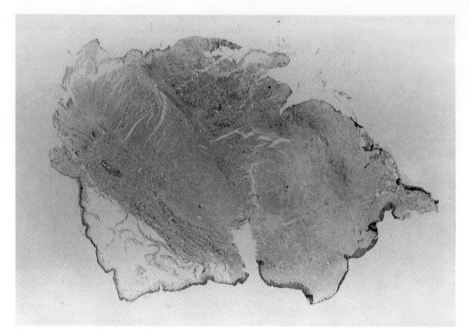

Fig. 4. Results of therapy for recurrent cancer in 40-year-old patient

done in radiated tissue and does not reach deeper layers without danger to the sphincter muscles.

With respect to tumor size, in the group of patients treated by abdominoperineal excision, two T1 tumors, four T2 tumors, and one T4 tumor with invasion of the vagina disappeared. Within the four patients with remaining tumors, two T2 tumors and one T3 tumor were clearly regressive, but a portion of the tumor was still present. On the other hand, of eight patients who had no local surgery but complementary radiation up to 60 Gy or radium, six apparently did not receive sufficient therapy; they developed recurrent tumors locally.

After therapy for recurrent cancer, it also remains difficult to say whether it is advisable to forge a radical abdominoperineal excision. This problem is elucidated by a specimen from a 40-year-old patient (Fig. 4). In the superficial tumor region the tumor had disappeared. The anoderm was healed both macroscopically and microscopically. The subdermal layers are also free of disease, but in the deeper layers tumor cells are still present. These remaining malignant cells would not have been detected by inspection, palpation, or probably even by superficial sphincter-saving excision. The same would be true for remaining perirectal lymph nodes.

Conclusion

From our limited experience we would conclude that preoperative radio-chemotherapy is indicated for carcinomas staged T_2 or higher. This therapy is also efficient as palliative treatment in advanced disease.

T1 tumors apparently respond well to all treatment modalities. All T1 tumors in our series had disappeared completely in the histologic specimen. We do not want to draw conclusions about tumor response with respect to tumor size if the tumor is staged T2 or higher. Also, we cannot draw conclusions with respect to the histological type or grade of differentiation, but this is because of our small number of patients.

A remission or regression can be expected in 90%–95% of cases. Some of the tumor may remain under a superficial scar tissue. As in the literature as well the number of 5-year observations is still limited, it remains open whether this treatment is safe enough to avoid sacrifice of the anal sphincter. From our results it can be concluded that by combining radio-chemotherapy with radical surgery the highest degree of radicality is achieved. We feel that it is too early to give up abdominoperineal excision routinely. But we do agree that more experience may make it possible to change this concept.

References

1. Cummings BJ, Roder WD, Harwood AR (1980) Combined treatment of squamous cell carcinoma of the anal canal. Dis Colon Rectum 23: 389
2. Flam MS, John M, Lovalvo LJ, Mills RJ, Romalho LD, Prather C, Mowry PA, Morgan DR, Lan BP (1983) Definitive nonsurgical therapy of epithelial malignancies of the anal canal. Cancer 51: 1378
3. Michaelson RA, Magill GB, Quan SHQ, Leaming RH, Nikrui M, Stearens MW (1983) Preoperative chemotherapy and radiation therapy in the management of anal epidermoid carcinoma. Cancer 51: 390
4. Nigro ND, Vaitkevicius VK, Considine B (1974) Combined therapy for cancer of the anal canal. A preliminary report. Dis Colon Rectum 17: 354
5. Nigro ND (1984) An evaluation of combined therapy for squamous cell cancer of the anal canal. Dis Colon Rectum 27: 763
6. Sischy B, Remington JH, Sobel SH, Savlov ED (1980) Treatment of carcinoma of the rectum and squamous carcinoma of the anus by combination chemotherapy, radiotherapy and operation. Surg Gynecol Obstet 151: 369
7. Veidenheimer MC (1984) Discussion. Am J Surg 147: 48

Combined Modality Treatment of Anal Carcinoma

W. Dobrowsky and E. Dobrowsky

Klinik für Radiotherapie und Radiobiologie, Universität Wien, Alser Straße 4, 1090 Wien, Austria

Introduction

There are two main problems in the treatment of anal cancer. Obviously, it is important to achieve local tumor control and a high survival rate, and, if possible, treatment should be conservative to retain normal anal function. This cancer should not be treated by surgery only or by percutaneous radiotherapy only for the following reasons:

1. Anal carcinomas are accessible to interstitial radiotherapy.
2. The tumor and lymph node secondaries are highyl radiosensitive but regression is slow.
3. There is a high frequency of sequelae (radionecrosis) when the perineal region receives high doses of radiation.
4. Permanent colostomy is necessary for a majority of surgically treated patients.

In the past, surgery was the main treatment modality, but a change in the treatment strategy has been noted during the past few years. Radiotherapy has attracted increasing interest, especially since the introduction of combined radio-chemotherapy with mitomycin C (MMC) and 5-fluorouracil (5-FU). This new treatment regime was initiated by Nigro et al. [13], Newman [12], Quan et al. [16], Sischy [21], and Papillon [15].

Radio-chemotherapy is now an established treatment modality in anal cancer and is considered the treatment of choice [3, 6, 15] even by surgeons who formerly proposed surgery as the primary treatment [2]. One of the reasons for this changed policy is that even radical surgery obviously does not further increase local control rates and survival [15, 23]. Another reason for the change in the treatment regime is the encouraging results of combined radio-chemotherapy that have been reported [8, 14, 20, 21].

The conservative treatment modality (radio-chemotherapy) employed at the Dept. of Radiotherapy and Radiobiology of the University of Vienna is presented here.

Recent Results in Cancer Research, Vol. 110
© Springer-Verlag Berlin · Heidelberg 1988

Patients and Method

During 1986, six patients with squamous cell cancer of the anal canal were treated by combined modalities (radio-chemotherapy). Five patients were female and one was male. The mean age of the patients was 62 years (range 44–74 years).

All patients were staged clinically (UICC) and by endocavitary sonography: three patients were classified T2N0, two were T3N0 and one was T2N1.

The combined-modality treatment consists of concomitant radio-chemotherapy as follows: day 1 – 15 mgMMC/m^2 (i.v. bolus) and days 1–5 750 mg 5-FU/m^2/24 h (infusion), with radiotherapy starting simultaneous with the beginning of the chemotherapy. Radiotherapy was performed either with a telecobalt unit (Gammatron) or 42-MeV Betatron (both by Siemens).

We use the same technique as Papillon et al. [14] with cobalt 60, with one perineal field and sacral arc therapy. When treating with the 42-MeV Betatron we used one perineal electron beam of 25 MeV and one sacral (wedged) photon field (isodose Fig. 1). The dose delivered to the tumor region was 50 Gy in 4 weeks (single dose 2.5 Gy). Six weeks after completion of the percutaneous radiation implantation of iridium 192 was performed. We use a method quite similar to that of Papillon et al. [14]. The dose delivered to the residual tumor volume is 20 Gy. The implantation itself is performed with the patient under general anesthesia, using fluoroscopy to control the parellelism of the implanted needles (isodose of implantation, Fig. 2). The inguinal region was radiated only in the patient with N1 (dose 50 Gy) after removal of enlarged lymph nodes.

In addition to treatment, a roentgenogram of the lung was made, sonography of the abdomen was performed, and blood tests were done.

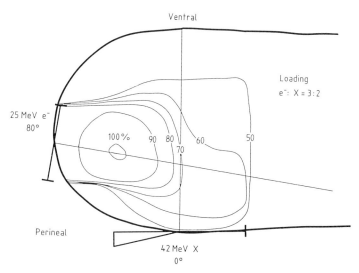

Fig. 1. Isodose of percutaneous radiotherapy (perineal electron beam – 25 MeV, sacral photon wedged beam – 42 MeV)

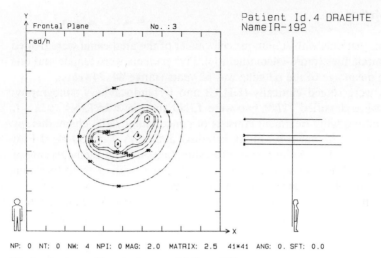

NP: 0 NT: 0 NW: 4 NPI: 0 MAG: 2.0 MATRIX: 2.5 41*41 ANG: 0. SFT: 0.0

Fig. 2. Isodose of brachytherapy (iridium 192)

Results

All patients showed complete remission of their tumor. Except for a slight moist desquamation in the perianal region in three patients, there were no local side effects of treatment. The chemotherapy was well tolerated; none of the patients had a white blood cell count below $1500/mm^3$ or fewer than 150000 thrombocytes/ mm^3. Also, nausea and diarrhea were minimal.

Discussion

In treatment of anal cancer efforts are made to increase the cure and survival rates as well as to use a conservative method to avoid a permanent colostomy.

The combined-modality treatment takes into consideration, the biology of squamous cell carcinomas and cloacogenic carcinomas. These tumors are highly radiosensitive, though the regression of the tumor seems slow. Due to the split-course technique, with 6 weeks between the percutaneous radiotherapy and the brachytherapy the tumor size is reduced so that the remaining tumor volume can easily be treated by an implant of iridium 192.

By limiting the percutaneous radiotherapy to 50 Gy/4 weeks, side effects such as radionecrosis or severe fibrosis can be avoided. Six weeks after completion of the teleradiotherapy the implantation of iridium 192 is performed. This provides a high tumor dose without radiation to the perineal skin.

In the operation specimens from patients who received combined treatment preoperatively (MMC + 5-FU + radiotherapy) often no tumor was found histologically, even if quite low doses of radiation had been delivered. Buroker et al. [4] found no tumor in 14/19 patients treated by preoperative radio-chemotherapy.

Quan [17] found no tumor in 50% (11/22) of preoperatively treated patients, though the radiated dose was as low as 30 Gy, which cannot be considered a tumoricidal dose. Sischy et al. [22] report 100% complete remission of all patients who received combined treatment. John et al. [8] found residual tumor in only three of 22 patients who were treated by combined modalities (radiated dose 30–45 Gy). All three patients showed a complete response after an additional 9 Gy. Thus, all 22 patients showed a complete response to radio-chemotherapy and had normal anal function.

Sischy [21] achieved local tumor control in 89.6% of patients with combined treatment. Papillon et al. [14] report on significantly lower recurrence rates after combined-modality treatment compared with radiotherapy as the only treatment. They further report that normal anal function is preserved in 85% of surviving patients in the very large series of Centre Léon Bérard.

By combining radiotherapy with concomitant chemotherapy, the radiation effect is reported to be enhanced.

The exact way in which chemotherapy and radiotherapy interact is not yet clear. In vivo MMC shows a markedly enhanced radiation response if administered 15 min before compared with 4 h after irradiation [11]. Besides this radiosensitizing effect, MMC shows an increased cytotoxicity to hypoxic cells (less radiosensitive) rather than to cells with normal oxygen content, thus supplementing radiotherapy.

Several investigators [1, 5, 10] have reported on 5-FU as a radiosensitizing agent. To optimize the enhancing effect, the drug should be administered after irradiation for a least 48 h [20]. A 120-h infusion is in accordance with the pharmacological requirements found by Byafield et al. [5] in vitro with infusion of 5-FU the side effects (nausea, bone marrow toxicity) are reduced compared with bolus administration [19]. We have maximized the total dose of 5-FU to 1.5 g/24 h, though others [7] report on higher dose tolerance when allopurinol is added.

Both radiotherapy and chemotherapy are tolerated very well by patients. Concomitant radio-chemotherapy is by now an established potent therapy modality which has shown remarkable results in the treatment of squamous cell cancer of other regions. Keane et al. [9] report a significant increase in local tumor control in esophageal carcinoma with combined radio-chemotherapy as compared with radiotherapy alone. In a pilot study, Thomas et al. [24] showed complete remission in 74% of patients with advanced (IIIB or IVA) cervical cancers.

Large tumors which initially are not controlled by radio-chemotherapy should be referred to surgery, which can be performed without any (preoperative) treatment-induced complications. An increased operation complication rate is not expected.

Combined radio-chemotherapy is recommended as the treatment of choice for anal cancer for the following reasons:

1. Radiotherapy is enhanced by a well-tolerated chemotherapy.
2. By combining a percutaneous radiotherapy with an interstitial brachytherapy the perineal skin is spared, even with a high tumor dose.
3. There is a high rate of cure combined with normal anal function.

References

1. Bagshaw MA (1961) Possible role of potentiators in radiation therapy. Am J Roentgenol 85: 822–833
2. Beahrs OH (1979) Management of cancer of the anus. Am J Roentgenol 133: 790–795
3. Beahrs OH (1985) Management of squamous cell carcinoma of the anus and adenocarcinoma of the lower rectum. Int J Radiat Oncol Biol Phys 11: 1741–1742
4. Buroker T, Nigro N, Considine B, Vaitkevicius VK (1979) Mitomycin C, 5-fluorouracil, and radiation therapy in squamous (epidermoid) cell carcinoma of the anal canal. In: Carter SK, Crooke ST (eds) Mitomycin C, current status and new developments. Academic, New York, pp 183–188
5. Byfield JE, Barone R, Mendelsohn J, Frankel S, Quinol L, Sharp T, Seagren S (1980) Infusional 5-fluorouracil and X-ray therapy for non-resectable esophageal cancer. Cancer 45: 703–708
6. Cummings BJ (1982) The place of radiation therapy in the treatment of carcinoma of the anal canal. Cancer Treat Rev 9: 125–147
7. Howell SB, Wung WE, Taetle R, Hussain F, Romine JS (1981) Modulation of 5-fluorouracil toxicity by a allopurinol in man. Cancer 48: 1281–1289
8. John M, Flam M, Podolsky W, Ager Mowry P (1985) Feasibility of non-surgical definitive management of anal canal carcinoma (Abstr.) Int J Radiat Oncol Biol Phys 11 Suppl 1: 109
9. Keane TJ, Harwood AR, Rider WD, Cummings BJ, Thomas GM (1984) Concomitant radiation and chemotherapy for squamous cell carcinoma (scc) esophagus. (Abstr.) Int J Radiat Oncol Biol Phys 10 Suppl 2: 89
10. Lo TCM, Wiley AL, Ansfield FJ, Brandenburg JH, Davis Jr HL, Gollin FF, Johnson RO, Ramirez G, Vermund H (1976) Combined radiation therapy and 5-fluorouracil for advanced squamous cell carcinoma of the oral cavity and oropharynx: a randomized study. Am J Roentgenol 126: 229–235
11. Maase von der H, Overgaard J (1985) Interactions of radiation and cancer chemotherapeutic drugs in a C3H mouse mammary carcinoma. Acta Radiol [Oncol] 24: 181–187
12. Newman HK, Quan SHQ (1976) Multi-modality therapy for epidermoid carcinoma of the anus. Cancer 37: 12–19
13. Nigro ND, Vaitkevicius VK, Buroker T, Bradley GT, Considine B (1981) Combined therapy for cancer of the anal canal. Dis Colon Rect 24: 73–75
14. Papillon J, Montbarbon JF, Ardiet JM, Pipard G (1987) Epidermoid carcinoma of the anal canal. Dis Colon Rect 30: 324–333
15. Papillon J (1982) In: Rectal and anal cancers. Springer, Berlin Heidelberg New York
16. Quan SHQ, Magill GB, Leaming RH, Hajdu SI (1978) Multidisciplinary preoperative approach to the management of epidermoid carcinoma of the anus and anorectum. Dis Colon Rect 21: 89–91
17. Quan SHQ (1979) Squamous cancer of the anorectum. (Abstr.) Int J Radiat Oncol Biol Phys 5: 63
18. Rauth AM, Mohindra JK, Tannock IF (1983) Activity of mitomycin C for aerobic and hypoxic cells in vitro and in vivo. Cancer Res 43: 4154–4158
19. Seifert P, Baker LH, Reed ML, Vaitkevicius VK (1975) Comparison of continuously infused 5-fluorouracil with bolus injection in treatment of patients with colorectal adenocarcinoma. Cancer 36: 123–128
20. Shank B (1985) Treatment of anal canal carcinoma. Cancer 55: 2156–2162
21. Sischy B (1985) The use of radiation therapy combined with chemotherapy in the management of squamous cell carcinoma of the anus and marginally resectable adenocarcinoma of the rectum. Int J Radiat Oncol Biol Phys 11: 1587–1593
22. Sischy B, Remington JH, Sobel SH, Sarlov ED (1980) Treatment of carcinoma of the rectum and squamous carcinoma of the anus by combination chemotherapy, radiotherapy and operation. Surg Gynecol Obstet 151: 369–371

23. Stearns MW, Quan SHQ (1970) Epidermoid carcinoma of the anorectum. Surg Gynecol Obstet 131: 953–957
24. Thomas G, Dembo A, Beale F, Bean H, Bush R, Herman J, Pringle J, Rawlings G, Sturgeon J, Fine S, Black B (1984) Concurrent radiation, Mitomycin C and 5-fluorouracil in poor-prognosis carcinoma of cervix: preliminary results of a phase I–II study. Int J Radiat Oncol Biol Phys 10: 1785–1790

Current Therapeutic Concepts in Management of Carcinoma of the Anal Canal

J. Papillon

Department of Radiotherapy, Centre Léon Berard, 69008 Lyon, France

Radical surgery as initial treatment has been abandoned or questioned in most institutions in favor of a radio-chemotherapy approach, followed or not by surgery. The use of radiosensitizers such as 5-FU and mitomycin C during the first days of radiotherapy has been demonstrated as effective. Today the main problem consists in defining the most efficient protocol of radiotherapy able to give the highest chance of both tumor control and anal preservation.

Two types of protocols of radiotherapy have been suggested:

1. An external-beam irradiation, regularly fractionated, delivering a homogeneous dose of 5000 rads in 5–6 weeks to the whole pelvis by two opposed AP-PA portals, plus a booster dose to the anal area. The overall treatment time is 7–8 weeks.
2. A split-course regimen combining a short-term external-beam irradiation and an interstitial curietherapy after a 2-month rest (Fig. 1). The first stage is aimed at delivering a minimum tumor dose of 3000 rads in 19 days through perineal and sacral fields to a target volume which includes the anal area and most pelvic lymphatic drainage areas tributary to the anal area. The one-plane iridium-192 implant is aimed at giving a booster dose of 1500–2000 rads to the bed of the anal tumor, taking advantage of the tumor regression during the free interval

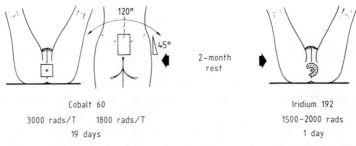

Fig. 1. Split-course irradiation with cobalt 60 and iridium 192 is justified by the slow regression rate of anal canal epidermoid carcinoma. The moderate dosage of irradiation used is aimed at reducing the incidence of radionecrosis

Recent Results in Cancer Research, Vol. 110
© Springer-Verlag Berlin·Heidelberg 1988

between the two stages. The split-course technique is well adapted to the accessibility of the primary tumor, to the site of lymphatic chains at risk, and to the slow shrinkage of large tumors after irradiation, as well as to the proneness of anal and perineal structures to radionecrosis. In case of palpable pelvic metastatic lymph nodes, a booster dose by fixed field is given to a limited pelvic area.

Split-course irradiation was initiated in Lyon at the Centre Léon Bérard in 1971. Since that time it has been applied to 222 patients with resectable tumors suitable for conservation, among a whole group of 275 patients followed up for more than 3 years, which includes 33 patients with unresectable or disseminated tumors and 21 patients with resectable tumors not suitable for anal conservation because of involvement of the entire anal circumference or of vaginal mucosa.

Pretreatment evaluation included endoscopy, biopsy, rectal – and vaginal – examination, and a systematic search for pelvic metastatic lymph nodes by palpation and CT scan, as well as inguinal palpation and general examination.

The efficacy of a treatment may be assessed on the basis of three criteria: tolerance, tumor control and anal preservation. Immediate tolerance is good, with a short period of proctitis and irritation of the anal area without moist desquamation that is easily controlled medically. With regard to late side effects, it must be emphasized that there is never any perineal fibrosis. The perineal skin and soft tissues remain supple without any change in consistency. This demonstrates the perfect tolerance of perineal irradiation at a dose of 3000 rads calculated at 5 cm in ten fractions within 17 days. Five patients developed severe anal radionecrosis requiring AP resection or colostomy. Two patients developed major rectal bleeding due to faulty technique or to a high dose to the pelvic mass. One underwent an AP resection, one had a colostomy. Altogether the rate of severe complications is 3.1%. Benign painful necrotic ulcerations spontaneously curable in less than 3 months were observed in 15 cases (6.7%). Intermittent benign bleeding related to telangiectasia of the rectal mucosa was mentioned in 15% of cases. The long-term results are given in Table 1. The survival rates and death rates at 3 and 5 years are similar. This suggests that patients who are disease free at 3 years have the best chance of being definitively controlled. These data contrast with the results of external-beam irradiation alone, which show a significant increase in the death rate between the 3rd and the 5th year, so that the comparison of efficacy of both techniques must be made at 5 years (Table 2).

It must be emphasized that among the 222 patients followed up for more than 3 years, and among the 159 followed up for more than 5 years, the rate of death from cancer or postoperatively is less than 21% and that the disease-free survival rates are 65.7% and 65.4%, the rate of patients who died of intercurrent disease being almost the same.

This shows that for approximately 80% of patients the tumor has been controlled and 90% of the patients whose tumor was controlled had normal anal function.

Table 2, which compares the results of external-beam irradiation alone with those of split-course cobalt 60 + iridium 192, shows a significant difference in the death rate from cancer, in disease-free survival, in severe complications, and in the rate of anal preservation, especially for large infiltrating tumors. These data dem-

Table 1. Results at 3 and 5 years of split-course irradiation (cobalt 60 and iridium 192) to resectable tumors in cancer of the anal canal

	No. of cases	Alive and well	Dead of interc. dis	Dead of cancer	Post-op. deaths
At 3 years	222	146[a] (65.7%)	31 (14%)	42 (18.9%)	3 (1.3%)
At 5 years	159	104[a] (65.4%)	24 (15.1%)	29 (18.2%)	2 (1.2%)

[a] Anal preservation: at 3 years, 91.8%
　　　　　　　　　　 at 5 years, 89.5%.

Table 2. Carcinoma of the anal canal – comparison of results at 5 years according to the radiotherapy technique

	5-years survival	Dead from cancer or post-op.	Severe complica- tions	Alive with anal preservation		
				T_1-T_3	$T \leqslant 4$ cm	$T > 4$ cm
Split-course[a] Co60 + Ir192	65%	21%	3.1%	58%	67%	52%
External-beam irradiation[b]	31%–55%	31%	6%–22%	26%–41%	58%	22%

[a] Centre Léon Bérard [1]　　　　　　　　　　　　　　　　　　　　　159 cases
[b] Institut Curie, Paris [2]　　　　　　　　　　　　　　　　　　　　　169 cases
　　Hopital Tenon, Paris (M. Schlienger, personal communication)　　　122 cases
　　Institut Gustave Roussy, Villejuif [3]　　　　　　　　　　　　　　　64 cases

onstrate that the split-course regimen is better adapted to the clinical behavior and radiation response of epidermoid carcinoma of the anal canal than is external-beam irradiation alone.

Among the 33 patients with unresectable or disseminated tumors, 27 died of cancer and three of intercurrent disease, and three are alive and well with their tumor clinically controlled in spite of the extent of the disease; one of them has a colostomy, performed because of complete anal obstruction, and two have normal sphincter function.

Among the 21 patients with huge resectable tumors not suitable for anal conservation, who were treated by radio-chemotherapy followed by abdominoperineal resection 2 months later, seven (33%) died of cancer, eleven are alive and disease free, and three died of intercurrent disease.

So far, the role of chemotherapy used as a radiosensitizer during the first days of radiotherapy is not generally accepted. However, sufficient data have been reported demonstrating the efficacy of the Nigro protocol in enhancing the action of radiotherapy and increasing the rate of local control [4]. At the Centre Léon Bérard since 1977, chemotherapy has not been used systematically for large T_3 tumors in patients not older than 70. A retrospective study of 77 patients with T_3 tumors treated by irradiation alone and 70 patients treated by radio-chemotherapy showed a statistically significant increase in the local control rate at 3 years after the combined treatment. Since 1985 chemotherapy has been used systematically during the first 4 days of irradiation irrespective of the stage of disease and patients" status but the dosage do not exceed 5-FU 600 mg/m² per day and mitomycin C 12 mg/m² on day 1. In frail patients or patients older than 80, mitomycin C is not used and the dosage of 5-FU does not exceed 500 mg/m² per day for 4 days.

In conclusion, the split-course regimen of irradiation has demonstrated a real superiority over external-beam irradiation alone with regard to tolerance and efficacy. There are four key factors in the effectiveness of the split-course regimen: (a) The perineal field, applied with the patients in the lithotomy position, allows one to deliver a high dose to an area which includes the tumor and the proximal pelvic lymphatic chains with satisfactory protection of the vulva and bladder. It may be adapted exactly to the site and size of the primary tumor. Although a high dose is delivered to the perianal area, it does not give rise to any perineal fibrosis. (b) The sacral field, combined if necessary with a booster dose to the ipsilateral side of the pelvis, has proved to control not only most infraclinical metastatic lymph nodes but also clinically involved pelvic nodes, while achieving a satisfactory protection of the small bowel. (c) The long free interval between external-beam and interstitial irradiation allows the normal tissues time to recover and the clinician to take advantage of the tumor regression. (d) The booster dose given by the one-plane iridium-192 implant involves a very limited target volume, which represents the bed of the tumor, known to be less radiosensitive than the peripheral part of the lesion.

Finally, sufficient data concerning the role of radiosensitizer such as 5-FU and mitomycin C have been published to warrant systematic use of this method during the first days of radiotherapy.

In this protocol, radical surgery has no place in the initial treatment. However, groin dissection in case of clinically involved inguinal nodes and colostomy in case of complete anal obstruction are advisable before irradiation.

After such conservative treatment, applicable to 80% of patients with carcinoma of the anal canal, regular follow-up must be performed carefully to make sure that tumor control has been achieved and to detect a potential recurrence in the anal, inguinal, or pelvic areas.

One can state that such a strategy is able to control more than 75% of tumors suitable for conservation and to spare 90% of cured patients a permanent colostomy.

References

1. Papillon J (1982) Rectal and anal cancers. Conservative treatment by irradiation: an alternative to radical surgery. Springer, Berlin Heidelberg New York
2. Salmon RJ, Fenton J, Asselain B, Mathieu G, Girodet J, Durand JC, Decroix Y, Pilleron JP, Rousseau J (1984) Treatment of epidermoid anal canal cancer. Am J Surg 147: 43–48
3. Eschwege F, Lasser P, Chavy A, Wibault P, Kac J, Rougier P, Bognel C (1985) Squamous cell carcinoma of the anal canal: treatment by external beam irradiation. Radiother Oncol 3: 145–150
4. Nigro MD, Vaitkevicius VK, Considine BJ (1974) Combined therapy for cancer of the anal canal. A preliminary report. Dis Colon Rectum 17: 354

Approach of the Treatment of Colorectal Liver Metastases

A. Flowerdew and I. Taylor

Winchester Health Authority, Royal Hampshire County Hospital,
Winchester SO22 5DG, Great Britain

Introduction

Colorectal liver metastases have aroused ever increasing interest over the past
30 years. This is due to a number of factors. Firstly, better understanding of surgical anatomy and the limits of hepatic resection, accompanied by better anaesthetic
and postoperative support, has enabled far more extensive procedures to be undertaken with decreasing morbidity and mortality. Secondly, new cytotoxic drugs
have become available and been given by a variety of routes both alone and as
multiple regimens. Finally, technological advances in diagnostic modalities and
drug-delivery mechanisms have enabled earlier diagnosis and the implementation
of more sophisticated treatments.

Readers are referred to past critical reviews of the status of treating colorectal
liver metastases [1, 2] and to more recent extensive publications on all aspects of
liver metastases [3, 4]. Ensminger and Gyves [5] have recently reviewed the principles, and Sterchi [6] the results of hepatic arterial infusion. This review is primarily
directed at the current position on treating liver metastases, with special reference
to recent developments.

Natural History of Liver Metastases

Almost all treatments have been compared with retrospective historical controls,
although there has been one recent prospective study [23]. It has become increas-
ingly clear that hepatic metastases do not often occur in isolation but are part of a
more extensive disease process, although they are frequently the first to present
clinically. They almost certainly arise through haematogenous spread from the primary tumour by way of the portal venous system. Lymph node involvement in the
primary colonic resection is a significant poor prognostic factor in the presence of
liver metastases, presumable because selective treatment to the liver will have no
effect on systemic spread via the lymphatic sytem. Gilbert et al. [26] found that recurrence was limited to the liver in only 6.6% of patients at time of necropsy and
in 26% in an on-going clinical study of sites of recurrence following curative resec-

tions of colorectal cancer. It appears likely that the later clinical manifestation of distant, other than liver metastases may simply be a result of cells taking a longer time to transgress the lymphatic system prior to becoming established and overt. This natural behaviour of colorectal carcinoma must not be forgotten when many of the methods of selective treatment of hepatic metastases are being considered.

The results of several studies on the natural history of colorectal liver metastases are shown in Table 1 (most patients having had a resection of the primary tumour). Many reports of treatment have concluded that there has been a benefit in prolonging survival by selectively comparing the results with a retrospective study showing a low median survival. However, the untreated survival range extends from 4 to 24 months. Some of the longer survival figures reported more recently may be the result of earlier diagnosis with more sophisticated tumour markers such as CEA and radiological scanning techniques.

If historical control studies are used for comparing current treatments, some of the more recent reports should be referred to (Table 2). These studies have taken into account many prognostic aspects, including the extent of liver involvement, general performance status and extrahepatic disease. Almost all these studies have shown an inverse relationship between the extent of tumour burden and the length of survival. A proportion of solitary metastases seem to have a unique inherent biological tendency to remain localised and slow growing. However, they account for only about 5% of colorectal hepatic metastases.

The need for stratification or staging is now accepted. Different systems have been recommended according to clinical and biochemical parameters and the extent of liver involvement [27–29]. The revised version of the Lausanne international staging system, which recommends three stages, has a wide range of 25–75 percent hepatic replacement (PHR) encompassing stage II [30]. The presence of extrahepatic disease and general condition of the patients are poor prognostic factors [24] and should be clearly recorded.

Table 1. The overall natural history of patients with colorectal metastases in whom the primary tumour has been resected (–, no information)

Study		Survival (months)		Survival (%) Patients			
		Mean	Median	2-year	3-year	5-year	(n)
Modlin and Walker [7]	overall	11.2	8	18	–	0	17
Stearns and Binkley [8]	overall	18	11	–	–	–	22
Pestana et al. [9]	overall	9	–	–	–	–	353
Flanagan and Foster [10]	overall	5.5	4	4	–	0	26
Swinton et al. [11]	overall	13	–	17.5	10	–	40
Jaffe et al. [12]	overall	–	5	–	–	–	177
Bengmark and Hafstrom [13]	overall	7.8	–	–	–	–	173
Oxley and Ellis [14]	overall	–	10	–	–	–	76
Cady et al. [15]	overall	13	–	–	–	–	269
Baden and Andersen [16]	overall	–	10	–	–	3.8	105
Fischerman et al. [17]	overall	6.5	6	–	–	–	49
Goslin et al. [18]	overall	–	24	–	–	–	24

Table 2. The natural history of patients with untreated colorectal liver metastases related to the solitary nature or the extent of the tumours replacing the liver

Study	Extent of metastases	Survival months		Survival (%)			Pat-ients (n)
		Mean	Median	2-year	3-year	5-year	
Nielson et al. [19]	Few	18	–	–	–	–	20
	Several	9	–	–	–	–	5
	Multiple	7	–	–	–	–	7
Bengtsson et al. [20]	<25%	–	6.2	–	–	–	–
	25%–75%	–	5.5	–	–	–	–
	>75%	–	3.4	–	–	–	–
Wanebo et al. [21]	Overall-	–	7	–	–	–	149
	Solitary	–	19	–	–	–	18
Wood et al. [22]	Solitary	17	–	–	13.3	–	15
	(Sol. resectable)	25	–	–	28.5	–	7
	Several	11	–	–	9.9	–	11
Wood [23]	Solitary	–	–	–	–	16	15
Wagner et al. [24] 1 Lobe:	Solitary	–	21	–	20	3	39
	Multiple	–	15	–	–	–	31
Finan et al. [25]	Overall	–	10.3	–	–	–	90
	Solitary	–	15.5	–	–	–	–
	PHR<20%	–	16.4	–	–	–	–
	PHR 20%–80%	–	5.6	–	–	–	–
	Multiple	–	8	–	–	–	–

The PHR by tumour is assessed by radiological scans and at laparotomy. Scanning techniques have been found to be comparable in diagnosing liver metastases [31,32] but will often not identify many smaller tumour nodules [33]. The use of ethiodized oil emulsion as an enhancing contrast agent (limited in use to the United States) has been shown to be superior to standard intravenous agents used for this purpose, particularly in delineating small tumours [34]. Palpation of the liver at laparotomy may also be inaccurate, as it has been shown that occult metastases were identified by CT scanning in 29% of patients undergoing apparently curative resection for colorectal carcinoma [35]. The assessment of the PHR is principally subjective, although volume calculations from CT scan slices have been reported [36]. CT may be the most useful scan to measure an objective response in terms of tumour size, but the subjectivity of PHR assessment may make the cheaper and more practical isotope and ultrasound scans just as accurate for this purpose.

The one drawback of stratifying patients has been the accrual of small numbers into randomized trials more recently, and it is likely that sufficient numbers will be achieved only by coordinated multicenter trials.

Blood Supply of Liver Metastases

Experimental and Postmortem Studies

Many of the recent advances in treating multiple metastases have been advocated on the grounds that the tumours derive their blood supply almost entirely from the hepatic artery. This is worthy of reappraisal.

Experimental models have shown that liver tumours derive their blood supply from both the hepatic artery and the portal vein, with the artery being predominant [37, 38]. Others have shown tumours to be dependent entirely on the hepatic artery [39, 40]. Very few studies have been performed on human livers which enable the portal component of tumour blood flow to be evaluated. Four livers with colorectal metastases from a series studied by Breedis and Young [40] were injected with different coloured gelatin into the hepatic artery and portal vein. Tumours had to be excluded due to postmortem autolysis and intravascular clot blocking the passage of dye. Almost all tumours were less than 3 mm in size and most had an arterial blood supply. The portal vein supplied 25% and 5% of colorectal metastases in two livers respectively. The corrosion cast technique, which fills large vessels only, was used by Healey [41] to study metastases in livers from primary tumours draining into the portal vein. The tumours were invariably hypovascular, with arteries and bile ducts traversing the tumour nodules. Similar findings were made originally by Segall in 1923 [42]. More recent sophisticated methods have given a much clearer resolution of the small vessels. Coloured silicone rubber (Microfil) injected into the portal vein and hepatic artery showed that 71 of 83 metastases had a blood supply from both vessels [43]. It was also shown that there were many arterioportal anastomoses. However, there is a general consensus that colorectal metastases are hypovascular compared with normal liver tissue.

Angiography

Angiography is a very effective means of showing the arterial blood supply of tumours, but it is not suitable for the portal component due to poor resolution of the diluted contrast. However, it is a prerequisite for hepatic resecton or placement of an arterial catheter due to the frequency of morphological anomalies of the hepatic artery, the right arising from the superior mesenteric artery in 29% and the left hepatic from the left gastric artery in 25% of patients [44]. Portal flow must be ascertained prior to submitting patients to major resections and arterial and radiological dearterialisation procedures due to the hazards of infarcting normal liver.

Scintigraphy

Isotope scanning still plays a major role in the management of patients with colorectal liver metastases for diagnostic and staging purposes. Radionuclide catheter perfusion has been found to be a useful technique to evaluate catheter placement and the distribution of the infusate [45]. Dynamic liver scanning of the first pass of colloid through the liver following a rapid intravenous bolus of radiocolloid has been used to measure the relative arterial blood flow, from which an hepatic perfusion index (HPI) is derived [46]. It was found that 97% of patients with overt metastases had an HPI value higher than that of controls, and the investigation had a specificity of 72% and sensitivity of 96% in predicting liver metastases when there was a normal liver at the time of a primary resection. This technique is currently being evaluated in measuring liver tumour blood flow and the changes following hepatic arterial embolisation [91]. Xenon clearance techniques have shown that metastatic nodules have predominantly arterial blood supply [47, 48], but following hepatic artery ligation there is a significant increase in portal perfusion to the tumours [48].

Follow-up Screening of Patients

Liver function tests and liver scanning are performed to monitor any complicatoins of therapy and the response or progression of the disease. Liver enzyme levels must be carefully observed with long-term arterial chemotherapy due to the high incidence of chemical hepatitis and biliary sclerosis. However, they are of little use in measuring response. The non-specific tumour marker carcinoembryonic antigen (CEA) has been found to rise with expansion of tumour in the liver, but this is by no means consistent [49]. Liver scanning is the most reliable method of determining whether tumours have enlarged or responded, although each modality has its drawbacks. Ultrasound is limited by being operator dependent, and difficulty is experienced in duplicating previous views for estimating tumour size. CT and scintigraphy are free of these problems, but the former is expensive and the clarity of the tumour margins is indistinct in the latter. CT would seem to be the ideal technique, altough it may be academic as the important end point is prolonged survival. As initial response to chemotherapy is associated with prolonged survival [50], early sequential imaging could be valuable as a prognostic index.

Treatment Options

Many different forms of treatment have been used for colorectal liver metastases, including surgical resection, hepatic arterial ligation, embolisation or surgical dearterialisation, radiotherapy, a variety of cytotoxic regimens given by different routes, or often a combination of these therapeutic modalities. The only patients who may achieve 5-year survival are the highly selected group suitable for surgical resection.

Direct comparisons between studies are difficult due to variations in protocols, accrual of patients, and response criteria. However, the survival patterns can be compared with the accumulated knowledge of the natural history, giving some clarity as to the benefits or limitations experienced so far.

Hepatic Arterial Devascularisation

On the grounds that metastases derive their blood supply predominantly from the hepatic artery, it was hoped that hepatic artery ligation would prolong survival by causing tumour necrosis, as was found experimentally in rats. Tumour regression has been observed in man but survival has not been prolonged compared with historical controls [51]. This has been attributed to arterial collaterals seen angiographically soon after the procedure [52] and more recently to an increase in portal flow [48]. Surgical dearterialisation of the liver with division of all peritoneal and vascular connections apart from the hepatic and portal veins and common bile duct was adopted but was accompanied by a high mortality and mean survival of only 4.5 months for a mixture of primary and secondary tumours [53]. In view of the portal venous supply, 19 patients with colorectal secondaries underwent hepatic artery ligation combined with portal vein infusion of 5-fluorouracil for 5 days every month [54]. Some patients continued treatment for 12 months, and overall the median survival was 13 months.

Hepatic artery ligation with arterial infusion of cytotoxic drugs has also been used, but it was thought that arterial collaterals would supply the tumours without delivering the drugs. An alternative approach was to maintain the patency of the hepatic artery but perform repeated temporary occlusion with special slings in conjunction with cytotoxic infusion [55]. A more recent concept is that pulsed occlusion of the hepatic artery will result in the tumours being exposed to cytotoxic oxygen-derived free radicals which are released from cells subjected to temporary hypoxia, but no clinical results are available yet [56].

Surgical dearterialisation is useful for temporary palliation of symptoms from the carcinoid syndrome and capsular pain from rapidly enlarging deposits. However, the less invasive technique of radiological hepatic arterial embolisation is very effective [57].

Hepatic Arterial Embolisation

It is not possible to draw any conclusions about the therapeutic efficacy of hepatic arterial embolisation (HAE) for colorectal metastases from the small series reported [58, 59]. Median survival was 7.5 months and 11.5 months for metastases from various sites. The theoretical advantage of occluding the artery both distally and proximally would be to diminish the effects of arterial collateral formation, and hence the chances of early collateral formation reaching the tumours. An interesting study of resected specimens of liver containing recently embolised primary tumours has shown necrosis ranging from 54% to 99% [60]. Recanalisation of the occluded vessels may occur, but repeated procedures will not inconvenience patients. Serious morbidity is rare but potential hepatic abscess formation requires prophylactic antibiotics, and portal vein patency must be verified on angiography. Jaundice and extensive tumour replacement are only relative contraindications to embolisation.

The claim that intra-arterial chemotherapy followed by intentional or inadvertent occlusion is superior to arterial infusion alone when the median survival of

15 months is compared with 8 months is not wholly justified, as the former group contained more patients with poor prognostic factors [61].

Arterial Embolisation with Radioactive or Degradable Microspheres

Internal radiation emitted by Yttrium 90-labelled microspheres injected into the hepatic artery, either alone [62] or in combination with 5-FU infusion [63], have been reported. Serious side effects were experienced, with three deaths as a result of the treatment. However, 17 of 25 patients had objective remission in one study and in the other survival between 12 and 14 months was recorded. External radiation has been found to be useful mainly for relief of hepatic pain from large tumours [64].

A more recent concept involves mixing or encapsulating cytotoxic drugs within degradable microspheres. The microspheres act on two basic principles: tumour vessel embolisation and the slow release or increased saturation of tumours with cytotoxic drugs. Kato et al. [65] pioneered mitomycin encapsulation in ethylcellulose microspheres and applied them clinically to tumours of the liver. A number of studies with degradable starch microspheres which temporarily arrest arterial blood flow for 30 min have shown an increase in liver uptake of 5-FU experimentally [66] and decreased systemic exposure of a number of drugs not normally cleared by the liver. This adjunct to chemotherapy will hopefully enhance the therapeutic effect of arterial function (see below).

Chemotherapy

The most commonly used cytotoxic drugs are the fluoropyrimidines 5-FU and FUDR, given as bolus injection or infusion by a number of routes. Mitomycin as a bolus injection has often been included in regimens. However, almost all cytotoxic drugs have been tried, either alone or in different combinations, without any advantage over 5-FU. Unfortunately, 5-FU is only partially active against colorectal cancer and its pride of place is held principally by default. Colon cancers have been found to contain enzymes that convert the parent drug into its cytotoxic anabolic metabolites which block cellular DNA synthesis and mRNA. The advantage of FUDR is that it can be given in small volumes and is suitable for the small chambers of implantable infusion pumps as well as having pharmacokinetic benefits when given as an hepatic arterial infusion [67].

Systemic Chemotherapy. Systemic administration is of little benefit overall when treating colorectal metastases. The longer survival seen in responders my be partly related to the natural history of the disease. Response rates of 20% have been documented, with median survival seldom being more than 10 months. A good review of colorectal metastases treated by this route is given by Kemeny [68].

Hepatic Arterial Infusion. Earlier, infusion was carried out with radiologically or surgically placed catheters. If they were inserted into the hepatic artey directly, this was ligated. An alternative and what is generally practiced today, is placement into the gastroduodenal artery so that arterial flow to the liver is not impeded. Early studies are hard to evaluate in relation to the present context due to many variables not accounted for then. In general terms, the response rate was often about 50% but survival was not improved. In the Central Oncology Group randomized study [50] the mean survival with systemic chemotherapy was 15.4 months and with intra-arterial infusion, 13.5 months. Long-term administration was initially on an intermittent basis by radiologically or surgically placed catheter. Falk et al. [69] gave monthly infusion of 5-FU (mitomycin added in some cases) to 98 patients with colorectal carcinoma. The 1- and 2-year survival rates of those with metastases confined to the liver were 60% and 17% respectively, compared with 32% and 5% for patients with extrahepatic metastases as well. Pettavel and Morgenthaler [29] gave protracted arterial infusions through surgically placed catheters in the gastroduodenal artery for periods of up to 1 year in 57 patients with colorectal liver metastases from a total of 106 patients. Those patients with stage-II disease had a median survival of 18.5 months and those with stage III 9.6 months.

The development of reliable long-term infusion pumps in recent years has resulted in marked resurgence in treating colorectal liver metastases. The totally implantable subcutaneous Infusaid pump [70] has been extensively used and found to be reliable and requires refilling only every 1 or 2 weeks. It is expensive, and current randomised trials are in progress to see if its use is justified. The alternative is an external pump based on the Cormed system for hepatic arterial infusion. The advantages of this system are that the flow rate can be adjusted and that the pumps are interchangeable between patients, thus reducing the costs significantly.

A number of centres have now reported their experience with the Infusaid pump and survival figures are shown in Table 3. Two of the initial reports were very encouraging [71,72]. In both series there was a response rate in excess of 80%, although a fall in the CEA level was used as a marker. The measurement of sur-

Table 3. Review of survival data with long-term cytotoxic infusion alone

Study	Patients (n)	Median survival	
		From start of infusion (months)	From time of of diagnosis (months)
Balch et al. [73]	81	–	26[a]
Cohen et al. [74]	10	10	–
Kemeny et al. [75]			
Extrahepatic disease in all	11	12	–
Niederhuber et al. [71]			
Liver involvement only	50	18	25
Extrahepatic disease also	43	9	14
Weiss et al. [76]	21	13	17
Schwartz et al. [77]	18	10*	21[a]
Shepard et al. [78]			
Liver involvement only	53	17	

[a] Mean survival.

vival from time of diagnosis rather than from insertion of the catheter gives a somewhat favourable bias. Other more recent reports are not quite so encouraging (Table 3). These studies used FUDR for the infusion, often with intermittent bolus injections of mitomycin. Didolkar et al. [79] treated 30 patients, three of whom had carcinoid metastases, with long-term 5-FU and the external Cormed pump, resulting in a median survival of 21 months. Fourteen patients in one series were given weekly 5-FU into Infusaid pumps and although the benefits cannot be evaluated, two patients had serious haemorrhage from duodenal ulcers [81].

Additional procedures in conjunction with long-term infusion have been reported recently. One prospective randomised trial compared infusion with resection with infusion alone and found little difference in survival – 19 and 20 months respectively [75]. However, Hodgson et al. combined infusion with resection in one group, arterial embolisation and portal vein branch ligation in another, and all manipulations in another [81]. The overall median survival was 18 months and showed a trend suggesting that the more radical the treatment, the better the results.

The minimal compliction rate reported initially [71, 72] has not been experienced more recently. Gastritis and chemical hepatitis with abnormal liver function tests are common [82]. A more ominous problem is the development of strictures in the bile ducts – a form of biliary sclerosis [83]. An incidence of 17.4% with FUDR infusion was reported by Kemeny et al. [84]. The junction of the common hepatic ducts is a common site but intrahepatic strictures are also frequent. It is not clear whether this is due to toxicity to FUDR alone or to a combination of factors. The condition is potentially fatal but may be partially resolved by reducing or omitting therapy. Catheter occlusion and displacement are not common, but catheters have been seen to infuse into the duodenum, having eroded into the base of a duodenal ulcer.

Hepatic Resection

It is almost a century since the first hepatic resection for a tumour was performed, which was coincidentally the same time that Paget observed the liver as a preferential site for metastases and drew up the seed and soil hypothesis [85]. Resection of colorectal metastases became much more common-place following the review by Flanagan and Foster [86] of 45 patients who had undergone hepatic resection; the overall 5-year survival was 23%. In retrospect, this was superior to the expected natural history (Table 2). Since that time, reports have been directed at how to identify those patients who will benefit from resection and how to reduce the high morbidity and mortality previously associated with the more extensive procedures. Mortality is seldom greater than 5% and is often less, due to better surgical expertise, awareness of vascular anatomy, temporary control of vessels and more sophisticated postoperative support.

The general feeling is that resection of solitary metastases is worthwhile, as 5-year survival has been recorded in the region of 30%–40% [87–90]. However, the attitude towards multiple metastases has been against surgery. Nevertheless, there are a number of reports showing that selected patients with multiple deposits fare as well as those having solitary resections. Cady and McDermott [90] recently suggested that when there were less than four deposits the median survival was 24 months but in the presence of more than this number the survival was 10 months. Five-year survival was 40% and 0% respectively. August et al. [91] reported survivals of 44 months vs. 20 months using the same criteria. This latter study incorporated intraperitoneal 5-FU administered through a Tenckhoff catheter in some patients, but due to the disparity between the two groups it was not possible to ascertain what benefit occurred. Prognosis is affected by the leaving of residual tumour in the liver but there is some controversy regarding the extent of tumour that should be resected. It appears that resection should be limited to removal of the tumour with a small cuff of normal liver tissue, making a resection range from a simple wedge to a major formal lobectomy or trisegmentectomy.

Although it is reasonable to advocate resection of solitary metastases in fit individuals, it should be remembered that approximately 70% of this small subgroup of patients are unlikely to benefit from the procedure. This is usually due to the remaining apparently normal liver harbouring occult tumours, unidentifiable on scanning or at laparotomy. In order to verify the true solitary nature it may be wise to defer resection for a few months, unless, of course, there is a small deposit that can be simply removed by wedge resection.

Conclusion

The appraisal of any treatment for colorectal liver metastases must be viewed critically against the overall knowledge of the natural history, which has now been well established by many studies. The role of the portal venous supply to metastases may have been underestimated in the past and hence selective arterial therapy may be limited. The benefit in terms of survival appears limited, even using long-term infusion with modern implantable pumps. Although technological advances have made it attractive, the main obstacle is the limited effect of present-generation cytotoxic drugs and their inability to penetrate these frequently avascular tumours. Surgical resection will help only a very small proportion of patients, and radiological embolisation gives good palliation for pain. However, our knowledge has been achieved only through active treatment of this condition, and avenues must continue to be explored both in the prevention and in the treatment of colorectal liver metastases.

References

1. Taylor I (1985) Colorectal liver metastases – to treat or not to treat? Br J Surg 72: 511–516
2. Taylor I (1982) A critical review of the treatment of colorectal liver metastases. Clin Oncol 8: 109–114
3. Weiss L, Gilbert HA (eds) (1982) Liver metastasis. Hall, Boston
4. van de Velde CJH, Sugarbaker PH (eds) (1984) Liver metastases. Nijhoff, The Hague
5. Ensminger WD, Gyves JW (1984) Regional cancer chemotherapy. Cancer Treat Rep 68: 101–115

6. Sterchi JM (1985) Hepatic artery infusion for metastatic neoplastic disease. Surg Gynecol Obstet 160: 477–489
7. Modlin J, Walker HSJ (1949) Palliative resection in cancer of colon and rectum. Cancer 2: 767–776
8. Stearns MW, Binkley GE (1954) Palliative surgery for cancer of the rectum and colon. Cancer 7: 1016–1019
9. Pestana C, Reitemeier RJ, Moertel C (1964) The natural history of carcinoma of the colon and rectum. Am J Surg 108: 826–829
10. Flanagan L, Foster JH (1967) Hepatic resection for metastatic cancer. Am J Surg 113: 551–557
11. Swinton NW, Samaan S, Rosenthal D (1967) Cancer of the rectum and sigmoid. Surg Clin North 47: 657–662
12. Jaffe BM, Donnegan WL, Watson F (1968) Factors influencing survival in patients with untreated hepatic metastases. Surg Gynecol Obstet 127: 1–11
13. Bengmark S, Hafstrom L (1969) The natural history of primary and secondary malignant tumors of the liver. Cancer 23: 198–201
14. Oxley EM, Ellis H (1969) Prognosis of carcinoma of the large bowel in the presence of liver metastases. Br J Surg 56: 149–152
15. Cady B, Monson DO, Swinton NW (1970) Survival of patients after colonic resection for carcinoma with simultaneous liver metastases. Surg Gynecol Obstet 131: 697–700
16. Baden H, Andersen B (1975) Survival of patients with untreated liver metastases from colorectal cancer. Scan J Gastroenterol 10: 221–223
17. Fischerman K, Petersen CF, Lindkaer Jensen S, Christensen KC, Elfsen F (1976) Survival among patients with liver metastases from cancer of the colon and rectum. Scand J Gastroenterol 11 [Suppl 37]: 111–115
18. Goslin R, Steele G, Zamcheck N, Mayer R, MacIntyre J (1982) Factors influencing survival in patients with hepatic metastases from adenocarcinoma of the colon and rectum. Dis Colon Rectum 25: 749–754
19. Nielsen J, Balsev I, Jensen H (1971) Carcinoma of the colon with liver metastases. Acta Chir Scand 137: 463–465
20. Bengtsson G, Carlsson G, Hafstrom L, Jonsson P (1981) Natural history of patients with untreated liver metastases from colorectal cancer. Am J Surg 141: 586–589
21. Wanebo HJ, Semoglou C, Attiyeh F (1978) Surgical management of patients with primary operable colorectal cancer and synchronous metastases. Am J Surg 135: 81–84
22. Wood CB, Gillis CR, Blumgart LH (1976) A retrospective study of the natural history of patients with liver metastases from colorectal cancer. Clin Oncol 2: 285–288
23. Wood CB (1984) Natural history of liver metastases. In: van de Velde CJH, Sugarbaker PH (eds) Liver metastases. Nijhoff, The Hague, pp 47–54
24. Wagner JS, Adson MA, Van Heerden JA, Adson MH, Ilstrup DM (1984) The natural history of hepatic metastases from colorectal cancer. Ann Surg 199: 502–507
25. Finan PJ, Marshall RJ, Cooper EH, Giles GR (1985) Factors affecting survival in patients presenting with synchronous hepatic metastases from colorectal cancer: a clinical and computer analysis. Br J Surg 72: 373–377
26. Gilbert JM, Jeffrey I, Evans M, Kark AE (1984) Sites of recurrent tumour after curative colorectal surgery: implications for adjuvant therapy. Br J Surg 71: 203–205
27. Fortner JG, Kim DK, Maclean BJ et al. (1978) Major hepatic resection for neoplasia: personal experience in 108 patients. Ann Surg 188: 363–371
28. Gennari L, Doci R, Bozzetti F, Bignami P (1986) Surgical treatment of hepatic metastases from colorectal cancer. Ann Surg 203: 49–54
29. Pettavel J, Morgenthaler F (1978) Protracted arterial chemotherapy of liver tumors: an experience of 107 cases over a 12-year period. In: Ariel IM (ed) Progress in clinical cancer, vol 7. Grune and Stratton, New York, pp 217–223
30. Pettavel J, Leyvraz S, Douglas P (1984) The necessity for staging liver metastases and standardizing treatment-response criteria. The case of secondaries of colorectal origin.

In: van de Velde CJH, Sugarbaker PH (eds) Liver metastases. Nijhoff, The Hague, pp 154–168

31. Smith TJ, Kemeny MM, Sugarbaker PH, Jones AE, Vermess M, Shawker TH, Edwards BK (1982) A prospective study of hepatic imaging in the detection of metastatic disease. Ann Surg 195: 486–491

32. Alderson PO, Adams DF, McNeil BJ, Sanders R, Siegelman SS, Finberg HJ, Hessel SJ, Abrams HL (1983) Computed tomography, ultrasound, and scintigraphy of the liver in patients with colon or breast carcinoma: a prospective comparison. Radiology 149: 225–230

33. Mittal R, Kowal C, Starzl T, Van Thiel D, Bron K, Iwatsuki S, Schade R, Straub W, Dekker A (1984) Accuracy of computerized tomography in determining hepatic tumor size in patients recieving liver transplantation or resection. J Clin Oncol 2: 637–642

34. Reed WP, Haney PJ, Elias EG, Whitley NO, Forsthoff C, Brown S (1986) Ethiodized oil emulsion enhanced computerized tomography in the preoperative assessment of metastases to the liver from the colon and rectum. Surg Gynecol Obstet 162: 132–136

35. Finlay IG, Meek DR, Gray HW, Duncan JG, McArdle (1982) Incidence and detection of occult hepatic metastases in colorectal carcinoma. Br Med J 284: 803–805

36. Brenner D, Whitley N, Theodore H, Aisner J, Wiernik P, Whitley J (1982) Volume determinations in computed tomography. JAMA 247: 1299–1302

37. Lien WM, Ackerman NB (1970) The blood supply of experimental liver metastases. II. A microcirculatory study of the normal and tumor vessels of the liver with the use of perfused silicone rubber. Surgery 68: 334–340

38. Honjo I, Matsumura H (1965) Vascular distribution of hepatic tumors. Experimental study. Rev Int Hepatol 15: 681–690

39. Fisher B, Fisher ER, Lee SH (1961) The effect of alteration of liver blood flow upon experimental hepatic metastases. Surg Gynecol Obstet 112: 11–18

40. Breedis C, Young G (1954) The blood supply of neoplasms in the liver. Am J Pathol 30: 969–977

41. Healey JE (1965) Vascular patterns in human metastatic liver tumours. Surg Gynecol Obstet 120: 1187–1193

42. Segall HN (1923) An experimental anatomical investigation of the blood and bile channels of the liver. Surg Gynecol Obstet 37: 152–178

43. Lin G, Lunderquist A, Hagerstrand I, Boijsen E (1984) Postmortem examination of the blood supply and vascular pattern of small liver metastases in man. Surgery 96: 517–526

44. Michels NA (1960) Newer anatomy of the liver variant blood supply and collateral circulation. JAMA 172: 125–132

45. Kaplan WD, D'Orsi CJ, Ensminger WD, Smith EH, Leven DC (1978) Intra-arterial radionuclide infusion: a new technique to assess chemotherapy infusion patterns. Cancer Treat Rep 62: 699–703

46. Leveson SH, Wiggins PA, Giles GR, Parkin A, Robinson PJ (1985) Deranged liver blood flow patterns in the detection of liver metastases. Br J Surg 72: 128–130

47. Gelin LE, Lewis DH, Nilsson L (1968) Liver blood flow in man during abdominal surgery. II. The effect of hepatic artery occlusion on the blood flow through metastatic tumor nodules. Acta Hepatogastroenterol 15: 21–24

48. Taylor I, Bennett R, Sherriff S (1979) The blood supply of colorectal liver metastases. Br J Cancer 39: 749–756

49. Broustein BR, Stede GD, Ensminger W, et al. (1980) The use and limitation of serial plasma carcinoembryonic antigen (CEA) levels as a monitor of changing metastatic liver tumor volume in patients receiving chemotherapy. Cancer 46: 266–272

50. Grage TB, Vassilopoulos, Shingleton WW, et al. (1979) Results of a prospective randomized study of hepatic artery infusion with 5-fluorouracil in patients with hepatic metastases from colorectal cancer: a Central Oncology Group study. Surgery 86: 550–555

51. Nilsson LV (1966) Therapeutic hepatic artery ligation in patients with secondary liver tumours. Rev Surg 23: 374–376

52. Bengmark S, Rosengren K (1970) Angiographic study of the collateral circulation to the liver after ligation of the hepatic artery in man. Am J Surg 119: 620–624

53. Almersjo O, Bengmark S, Rudenstam CM, Hafstrom L, Nilsson LAV (1972) Evaluation of hepatic dearterialization in primary and secondary cancer of the liver. Am J Surg 124: 5–9

54. Laufman LR, Nims TA, Guy JT, Guy JF, Courter S (1984) Hepatic artery ligation and portal vein infusion for liver metastases from colon cancer. J Clin Oncol 2: 1382–1388

55. Bengmark S, Nobin A, Jeppsson B, Tranberg KG (1983) Transient repeated dearterialization combined with intra-arterial infusion of oncolytic drugs in the treatment of liver tumours. In: Schwemmle K, Aigner K (eds) Vascular perfusion in cancer therapy. Springer, Berlin Heidelberg, New York, pp 68–74 (Recent results in cancer research, vol 86)

56. Bengmark S, Puntis M, Jeppsson (1986) Hepatic dearterialization in cancer: new perspectives. Eur Surg Res 18: 151–158

57. Odurny A, Birch SJ (1985) Hepatic arterial embolisation in patients with metastatic carcinoid tumours. Clin Radiol 36: 597–602

58. Allison DJ, Jordan H, Hennessy (1985) Therapeutic embolisation of the hepatic artery: a review of 75 procedures. Lancet I: 595–599

59. Chuang VP, Wallace S (1981) Hepatic artery embolization in the treatment of hepatic neoplasms. Radiology 140: 51–58

60. Hsu H-C, Wei T, Tsang Y, Wu M, Lin Y, Chuang S (1986) Histological assessment of resected hepatocellular carcinoma after transcatheter hepatic arterial embolization. Cancer 57: 1184–1191

61. Patt YZ, Wallace S, Freireich EJ, Chuang VP, Hersh EM, Mavligit GM (1981) The palliative role of hepatic arterial infusion and arterial occlusion in colorectal carcinoma metastatic to the liver. Lancet I: 349–351

62. Grady ED (1979) Internal radiation therapy of hepatic cancer. Dis Colon Rect 22: 371–375

63. Ariel IM, Padula G (1978) Treatment of symptomatic metastatic cancer to the liver from primary colon and rectal cancer by intra-arterial administration of chemotherapy and radioactive isotopes. In: Ariel IM (ed) Progress in clinical cancer, vol 7. Grune and Stratton, New York, pp 247–254

64. Sherman DM, Weichselbaum RR (1982) Hepatic metastasis: the role of radiotherapy. In: Weiss L, Gilbert HA (eds) Liver metastasis. Hall, Boston, pp 337–347

65. Kato T, Nemoto R, Mori H, Takahashi M (1981) Arterial chemoembolization with mitomycin C microcapsules in the treatment of primary or secondary carcinoma of the kidney, liver, bone and intrapelvic organs. Cancer 48: 674–680

66. Teder H, Aronsen KF, Lindell B, Rothman U (1978) Studies in pharmacokinetics of 5-fluoro-uracil temporarily retrained in the rat liver by degradable microsphere embolization. Acta Chir Scand 144 [Suppl 487]: 71

67. Ensminger WD, Rosowsky A, Raso V, et al. (1978) A clinical-pharmacological evaluation of hepatic arterial infusions of 5-fluoro-2'-deoxyuridine and 5-fluorouracil. Cancer Res 38: 3784–3792

68. Kemeny N (1983) The systemic chemotherapy of hepatic metastases. Semin Oncol 10: 148–158

69. Falk RE, Grieg P, Makowka L, et al. (1982) Intermittent percutaneous infusion into the hepatic artery of cytotoxic drugs for hepatic tumours. Can J Surg 25: 47–50

70. Blackshear PJ (1979) Implantable drug-delivery systems. Sci Am 241: 66–73

71. Niederhuber JE, Ensminger W, Gyves J, Thrall J, Walker S, Cozzi (1984) Regional chemotherapy of colorectal cancer metastatic to the liver. Cancer 53: 1336–1343

72. Balch CM, Urist MM, McGregor ML (1983) Continuous regional chemotherapy for metastatic colorectal cancer using a totally implantable infusion pump. Am J Surg 145: 285–290

73. Balch CM, Urist MM, Soong S, McGregor M (1983) A prospective phase-II clinical trial of continuous FUDR regional chemotherapy for colorectal metastases to the liver using a totally implantable drug infusion pump. Ann Surg 198: 567–573
74. Cohen AM, Kaufman SD, Wood WC, Greenfield AJ (1983) Regional hepatic chemotherapy using an implantable drug-infusion pump. Am J Surg 145: 529–533
75. Kemeny M, Goldberg DA, Browning S, Metter GE, Miner GE, Terz JJ (1985) Experience with continuous regional chemotherapy and hepatic resection as treatment of hepatic metastases from colorectal primaries. Cancer 55: 1265–1270
76. Weiss GR, Garnick MB, Osteen RT, et al. (1983) Long-term hepatic arterial infusion of 5-fluorodeoxyuridine for liver metastases using an implantable infusion pump. J Clin Oncol 1: 337–344
77. Schwartz SI, Jones LS, McCune CS (1985) Assessment of treatment of intrahepatic malignancies using chemotherapy via an implantable pump. Ann Surg 201: 560–567
78. Shepard KV, Levin B, Karl RC, et al. (1985) Therapy for metastatic colorectal cancer with hepatic artery infusion chemotherapy using a subcutaneous implanted pump. J Clin Oncol 3: 161–169
79. Didolkar MS, Elias EG, Whitley N, et al. (1985) Unresectable hepatic metastases from carcinoma of the colon and rectum. Surg Gynecol Obstet 160: 429–436
80. Stephens FO, Crea P, Walker P (1986) The implantable Infusaid infusion pump: the Sydney experience using 5-fluorouracil. Med J Aust 144: 74–77
81. Hodgson WJB, Friedland M, Ahmed T, et al. (1986) Treatment of colorectal hepatic metastases by intrahepatic chemotherapy alone or as an adjuvant to complete or partial removal of metastatic disesae. Ann Surg 203: 420–425
82. Kemeny N, Daly J, Oderman P, Shike M, et al. (1984) Hepatic artery pump infusion: toxicity and results in patients with metastatic colorectal carcinoma. J Clin Oncol 2: 595–600
83. Melnick J, Hohn D, Stagg R, et al. (1983) Cholestasis and biliary sclerosis in patients receiving hepatic arterial chemotherapy. Hepatology 3: 844
84. Kemeny M, Battifora H, Blayney DW, et al. (1985) Sclerosing cholangitis after continuous hepatic artery infusion of FUDR. Ann Surg 202: 176–181
85. Paget S (1889) The distribution of secondary growths in cancer of the breast. Lancet I: 571–573
86. Flanagan L, Foster JH (1967) Hepatic resection for metastatic cancer. Am J Surg 113: 551–557
87. Fortner JG, Silva JS, Golbey RB, et al. (1984) Multivariate analysis of a personal series of 247 consecutive patients with liver metastases from colo-rectal cancer. Ann Surg 199: 306–316
88. Kortz WJ, Meyers WC, Hanks JB, Schirmer BD, Jones RS (1984) Hepatic resection for metastatic cancer. Ann Surg 199: 182–186
89. August DA, Sugarbaker PH, Ottow RT, Gianola FJ, Schneider PD (1985) Hepatic resection of colorectal metastases. Ann Surg 201: 210–218
90. Cady B, McDermott WV (1985) Major hepatic resection for metachronous metastases from colon cancer. Ann Surg 201: 204–209
91. Flowerdew ADS, McLaren MI, Fleming JS, et al. (1987) Liver tumour blood flow and responses to arterial embolization measured by dynamic hepatic scintigraphy.Br J Cancer 55: 269–273

Patterns of Failure Following Surgical Resection of Colorectal Cancer Liver Metastases: Rationale for a Multimodal Approach

F. Bozzetti, R. Doci, P. Bignami, A. Morabito, and L. Gennari

Istituto Nazionale per lo Studio e la Cura dei Tumori, Via Venezian 1, 20133 Milan, Italy

Although the surgical resection of hepatic metastases from colorectal cancer has gained worldwide acceptance as the therapeutic modality in selected cases, there is little information regarding the natural history of the resected cases and the areas of failure following the hepatic resection.

This study analyzed the recurrence rate and patterns of failure after radical liver resection for hepatic metastases from a colorectal cancer at the *Istituto Nazionale Tumori* of Milan, Italy.

Patients and Methods

Forty-five patients admitted to the *Istituto Nazionale Tumori* of Milan from May 1980 to October 1984 underwent successful radical liver surgery for hepatic metastases from a previously resected colorectal cancer. Table 1 summarizes the main features of this series. Patients were initially classified according to the extent of liver involvement [1] and according to the staging system recently published by the same authors [2, 3] (Tables 2 and 3). The postoperative schedule included clinical examination, CEA test, liver function tests, and sonography or isotopic scan every 3–4 months. Barium enema or endoscopic examination, liver CAT, and chest roentgenography were performed twice yearly. Unless patients complained of specific symptoms, bone roentgenography total abdominal CAT, and brain scans were not routinely performed. The postoperative follow-up ranged from 4 to 45 months.

Results

Of the 45 patients, 28 (62%) had a relapse (Table 4). The site of extrahepatic relapse was intra-abdominal (peritoneum and previous intestinal anastomosis or retroperitoneal nodes) and extra-abdominal (lung and brain). Analysis of the recurrence rate by stage showed incidences of 47%, 52%, and 76% for stages I, II, and III respectively after a median period of 18 months. The difference was significant according to the Mantel-Haenszel test (Fig. 1).

Recent Results in Cancer Research, Vol. 110
© Springer-Verlag Berlin · Heidelberg 1988

Table 1. Main characteristics of patients in the series

Characteristic	No. of cases
Total number	45
Sex	27 M, 18 F
Median age (years)	53
Primary tumor	
Site:	
Rectum and sigmoid colon	31
Descending colon	8
Transverse colon	2
Ascending colon	4
Dukes' classification:	
B	14
C	21
Unknown	10
Differentiation:	
Good	3
Intermediate	19
Poor	6
Unknown	17

Table 2. Case distribution according to the classification of hepatic metastasis [1]

Category	Single (s)	Multiple (m)	Bilateral (b)	Total
H_1	21	4	2	27
H_2	2	7	1	10
H_3	3	3	2	8
Total	26	14	5	45 [a]

[a] Twelve synchronous, 33 metachronous (median interval 22 months).

Table 3. Distribution of surgical resections by stage and category [2]

Type of surgery	I H_1s	II H_1m-H_1b-H_2s	III H_2m-H_2b, H_3s-H_3m-H_3b	Total
Right lobectomy	2	2	13	17
Extended right lobectomy	–	2	1	3
Left lobectomy	1	–	–	1
Left lateral lobectomy	5	–	1	6
Sublobectomy	13	4	1	18
Total	21	8	16	45

Table 4. Patterns of recurrence after hepatic resection in 45 patients with median follow-up of 18 months

Site of failure	No.	%
Hepatic	11	24.4
Extrahepatic		
Intra-abdominal	6	13.3
Extra-abdominal	6	13.3
Hepatic + extra-abdominal	5	11.1
Total	28	62.2

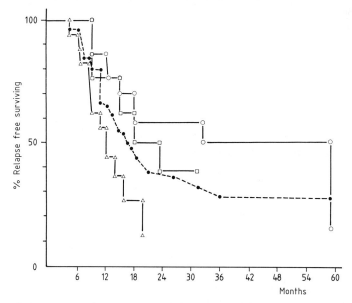

Fig. 1. Relapse-free survival by stage. ● overall series; ○ stage I; □ stage II; △ stage III

Discussion

The analysis of patterns of failure after hepatic resection for metastatic colorectal cancer showed that areas of failure included the liver, intra-abdominal extrahepatic structures and extra-abdominal organs. These data indicate that after failure of surgery on a primary large-bowel cancer, a second "local" approach on liver metastases will fail in a high percentage of patients.

To improve survival, an adjuvant therapy covering the potential areas of future relapses in the liver, abdomen, and distant sites is probably warranted in a phase in which microscopic residual disease could be present. Since only a few liver relapses after liver surgery are confined to the hepatic transection surface, the potential benefit of a *de principe* extended surgery should be minimal. However, since recent data [4] have shown that intraperitoneal administration of 5-fluorouracil achieves a portal venous level much higher than after intravenous dosing, intraperitoneal 5-fluorouracil or FUDR should be alternated with a systemic course of intravenous FUDR, which did not prove to be successful when administered alone [5].

References

1. Gennari L, Doci R, Bozzetti F, Veronesi U (1982) Proposal for a clinical classification of liver metastases. Tumori 68: 445–449
2. Gennari L, Doci R, Bozzetti F, Bignami P (1986) Proposal for staging liver metastases. In: Herfarth C, Schlag P, Hohenberger P (eds) Therapeutic strategies in primary and metastatic liver cancer. Springer, Berlin Heidelberg New York (Recent results in cancer research, vol 100: 80–84)
3. Gennari L, Doci R, Bozzetti F, Bignami P (1986) Surgical treatment of hepatic metastases from colorectal cancer. Ann Surg 203: 49–53
4. Sugarbaker PH, Gianda FJ, Speyer JC, Wesley R, Barofsky I, Meyers CE (1985) Prospective randomized trial of intravenous vs. intraperitoneal 5-FU in patients with advanced primary colon or rectal cancer. Surgery 98: 414–422
5. O'Connell MJ, Schutt AJ, Rubin J et al. (1985) Exploratory clinical trial of adjuvant chemotherapy following surgical resection of colorectal cancer liver metastases. Proc. AACR, No 657, Mayo Clinic, Rochester

Regional Chemotherapy of the Liver for Colorectal Malignancies

H. H. Gruenagel, E. Molzahn, U. Freund, and D. Groß

Chirurgische Abteilung, Evangelisches Krankenhaus Düsseldorf, Kirchfeldstraße 40, 4000 Düsseldorf, FRG

Prophylactic Liver Perfusion

Patients without metastases in the liver or other organs are perfused prophylactically. We follow the concept of Taylor [10], who perfused the liver via the umbilical vein starting immediately after resection of the primary tumor (1 g 5-FU/day for 7 days, continuously). The aim is to reduce the number of metachronous liver metastases and to achieve a better survival.

From October 1980 until January 1986 we had 428 patients with colorectal malignancies. Based on the criteria for inclusion only 132 patients were suitable for the study and control groups (Table 1). Postoperatively, we lost two patients from the study group (one cardiac infarction, one leukopenia) and one from the control group (lung embolism). Later we lost six patients from the study group and 13 from the control group. Liver metastases were found in five patients from the study group and in eight patients from the control group (Table 2). Regarding the survival time and the progression of the disease the figures for the study group were about 14% higher than those for the control group (Figs. 1 and 2; n.s.). Both groups were statistically equal in the distribution of age, sex, and localization and staging of the tumor (BMDP)[1]. Although the preliminary results are not statistically significant, we see an encouraging tendency and will therefore continue with the study.

Palliative Liver Perfusion

As liver metastases are nourished mainly by the arterial route [6] we inserted an arterial catheter into the hepatic artery via the gastroduodenal artery (Port-A-Cath) in 11 patients with nonresectable liver metastases. We administered cyclic chemotherapy with mitomycin (10 mg/m^2) as a bolus and 5-FU (1 g/m^2) continuously for 7 days, if possible every 6 weeks (Fig. 3).

---

[1] We thank Prof. Dr. W. Richter, Agricultural Faculty of the University of Bonn, Dept. of Statistics and Mathematics, for the biostatistical procedures.

Table 1. Distribution of patients ($n = 428$) with colorectal malignancies between October 1980 and January 1986: of 95 receiving an umbilical catheter, those with Dukes A or complications were excluded from the study group

	No. of patients
Study group Dukes B and C	62
Control group Dukes B and C	70

Table 2. Preliminary results in study involving prophylactic liver perfusion

Group	No. of patients with liver metastases	No. of patients lost to study
Study ($n = 62$)	5	2 (postoperatively) 6 (later)
Control ($n = 70$)	4 (ultrasound) 4 (ultrasound, suspicious)	1 (postoperatively) 13 (later)

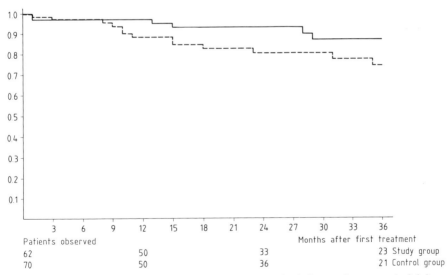

Patients observed			
62	50	33	23 Study group
70	50	36	21 Control group

Fig. 1. Survival curves according to Kaplan-Meier method for study group (*solid line; n = 62*) and control group (*broken line; n = 70*) of patients with Dukes B and C colorectal malignancies

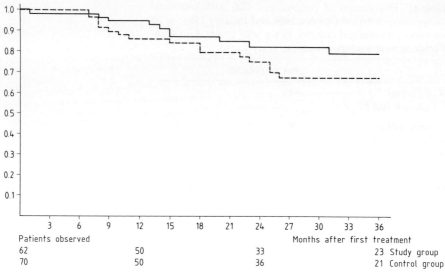

Fig. 2. Progression of disease according to Kaplan-Meier in study group *(solid line)* and control group *(broken line)*

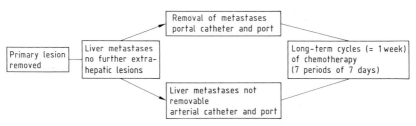

Fig. 3. Rationale for regional chemotherapy for liver metastases

Figure 4 shows the individual survey of our first patient with metachronous liver metastases. The improvement of her general condition even during the first cycle of chemotherapy was most impressing.

Figure 5 gives the follow-up of all patients with non-resectable liver metastases. There was no operative death. The evaluation of the therapy is difficult. The survival time alone is not convincing, but there is a remarkable improvement of the general condition and relief of pain. The therapy is well tolerated. Occasionally there is only slight upper abdominal pain and nausea.

Pat. L., H., 77 a

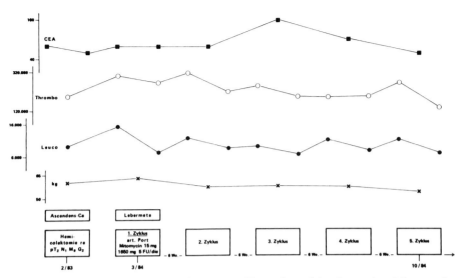

Fig. 4.   Individual survey of first patient (H. L., 77 years) receiving i.a. regional liver perfusion as palliative therapy for metachronous liver metastases

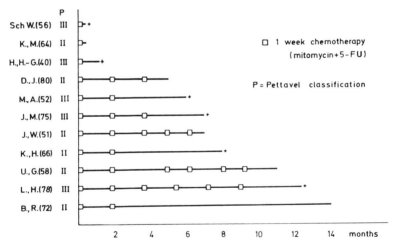

Fig. 5. Follow-up of 11 patients with non-resectable liver metastases who received palliative liver perfusion

Liver Perfusion After Removal of Metastases

The survey in Fig. 6 demonstrates the laboratory parameters during seven chemotherapeutic cycles. The patient is doing well now, 3.5 years after the removal of five liver metastases.

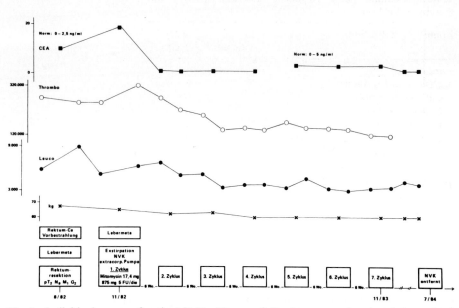

Fig. 6. Individual survey of patient D. H., 48 years, following repeated regional chemotherapy of the liver after removal of synchronous liver metastases

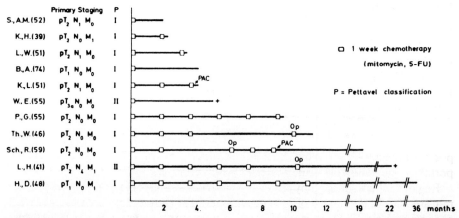

Fig. 7. Follow-up of 11 patients who underwent liver perfusion as regional chemotherapy after removal of metastases

Of 11 patients who underwent removal of the liver metastases we lost two: one due to the progression of pulmonary metastases and the second due to hemolytic-uremic disease (Fig. 7). At autopsy no intra- or extrahepatic tumor tissue could be found. Since this complication occurred we have stopped giving mitomycin at the maximum dose of 50 mg. Second operations were due to complications with the

Table 3. Complications in 70 patients receiving regional chemo-therapy of the liver

Route – complication	No. of patients	No. of cycles
Intra-arterial		
Dislocation to duodenum	1[a]	3
Catheter thrombosis	1	3
Catheter kinking	1	3
Perfusion of only one lobe	2	2
Liver coma (progression of cancer)	1	1
Subcutaneous drug infiltration	1	3
Total	7	
Portal or umbilical vein		
Dislocation	4	2, 2, 4, 6
Catheter thrombosis	1	3
Subcutaneous drug infiltration	1	1
Leukopenia, thrombocytopenia	1	1
Total	7	

[a] Implantofix used; all other systems were Port-A-Cath.

Table 4. Position of catheter in 165 long-term liver perfusions (including repeated treatments) for regional chemotherapy of the liver

Position of catheter	No. of patients
Hepatic artery Metastases not removed	11 (32 cycles)
Portal vein Metastases removed	11 (38 cycles)
Umbilical vein No metastases, prophylactic	95 (95 cycles)

portal catheter. (After removal of metastases liver perfusion is always done via the portal system, as in the randomized study of prophylactic liver perfusion.)

Regional chemotherapy by i.v. or i.a. catheters via the port system is easy to administer, but in the course of repeated chemotherapy numerous complications are observed (Table 3). There is no difference between the arterial and venous catheters concerning the number and the quality of complications (Table 4). They occur in about 20% of the applied chemotherapies.

Conclusions

Regarding the total number of 165 cycles of regional chemotherapy, of the liver we can say that it is well tolerated: the complications on the patient's side are minimal; the numerous complications with the catheter system should be reduced.

In the group of patients who received intra-arterial palliative treatment a prolongation of the survival time cannot be proved, but the quality of life was improved for all.

The study group who underwent prophylactic liver perfusion shows a tendency to better survival time. Following this observation, chemotherapeutic liver perfusion after removal of metastases should be a logical consequence.

References

1. Bengmark S, Hafström L, Jeppson B (1982) Metastatic disease in the liver from colorectal cancer: an appraisal of liver surgery. World J Surg 6: 61
2. Denck H (1984) Ergebnisse einer intraarteriellen intermittierenden Chemotherapie mit 5-FU bei Metastasenleber sowie inoperablen Tumoren des Gastrointestinal- und Urogenitaltrakts. Onkologie 7: 167
3. Gall FP, Scheele J, Herfarth C, Rothmund M, Funovics J, Siewert JR (1985) Therapiekonzept bei Lebermetastasen. Langenbecks Arch Chir 365: 219
4. Ghussen F, Grundmann R, Nagel K, Pichlmaier H (1985) Aktueller Stand der Therapie von Lebermetastasen kolorektaler Karzinome. Leber, Magen, Darm 15: 76
5. Hohenberger P, Schlag P, Herfarth C (1986) Zur Indikationsstellung operativer Verfahren bei primären und sekundären malignen Lebertumoren. Langenbecks Arch Chir 369: 789
6. Lien MW, Ackerman NB (1970) The blood supply of experimental liver metastases. II. A microcirculatory study of the normal and tumor vessels of the liver with the use of perfused silicone rubber. Surgery 68: 334
7. Metzger U, Schneider K, Largiadèr UF (1982) Adjuvante Therapie des Kolon- und Rektumkarzinoms. Onkologie 5: 228
8. Metzger U (1985) Prevention of liver metastases of colorectal carcinoma. In: Herfarth C, Schlag P, Hohenberger P (eds) Therapeutic strategies in primary and metastastic liver cancer. Springer, Berlin Heidelberg New York Tokyo (Recent results in cancer research, vol 100)
9. Schlag P (1985) Die Chemotherapie im Rahmen der operativen Primär- und Rezidivbehandlung des colorectalen Karzinoms. Onkol Forum 3: 5
10. Taylor J, Rowling JT (1979) Adjuvant cytotoxic liver perfusion for colorectal cancer. Br J Surg 66: 833
11. Wolff H, Lippert H, Sperling P (1985) Die chirurgische Therapie von Lebertumoren. Klinikarzt 14: 610

Interim Results of Intra-Arterial 4'-Epi-Doxorubicin for Liver Metastases

G. Simoni, M. T. Nobile, M. Repetto, P. L. Percivale, S. Razzi, R. Tatarek, M. G. Vidili, M. Muggianu, and D. Civalleri

Istituto di Patologia Chirurgica, Universita di Genova, Via le Benedetto XV/10, 16132 Genova, Italy

The results of systemic i.v. chemotherapy of unresectable colorectal cancers metastatic to the liver have so far been disappointing. Response rates from 10% to 30% have been reported with either mono- or combination chemotherapy [1, 2].

In contrast, objective response rates ranging from 40% to 80% have been reported in patients with colorectal metastases confined to the liver undergoing continuous intra-arterial FUDR infusion [3–5].

The clinical value of those promising results, however, has been limited by the high rates of both systemic progression and severe hepatic toxicity. The latter is represented mainly by sclerosing cholangitis (4%–56%), which can become a progressive disease causing death independent of the evolution of the neoplastic disease. Therefore, a regional treatment with a comparable effect on liver disease but with lower toxicity seems to be desirable. Though anthracyclines have exhibited only marginal activity in colon cancer when administered intravenously, their pharmacokinetic characteristics provide a rationale for intrahepatic administration.

The new anthracycline analogue 4'-epi-doxorubicin (4'-EpiDX) exhibits a similar antitumoral activity but lower cardiac toxicity in comparison with its parent compound doxorubicin (DX) [6, 7].

It has been shown that 4'-EpiDX disappears more rapidly from the serum than DX [8, 9]; the primary excretion of anthracyclines appears to occur through hepatic metabolism and biliary clearance. In fact, during the first 72 h following i.v. EpiDX infusion, 40% of the administered dose was found in bile in contrast to 10%–12% in urine [10, 11].

Furthermore, the systemic levels of DX during i.a. hepatic infusion are 25% lower than corresponding systemic levels after peripheral venous infusion.

Hepatic venous anthracycline levels, which are a measure of intrahepatic drug concentration, both in the tumor and hepatic capillary bed, are consistently higher when the drug is given by the hepatic arterial route [12]. In addition, patients with liver metastases who received intra-arterial 4'-EpiDX showed an higher clearance from plasma and high concentrations in the liver and the gallbladder with no side effects [9].

Based on this rationale, a phase I–II study has been activated to evaluate the efficacy of the arterial bolus administration of 4'-EpiDX in both pretreated and non-pretreated patients with unresectable, measurable, and histologically confirmed primary liver cancer or colorectal liver metastases.

Patients eligibility criteria further included: age less than 75 years, performance status (PS; ECOG ≤ 3), WBC > 3000, Hb > 10 g/100 ml, platelets > 120000, adequate liver function, and no heart disease. Response and toxicity have been evaluated according to UICC criteria.

Since March 1985, 20 patients (14 men and six women), median age 63 (range 40–75) and median PS = 0 (0–2) have entered the study. Five patients had primary liver cancer (four with hepatocellular carcinoma and one with cholangiocarcinoma) (PT) and 15 colorectal metastases (MT) with primary resected. In all cases the degree of liver involvement ranged from 25% to more than 50%. One PT and two MT patients had extrahepatic deposits (hilar nodes, lung, and pelvis respectively), and three MT patients had been pretreated with systemic chemotherapy (5-FU).

Regional access is obtained by means of a surgically implanted system (Infuse-A-Port, Port-A-Cath) with the catheter inserted through the gastroduodenal artery, up to but not into the hepatic artery [13, 14]. Starting 15 days after the operation, 4'-EpiDX is administered weekly as a 30-mg standard, i.a. bolus, up to progression or severe toxicity.

Neither major operative complications nor operative mortality has been observed so far; moreover, no treatments have had to be stopped for complications related to the access device.

Until now the total number of cycles is 213, with a median of 9 (range 1–26). The cumulative dosage is 6390 mg with a median of 270 mg.

All the patients have been evaluated for toxicity. Four patients (20%) experienced grade-1 to -2 epigastric pain following drug administration, nine had (45%) grade-1 to -4 nausea and vomiting, four (20%) developed grade-2 to -3 hyperbilirubinemia, and one (5%) grade-2 cardiac toxicity. Neither myelosuppression nor alopecia has been detected.

The treatment was stopped after 13 and 20 cycles, i.e., after a cumulative dose of 390 and 600 mg respectively, in the two patients who developed grade-4 G.I. toxicity and grade-2 cardiac toxicity.

Fourteen MT and four PT patients are fully evaluable for the response. One complete response (CR; 7.1%), four partial responses (PR; 28.5%), five stable disease (SD; 35.7%) and four progressions (P; 28.5%) have been observed in patients with colorectal metastases, while all patients with primary tumors showed SD. It is interesting that all responders had liver involvement less than 50%. The response duration for CR and PR is 29+, 54, 39, 33, 32+ weeks respectively.

The median time to progression has been 39 and 36 weeks for the CR + PR and SD groups respectively. Only two patients in the MT group (14.3%) showed extrahepatic progression, both to the lung. The overall median survival from the implant of the arterial access device has been 57.5+ weeks, while median survival of responders has been 58+ weeks. Our results suggest that the i.a. bolus administration of 4'-EpiDX is well tolerated, with mild and transient toxicity. The response rate and the low toxicity are encouraging and promising of better results, likely with higher doses, in more selected patients with colorectal liver metastases.

References

1. Ramirez G, Ansfield FJ (1982) Chemotherapy of liver metastases. In: Weiss L, Gilbert HA (eds) Liver metastases. Hall, Boston
2. Kemeny N (1983) The systemic chemotherapy of hepatic metastases. Semin Oncol 10: 148–158
3. Niederhuber JE, Ensminger W, Gyves J, Thrall J, Walker S, Cozzi E (1984) Regional chemotherapy of colorectal cancer metastases to the liver. Cancer 53: 1336–1343
4. Balch CM, Urist MM, Soong S, McGregor M (1983) A prospective phase-II clinical trial of continuous FUDR regional chemotherapy for colorectal metastases to the liver using a totally implantable drug-infusion pump. Ann Surg 198: 567–573
5. Kemeny MM, Battifora H, Blayney DW, Cecchi G, Goldberg DA, Leong LA, Margolin KA, Terz JJ (1985) Sclerosing cholangitis after continuous hepatic artery infusion of FUDR. Ann Surg 202: 176–181
6. Natale M, Brambilla M, Luchini S, Martini A, Moro E, Pacciarini MA, Tamassia V, Vago G, Trabattoni A (1981) 4'-Epi-doxorubicin and doxorubicin: toxicity and pharmacokinetics in cancer patients. In: Current chemotherapy and immunotherapy. The American Society for Microbiology, Washington DC, pp 1447–1449
7. Weenen H, Lankelma JP, Penders PGM, McVie JG, Ten Bokkel Huinink WW, De Planque MM, Pinedo HM (1983) Pharmacokinetics of 4'-epi-doxorubicin in man. Invest New Drugs 1: 59–64
8. Camaggi CM, Strocchi E, Tamassia V, Martoni A, Giovanni M, Lafelice G, Canova N, Marraro D, Martini A, Pannuti F (1982) Pharmacokinetic studies of 4'-epi-doxorubicin in cancer patients with normal and impaired renal function and with hepatic metastases. Cancer Treat Rep 66: 1819–1824
9. Strocchi E, Camaggi CM, Angelelli B, Monari P, Martoni A, Pannuti F (1983) 4'-Epi-doxorubicin in loco-regional therapy: pharmacokinetic study after intrahepatic arterial and intraperitoneal administration. IV NCI-EORTC symposium on new drugs in cancer therapy, Brussels, December 14–17 (Abstract 18)
10. Weenen H, Van Maanen JMS, McVie JG, De Planque MM, Pinedo HM (1984) Metabolism of 4' modified analogues of doxorubicin. Unique glucuronidation pathway for 4'-epi-doxorubicin. Eur J Cancer Clin Oncol 20 (7): 315–318
11. Cassinelli G, Penco S, Arcamone F (1983) Human urinary metabolites of epirubicin and idarubicin. IV NCI-EORTC symposium on new drugs in cancer therapy, Brussels, December 14–17 (Abstract 16)
12. Garnick MB, Ensminger W, Israel M (1979) A clinical pharmacological evaluation of hepatic arterial infusion of adriamycin. Cancer Res 39: 4105–4110
13. Niederhuber JE, Ensminger W, Gyves JW, Liepman M, Doan K, Cozzi E (1982) Totally implanted venous and arterial access system to replace external catheters in cancer treatment. Surgery 92: 706–712
14. Bothe A jr, Piccione W, Ambrosino J, Benotti PN, Lokich JJ (1984) Implantable central venous access system. Am J Surg 147: 565–569

The Use of an Implantable Vascular Occluder in the Treatment of Nonresectable Hepatic Malignancies

B. Persson, B. Jeppsson, M. C. A. Puntis, H. Ekberg, K. Tranberg, and S. Bengmark

Institutionen för Kirurgi, Lunds Universitet, 22185 Lund, Sweden

Since the pioneering work of Segall [1] and the introduction of hepatic artery ligation by Markowitz [2] occlusion of the hepatic artery has been used as a means to induce regression in liver tumors.

Different procedures are being practiced: Hepatic artery ligation with or without dearterialization, intermittent transient dearterialization, nonsurgical permanent embolisation with non-degradable micromaterial, and transient embolization with degradable microspheres. Transient occlusion of the hepatic artery has shown some favorable results in the treatment of malignant carcinoid disease. On the whole, however, the tumor reduction is short lived, partly due to a rapid formation of arterial collaterals which, within a few days, supply the tumors with new arterial flow.

Despite this, we think that manipulation of the tumor blood supply is an intresting principle to pursue in order to decrease the formation of collaterals. This is based on clinical observations. In 1978 Taylor [3] showed that regional infusion combined with hepatic artery ligation was associated with prolonged survival. In 1981 Patt et al. [4] showed an almost doubled survival after both intentional and nonintentional occlusion of the hepatic artery in patients receiving hepatic artery infusion of FUDR and mitomycin C. In 1986 Ekberg, Tranberg and others from our own department [5] showed a prolonged survival for patients developing hepatic artery thrombosis during hepatic artery infusion of 5-FU.

Therefore, we think that manipulation of the arterial supply might have a place in the treatment of nonresectable liver cancer. During the past 5 years we have developed a totally implantable device with which the hepatic artery can be occluded for a variable length of time [6]. The device consists of a silicone tourniquet connected to a subcutaneous injection reservoir. The tourniquet is placed around the hepatic artery, which can be compressed by the injection of 2–3 ml saline into the port. In animal experiments we have shown that brief (less than 2–3 h) daily occlusions prevent the formation of arterial collaterals and that permanent occlusion does not.

Hepatic dearterialization induces ultrastructural changes in the normal liver even after only 1 h. The cytological changes concerns the cytoplasmatic organelles, mainly the mitochondria. These changes might be expected to be more pro-

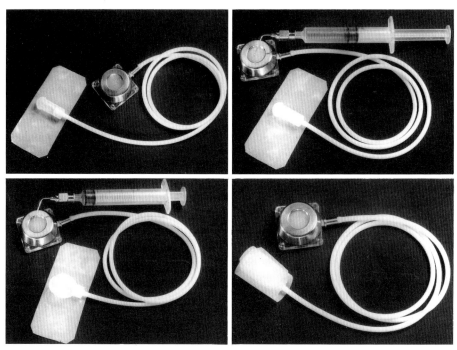

Fig. 1. *Top left:* Vascular occluder of silicone connected to a subcutaneous injection port. *Top right:* Angled Huber needle inserted through the self-sealing silicone membrane. *Bottom left:* Injection of 2 ml normal saline expands the balloon. *Bottom right:* Balloon expanded inside the ring created by connecting the sleeves around the vessel, which is occluded. (Device made by A. B. Nolato, Torekov, Sweden)

nounced in liver tumors, as these are supplied mainly by the hepatic artery. The origin of this damage is not known, but there is increasing evidence that the early changes are due to the oxygen reduction and the generation of free radicals. The DNA and its chromatin structure are target organs for free radicals which can induce single or double DNA strand breaks, cross links, or miscellaneous forms of base damage. We have found that genotoxic free radicals can be detected almost immediately after clamping of the hepatic artery in a rat model [7]. The reason for this is the dual blood supply of the liver, the oxygen supply from the portal vein being sufficiently high to allow immediate production of oxygen free-radical species.

In a rat tumor model with a transplanted adenocarcinoma we studied the DNA synthesis after 1 h of dearterialization by measuring incorporation of labeled thymidine [8]. We found that upon release of the circulation there was increased DNA synthesis and a high labeling of tumor cells. This might reflect a possible synchronization of the tumor cells after ischemia or reparative processes after DNA damage.

The effect of a cell-phase-dependent chemotherapeutic agent will be different on various phases of the cell cycle. It might be expected that the efficacy of a given treatment protocol would depend on the possibility to synchronize the cell cycle.

The device is now being used in patients with liver secondaries from colorectal cancers. Occlusions for 60 min two or three times daily are combined with intraperitoneal infusion of 5-FU at 6-week intervals. Four patients have been treated so far. The observation period is still too short to allow any conclusions to be made about the effect on tumor reduction. The implantation seems easy to perform, with fewer complications, which can be expected as the artery is not permanently ligated. The patients' compliance has been excellent: they have been able to perform the occlusions by themselves at home. If pain has been intolerable despite the use of analgetics they have been instructed to stop the occlusion.

During surgery for implantation of the occluder we have observed the changes in blood flow in the tumor deposits while the occluder was being inflated by means of a duplex ultrasound probe (Angioscan II). We have also measured the change in oxygen tension on the surface of the normal liver and on the tumor deposits. The oxygen tension declined steadily over 1–2 min following occlusion. Postoperatively, using a Diasonics ultrasound apparatus, we have been able to localize large tumor deposits in the liver by percutaneous ultrasound and then to demonstrate the decrease in flow on inflating the tourniquet around the hepatic artery. Reestablishment of flow is marked by a period of reactive hyperemia.

Degradable microspheres are now being used to obtain repeated tumor ischemia in combination with cytostatic infusion, with some promising results. The implantable vascular occluder offers a simple way to obtain repeated short-term ischemia, and implantation is a fairly simple procedure. We therefore would like to propose that the implantable vascular occluder be used in future trials on the treatment of liver secondaries in combination with either intra-arterial, intraportal, or intraperitoneal infusion of chemotherapeutic agents.

References

1. Segall MN (1923) An experimental anatomical investigation of the blood and bile channels of the liver. Surg Gynecol Obstet 37: 152
2. Markowitz J, Rappaport AM, Scott AC (1949) Prevention of liver necrosis following ligation of the hepatic artery. Proc Soc Exp Biol Med 70: 305
3. Taylor I (1978) Cytotoxic perfusion for colorectal liver metastases. Br J Surg 65: 109
4. Patt YZ, Chuang VP, Wallace S, et al. (1981) The palliative role of hepatic arterial infusion and arterial occlusion in colorectal carcinoma metastatic to the liver. Lancet 1: 349
5. Ekberg H, Tranberg KG, Lundstedt C, Hanff G, Ranstam J, Jeppsson B, Bengmark S (1986) Determinants of survival after intra-arterial infusion of 5-fluorouracil for liver metastases from colorectal cancer. J Surg Oncol 31: 246
6. Persson BG, Andersson L, Jeppsson B, Ekelund L, Strand SE, Bengmark S (1987) Prevention of collateral circulation after repeated transient occlusion of the hepatic artery in pigs. World J Surg 11: 672
7. Puntis MCA, Persson BG, Jeppsson B, Jonsson G, Pero RN, Bengmark S (1987) Free radical productin in the ischemic rat liver. Surg Res Comm 1: 17
8. Persson BG, Jeppsson B, Bengmark S (1987) Effects on DNA synthesis after temporary dearterialization of a rat liver tumor. Surg Res Comm

Hepatic Arterial Ligation with and Without Portal Infusion in Metastatic Colorectal Cancer

A. Gerard, O. Dalesio, N. Duez, H. Bleiberg, J. C. Pector, M. Lise, D. Nitti, G. Delvaux, G. Willems, G. Depadt, J. P. Arnaud, and P. Schlag*, **

Institut Jules Bordet, Rue Héger Bordet 1, 1000 Brussels, Belgium

If liver metastases are diffuse and spread out in both lobes of the liver, the question is: Which treatment should be given? Until now, no therapy has been proven to increase the survival rate of patients with these diffuse metastases. Liver tumors are irrigated mainly by arterial supply. Indeed, the blood flow of liver metastases decreases by 90% in the tumor after hepatic artery ligation. Under the same conditions, it decreases by only 35% in normal liver parenchyma. Unfortunately, the decrease in arterial flow in the liver after interruption of the blood supply is temporary. Within 3 weeks, a revascularization is visible through the lesser omentum and the greater omentum, as well as through the celiac axis and the inferior phrenic artery.

Nevertheless, it must be kept in mind that hepatic artery ligation is followed by a selective necrosis of the tumor with nearly no damage to the liver parenchyma. On the other hand, it is known that depriving the tumor of its arterial circulation is not sufficient to achieve a complete cure, since the portal blood supply will always save a rim of neoplastic cells around the area of necrosis. Furthermore, Lindell [1] showed that repeated embolization of the hepatic artery causes an increase in the portal vein blood flow, probably because of increased preportal arteriovenous shunting. One could postulate that tumor growth, which initially diminishes following hepatic artery ligation, subsequently increases as perfusion via the portal vein increases. Therefore, a combined therapy is necessary to treat tumor cells surviving the dearterialization, i.e., perfusion of the liver with a cytotoxic drug via the portal vein.

In February 1981, the Gastrointestinal Tumor Group of the European Organization for Research and Treatment of Cancer (EORTC) began a randomized comparative study with the aim of evaluating the effectiveness of hepatic artery ligation and portal infusion of 5-FU versus a surgical procedure which apparently has no influence on survival and is symptomatic, as is hepatic artery ligation alone. Patients with a resected colorectal primary tumor and unresectable liver metas-

---

* Trial of the Gastrointestinal Tract Cancer Cooperative Group of the European Organization for Research and Treatment of Cancer (EORTC).
** The authors thank Mrs. S. Devaux for her secretarial help.

tases are stratified according to the measurability of the lesions and the presence or absence of symptoms at the time of entry in the trial.

Material and Methods

Criteria for patient selection:

1. Karnofsky performance status of 60 or more
2. Less than 70 years old
3. Patients in the immediate postoperative period of primary tumor resection and patients relapsing primarily in the liver

Criteria for tumors:

1. Metastases of colorectal carcinoma proven by liver biopsy
2. Diffuse and non-resectable liver metastases
3. Primary colorectal adenocarcinoma resected during a previous surgical operation

Patients in the asymptomatic group are excluded if they have hepatic pain or have lost more than 10% of their normal body weight. In this group, bilirubin has to be less than 2 mg%. Patients must have less than 25% involvement of liver parenchyma, as estimated by the surgeon during laparotomy. Symptomatic patients present hepatic pain, weight loss of over 10%, bilirubin of over 2 mg%, or an involvement of over 25% of the liver parenchyma.

A measurable tumor is defined as a known mass that can be clearly measured at the surface of the liver by a ruler or a caliper. Hepatomegaly may be accepted as a measurable disease if the liver edge is clearly defined, extending at least 5 cm below the costal margin or the xiphoid process, with calm respiration. A liver scan, ultrasonography, or computed tomography must be used for the evaluation of tumor invasion and as the primary indicator of tumor response. The same method of measurement must be used to evaluate response to therapy. A schema of the trial is shown in Fig. 1.

Patients are randomized into two groups. The first group of patients are treated

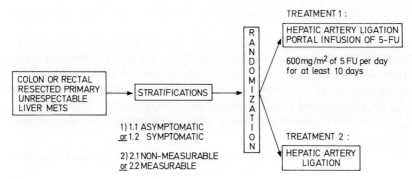

Fig. 1. Study scheme to evaluate hepatic artery ligation with and without portal infusion

by hepatic artery ligation (HAL) and portal infusion (PI) of 5-FU for at least 10 days. Courses of 10 days are repeated every 6 weeks until progression of the disease. The second group of patients undergo HAL alone.

During laparotomy, the hepatic artery and its left and right branches are dissected, double ligated with No. 00 silk sutures, and sectioned as close to the liver as possible. So are any of the accessory hepatic arteries which may have been demonstrated by preoperative angiography. The lesser omentum, triangular ligaments, and falciform ligaments are transected in an attempt to retard the development of collateral arterial circulation to the liver. The middle colic vein is identified and tied distally. A catheter is threaded cephalad until its tip lies in the portal vein. The efficacy of the perfusion is checked by fluorescein intraoperatively. To avoid infection of the catheter and to provide repeated access to the vascular system without trauma or complications, an Infuse-A-Port or Port-A-Cath is placed subcutaneously. This device is totally implantable. Patients are not subject to the frequent heparin flushes or dressing changes, nor are their normal activities restricted. Continuous infusions are connected through a pump system to provide adequate pressure in the portal system. During surgery, a rough estimation of the percentage of invaded liver parenchyma should be made. Also, the volume and the number of the metastases must be evaluated with the greatest accuracy possible. The size of the largest metastases must be measured with a caliper.

The patients treated by HAL and PI receive 600 mg/m^2 5-FU/day for 10 days per course. These courses of infusion are repeated every 6 weeks. The 5-FU is given as a continuous infusion in 5% dextrose. Heparin can be added to this solution. Portograms are performed by injecting contrast medium into the catheter before the first day of infusion.

A liver function test and a full hematological investigation are performed daily during the first course of infusion. The 5-FU infusion should be stopped in the case of disease progression, catheter complications (displacement, obstruction, infection), severe hematological toxicity, i.e., leucocyte count of less than 2000 and platelet count of less then 100000, and other severe toxicities, such as diarrhea or acute mucositis.

Table 1. Distribution of patients according to the institutions participating in the study

Institution	No. of patients
J. Bordet – Brussels	20
AZ – VUB – Brussels	11
Cl. Chirurgica – Padua	11
O. Lambret – Lille	8
CMCO – Strasbourg	6
University of Heidelberg	5
CHU – Caen	3
L. Caty, CHU Brest, Cl. Zurich, St.-Russelsheim, Glasgow	6
	70

Participating Institutions

Until now, 70 patients have been registered. The list of participating institutions and number of registered patients by institution are shown in Table 1.

Patient Evaluation

Thirty-five patients have been registered in each group. Six patients were un-eligible, three in each group: three patients in the group treated by HAL + PI 5-FU had extrahepatic malignancies and two had resectable metastases in the group treated by HAL alone. The third patient had a hepatic vein thrombosis. Four patients were not evaluable because of the absence of any data, two in each group, and four patients were partially evaluable, three in the group treated by HAL and one in the group treated by HAL + PI 5-FU. To date, 39 patients are fully evaluable, 20 in the group treated by HAL + PI 5-FU and 19 in the group treated by HAL. With 17 patients it is too early for evaluation.

Table 2. Patients' characteristics

		HAL + PI 5-FU	HAL
Age (years)	Median	58	58
	Range	38–71	34–70
Sex	Male	19	13
	Female	9-	12
Primary tumor site			
	Ascending colon	2	3
	Transverse colon	2	0
	Descending colon	10	12
	Rectum	14	10
Total no. of patients		28	25

Table 3. Patients' characteristics

	HAL + PI 5-FU	HAL	Total
Symptomatic	3	10	13
Asymptomatic	15	15	30
Not measurable	5	3	8
Measurable	23	21	44
Amount of liver parenchyma invaded			
≤ 25%	7	7	14
> 25%	18	19	37
Liver metastases diagnosed			
– Before or during surgery	17	14	31
– After surgery	11	11	22

Patient Characteristics

The patients' characteristics are summarized in Tables 2 and 3. The distribution of the patients in the two groups is well balanced.

During surgery, the number of liver metastases were determined and the measure of the largest metastases were taken, and these data are reported in Table 4. The duration of hospitalization has been longer for patients treated by HAL and PI, since for most of the patients the first course of locoregional chemotherapy was approximately 20 days.

Complications of Treatment

The complications of treatment are summarized in Tables 5 and 6 following the WHO grading. It should be noted that four patients had relatively severe hepatic

Table 4. Data regarding surgery

	HAL + PI 5-FU	HAL
No. of metastases observed		
Median	6	4
Range	1–35	1–15
Largest diameter of metastases (cm)		
Median	7	6
Range	2–13	3–15
No. of days of hospitalization		
Median	21	12
Range	7–55	9–45

Table 5. Complications of treatment – WHO grading > 2

	HAL + PI 5-FU	HAL
Septicemia	1	–
G. I. bleeding	1	–
Hepatic failure	4[a]	–
Biliary fistula	1	1
Wound infection	1	–

[a] One death 7 days after surgery.

Table 6. Complications of chemotherapy – WHO grading 2

WBC	1
Nausea/vomiting	1
Cutaneous	1

failure. One of these was lethal and was explained by a portal thrombosis; this patient had a history of thromboembolism disease.

Results

Evaluation of Response

Of the 20 patients who were fully evaluable in the group treated by HAL + PI 5-FU, six had a partial response. Five partial responses were observed, lasting 9, 22, 24, 37, and 52 weeks. The sixth patient with a partial response is still alive after 4 months. No partial responses were observed in the group treated by HAL alone. Nine patients in each group presented no change in the size of their tumors for at least 3 months. Four HAL + PI and eight HAL only patients had progression of their liver metastases.

Survival

Median survival for the whole group was 12 months. To date, no difference in the duration of survival has been detected between the two randomized treatment groups.

Conclusion

Among the various treatments possibilities for liver metastases of colorectal cancer, an occlusion of the hepatic artery combined with a portal infusion of cytotoxic drug seems the most reasonable approach. Such a treatment must be administered with respect to careful patient selection criteria to avoid complications. HAL + PI 5-FU showed the possibility of a partial response rate but it is still too early for an evaluation of the impact on survival.

Reference

1. Lindell B (1977) Transient liver ischemia by intra-arterial injection of degradable microspheres. (Paper issued by the Experimental Department, the Department of Surgery, and the Department of Nuclear Medicine, Malmö General Hospital) University of Lund, Malmö

Basic Investigations on Interaction of 5-Fluorouracil and Tumor Ischemia in the Treatment of Liver Malignancies

B. Eibl-Eibesfeldt, V. Storz, J. Kummermehr, and A. Schalhorn

Chirurgische Klinik Innenstadt und Chirurgische Poliklinik, Universität München, Nußbaumstraße 20, 8000 München 2, FRG

Introduction

Pharmacokinetic considerations are the main rationale for locoregional treatment of hepatic malignancies with anticancer drugs [3, 6, 10]. The advantage of regional exposure of arterially infused drugs increases when the blood flow rate into the target region is reduced [6, 13]. Impairment of tumor blood flow and synchronous intra-arterial chemotherapy have been employed in various clinical studies using 5-fluorouracil (5-FU) [8, 9, 18]. The antimetabolite 5-FU is activated in the tumor cell, requiring several energy-dependent anabolic steps (Fig. 1). This applies to the drug's action on RNA as well as DNA synthesis [14, 17]. Whether active carrier-mediated transport into the tumor cell of 5-FU is also involved is still a matter of discussion [17].

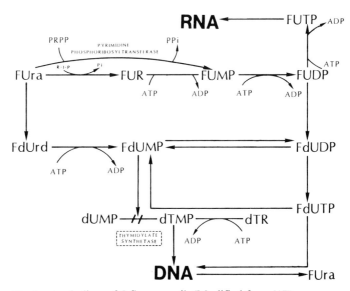

Fig. 1. Anabolism of 5-fluorouracil. (Modified from [17])

Recent Results in Cancer Research, Vol. 110
© Springer-Verlag Berlin · Heidelberg 1988

As transient ischemia through tumor blood flow reduction might impair these steps in the drug's activation [11], ischemia might actually have a protective effect for the tumor cell in spite of the pharmacokinetic advantages, and the pharmaco-dynamic response might consequently be reduced. On the other hand, the tumor cell might have an increased sensitivity to the drug in a phase of increased meta-bolic activity when blood flow is restored and cell-repair protein synthesis and cell reproduction are enhanced. We tested these two hypotheses in an animal model, using two different tumors in three series.

Method

Tumors

An undifferentiated mammary adenocarcinoma AT-7 and a differentiated mam-mary adenocarcinoma 284 were used in female isogenic C3H mice. Tumor cubes measuring 1×1 mm were transplanted subcutaneously using a cannula with a tro-car inserted through a cut on the right flank of the shaved animal. Tumor growth was regularly measured percutaneously using a stencil with round holes of in-creasing diameter. The measuring system had been correlated previously with the weight of the explanted tumor, and values were highly reproducible. Tumor growth was observed in 80% of the animals with transplants; five animals devel-oping more than one tumor were excluded (5/150, 3.3%).

When tumors had reached treatment size of 100 mg the animals were randomly allocated to the different treatment groups using a stratification schedule so that the groups were of roughly equal size. No group had more than two animals more than the other groups.

Chemotherapy

5-Fluorouracil was given intraperitoneal in a single dose of 100 mg/kg body weight.

Tumor Ischemia

Ischemia was reached by clamping the tumor percutaneously for 90 min under isothermic conditions (37 °C), similar to the method described by Thomlinson and Craddock [16]. This length of time was chosen because with longer ischemia times skin necrosis had been observed. For narcosis, intraperitoneal hexobarbital was given initially and after 60 min.

Treatment Groups

There were eight to ten animals per treatment groups. Group 1 received no treat-ment, group 2 received i.p. 5-FU only, and group 3 was treated by ischemia only. In groups 4–8 i.p. 5-FU was given, followed after time lapses of 20 min, 60 min,

4 h, 24 h, and 48 h by tumor ischemia. In groups 9–13 the sequences were reversed, with ischemia first and subsequent i.p. 5-FU treatment after 20 min, 60 min, 4 h, 24 h, and 48 h.

Tumors were measured every second day and regrowth delay (i.e., the time taken to reach one or two times pretreatment size beginning with 5-FU injection) was calculated. As the circadian rhythm might also play an important role on pharmacodynamic response, 5-FU was injected at 1 p.m. for all groups.

Pharmacokinetic Studies

Using high-pressure liquid chromatography after i.p. injection of 100 mg 5-FU/kg body weight, we ensured that peak serum drug levels had been reached at the time of subsequent ischemia (Fig. 2).

Results

Ischemia alone (group 3) leads to very slight tumor reduction. Treatment size had doubled after a mean of 5.6 days, whereas in the untreated group it had doubled after 4.6 days, which is significantly earlier ($P < 0.001$) (Fig. 3).

All groups showed marked tumor reduction after injection of 5-FU. However, there were marked and statistically significant differences between the groups. When groups receiving 5-FU prior to ischemia were compared with those receiving 5-FU alone, they showed earlier tumor regrowth to pretreatment and double pretreatment size. The inverse was observed with groups receiving 5-FU after the end of ischemia. They showed markedly more regrowth delay than those with 5-FU treatment alone. Consequently, the sequence ischemia–5-FU was much superior to 5-FU followed by ischemia, with P-values of < 0.0001 (Fig. 4). Differ-

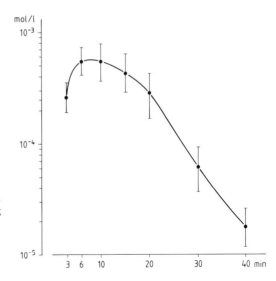

Fig. 2. Serum 5-fluorouracil levels after i.p. injection of 100 mg/kg body weight in C3H mice using high performance liquid chromatography; $n = 5$ animals for each measurement at 3, 6, 10, 20, 30, and 40 min. At 40 min 2 of the 5 had no detectable level

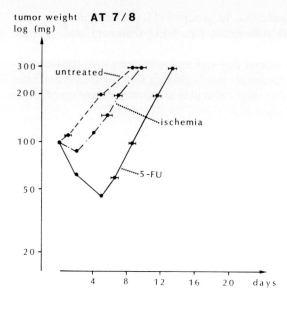

Fig. 3. Tumor growth (AT 7/8) in the three groups: untreated, ischemia alone, 5-fluorouracil *(FU)* given i. p.

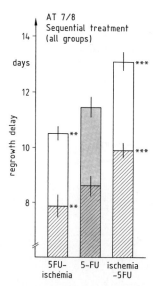

Fig. 4. Tumor regrowth delay (AT 7/8) after sequential treatment. *Hatched,* time to reach pretreatment size; *open,* time to reach twice pretreatment size; **$P<0.01$, ***$P<0.001$, compared with 5-fluorouracil alone

ences were most pronounced when the groups with 20-min time lapse to ischemia were compared (Fig. 5). Group 4 had reached pretreatment size (double pretreatment size) after 7.3 (10.7) days, compared with group 9 with 5-FU 20 min after ischemia with 11.9 (14.8) days. The values for 5-FU alone were 8.6 (11.5) days. Figures 6–8 demonstrate that the differences eventually become less pronounced, the longer the time lapse to ischemia. After 24 h (Fig. 7) there are still statistically significant differences, but at 48 h (Fig. 8) we found no differences between the

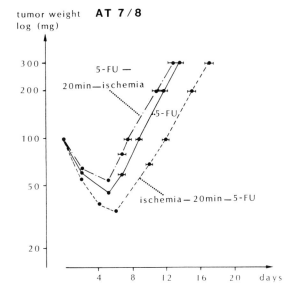

Fig. 5. Tumor growth (AT 7/8): *solid line*, 5-fluorouracil *(5-FU)* given i.p.; *dash and dotted line*, 5-FU i.p. given 20 min prior to ischemia; *broken line*, 5-FU i.p. given 20 min after ischemia

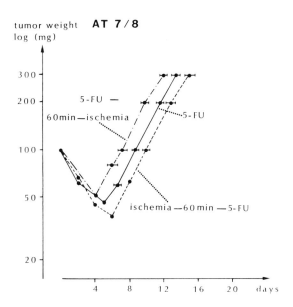

Fig. 6. Tumor growth (AT 7/8): *solid line*, 5-fluorouracil *(5-FU)* given i.p.; *dash and dotted line*, 5-FU i.p. given 60 min prior to ischemia; *broken line*, 5-FU i.p. given 60 min after ischemia

groups. Figure 9 summarizes the results in hierarchical order; the regrowth delays for 5-FU prior to ischemia, 5-FU alone, and ischemia followed by 5-FU are plotted.

The results were reproduced in another series with 15-min time lapse and the same tumors and with 10 min and a differentiated mammary adenocarcinoma 284. Again marked differences exist with little time lapse to ischemia and have disappeared when the time lapse to ischemia is 24 h.

tumor weight **AT 7/8**
log (mg)

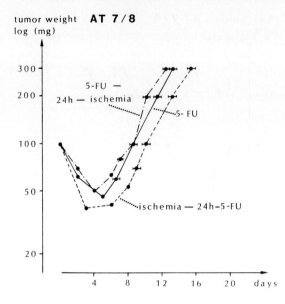

Fig.7. Tumor growth (AT 7/8): *solid line,* 5-fluorouracil *(5-FU)* given i.p.; *dash and dotted line,* 5-FU i.p. given 24 h prior to ischemia; *broken line,* 5-FU i.p. given 24 h after ischemia

tumor weight **AT 7/8**
log (mg)

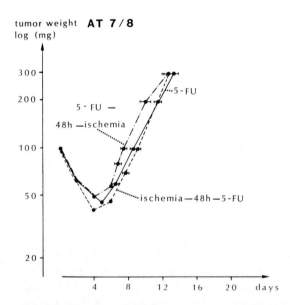

Fig.8. Tumor growth (AT 7/8): *solid line,* 5-fluorouracil *(5-FU)* given i.p.; *dash and dotted line,* 5-FU i.p. given 48 h prior to ischemia; *broken line,* 5-FU i.p. given 48 h after ischemia

Discussion

Even though animals treated by ischemia alone showed tumor growth retardation as compared with the untreated animals, the addition of ischemia after 5-FU is less effective than 5-FU alone. This sequence corresponds to synchronous 5-FU and ischemia application. The tumor is made ischemic at the time of maximum serum levels. At the time of ischemia the ability of the tumor to activate the drug is

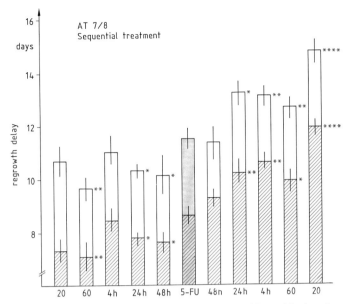

Fig. 9. Tumor regrowth delay (AT 7/8) after sequential treatment in hierarchical order: *hatched,* time to reach pretreatment size; *open,* time to reach twice pretreatment size; $*P<0.05$, $**P<0.01$, $***P<0.001$, $****P<0.0001$, compared with 5-FU i.p. alone

reduced, thus reducing clinical response. Laskin et al. [12] demonstrated that the differences of enzyme activity responsible for the metabolism of 5-FU correlate well with the differences in sensitivity to 5-FU. The longer the period between 5-FU and ischemia, the less pronounced are the differences in our study. In these cases the drug was able to act on a metabolically active cell for a longer period of time. Even though serum half-life of 5-FU is only 10 min, it is known that the active intracellular nucleotides FdUMP and FUTP have prolonged half-lives [2] of several days. The ternary complex formed between FdUMP, thymidilate synthetase, and N 5, N 10-methylentetrahydrofolate has a half-life of about 6 h [1, 17]. When 5-FU is given after 90 min of tumor ischemia, at a time when blood flow has been restored, there is a much longer regrowth delay than after 5-FU alone. Again, the differences were more pronounced, the shorter the time between the end of ischemia and 5-FU treatment. With restoration of tumor blood flow after ischemia, surviving tumor cells show increased metabolic activity. Protein synthesis, RNA and DNA synthesis, and repair mechanisms are enhanced. In a critical review, Tannock [15] showed that tumor sensitivity increases with the proliferation rate of the tumor. We consider this to be the reason for the increased vulnerability of the tumor cells in this phase and for the synergistic effect of the ischemia–5-FU sequence.

Cell protection through ischemia and increased sensitivity after ischemia account for the fact that although the administration of 5-FU in group 4 (5-FU – 20 min – ischemia sequence) and group 9 (ischemia – 20 min – 5-FU-sequence) lie only 130 min apart, group 4 reached pretreatment size after 7.3 ± 0.4 days, whereas the regrowth delay in group 9 was 11.5 ± 0.4 days. As early as 1971 DeVita [19] suggested

"What about altering cell cycles to our advantage? ... by using hormone or variations in nutrient supply, oxygen, or other growth promotors, a change may occur that renders the tumor more susceptible to drugs."

In planning multimodality treatment not only pharmacokinetic data have to be taken into account; tumor biology, cell kinetics, and drug metabolism also have to be considered. In the future, the measurement and monitoring of intracellularly activated metabolites of 5-FU under diverse metabolic conditions will become possible, thus refining and optimizing ways of conditioning tumors prior to antimetabolite treatment.

At present, it seems reasonable to give 5-FU therapy at a time when the tumor is not in a phase of ischemic reduction of metabolic activity. This policy has been followed and emphasized by our group since 1983. For the treatment of hepatic metastases using ischemic tumor damage we developed a method of temporary prolonged peripheral arterial microembolisation with enzymatically degradable starch microspheres [4, 5]. We have recently changed our approach, insofar as we now begin sequential intra-arterial 5-FU treatment as early as 1 h after the end of a 4-h period of transient arterial hepatic occlusion with degradable starch microspheres.

References

1. Chabner BA, Myers CE (1985) Clinical pharmacology of cancer chemotherapy. In: deVita V, Hellman S, Rosenberg SA (eds) Principles and practice of oncology, vol 1, 2nd edn. Lippincott, Philadelphia, pp 287–328
2. Chadwick M, Rogers WJ (1972) The physiological distribution of 5-fluorouracil in mice bearing solid L 1210 lymphocytic leukemia. Cancer Res 32: 1045–1056
3. Chen HSG, Gross JF (1980) Intra-arterial infusion of anticancer drugs: theoretic aspects of drug delivery and review of responses. Cancer Treat Rep 64: 31–40
4. Eibl-Eibesfeldt B, Brunner K, Pfeifer KJ, Schweiberer L, Geissler K (1984) Repeated ischemia and metachron cytostatic therapy in the treatment of liver metastases: a new application of degradable starch microspheres. Conference on therapeutic strategies in primary and metastatic liver cancer, Heidelberg, Sept. 17–19
5. Eibl-Eibesfeldt B, Pfeifer KJ, Wilker D, Hohner E, Bassermann R (1985) Starch microspheres embolisation and metachron cytostatic therapy: a new method of temporary liver dearterialisation. 2nd Int conf on advances in regional cancer therapy, Gießen, p 87 (Abstract)
6. Ensminger WD, Gyves JW (1983) Clinical pharmacology of hepatic arterial chemotherapy. Sem Oncol 10 (2): 176–182
7. Ensminger WD, Rosowsky A, RASO. V (1978) A clinical pharmacological evaluation of hepatic arterial infusion of 5-fluoro-2'-desoxyuridine and 5-fluorouracil. Cancer Res 38: 3784–3792
8. Hansen H (1984) Erste Ergebnisse der Therapie multipler Lebermetastasen durch passagere Leberdearterialisation und intraarterielle Chemotherapie. Langenbecks Arch Chir [Suppl Chir Forum]: 295–298
9. Helmer RE, Morettin LB, Costanzi JJ (1981) Hepatic artery occlusion with perfusion in the treatment of carcinoid syndrome. Oncology 38: 361–364

10. Howell SR (1985) Pharmacokinetic principles of intra-arterial therapy. 2nd Int Conf on advances in regional cancer therapy, Gießen, p 3 (Abstracts)
11. Jones DP (1981) Hypoxia and drug metabolism. Biochem Pharmacol 30: 1019–1023
12. Laskin JD, Evans RM, Slocium HK, Burke D, Hakala MT (1979) Basis for natural variation in sensitivity to 5-fluorouracil in mouse and human cells in culture. Cancer Res 39: 383–390
13. Lindberg B, Lote K, Teder H (1984) Biodegradable starch microspheres – a new medical tool. In: Davis SS, McVie JG, Tomlinson E (eds) Microspheres and drug therapy. Pharmaceutical, immunological and medical aspects. Elsevier, Amsterdam
14. Myers ChE (1981) The pharmacology of the fluoropyrimidines. Pharmacol Rev 33: 1–15
15. Tannock J (1978) Cell kinetics and chemotherapy: a critical review. Cancer Treat Rep 62: 1117–1133
16. Thomlinson RH, Craddock EA (1967) The gross response of an experimental tumor to single doses of X-rays. Br J Cancer 21: 107–123
17. Valeriote F, Santelli G (1984) 5-fluorouracil (FUra). Pharmacol Ther 24: 107–132
18. Wopfner F (1983) Intra-arterial chemotherapy of the liver with transient repeated hypoxia. In: Schwemmle K, Aigner K (eds) Vascular perfusion in cancer therapy. Springer, Berlin Heidelberg New York Tokyo, pp 75–82 (Recent results in cancer research, vol 86)
19. DeVita VT (1971) Cell kinetics and the chemotherapy of cancer. Cancer Chemother Rep 2: 23–33

Systemic Chemotherapy with Cisplatin, 5-Fluorouracil and Allopurinol in the Management of Advanced Epidermoid Esophageal Cancer

P. De Besi, V. Chiarion-Sileni, L. Salvagno, S. Toso, A. Paccagnella, V. Fosser, C. Tremolada, A. Peracchia, and M. V. Fiorentino

Divisione di Oncologia Medica, Ospedale Civile, Unitá Locate Socio Sanitaria N. 21, 35100 Padova, Italy

About 60% of patients with esophageal cancer have an advanced tumor at diagnosis, and for these patients neither surgery nor radiotherapy can offer anything more than palliation. This fact has led, in the past 10 years, to an increase in the number of studies of chemotherapy as a possible alternative treatment.

In 1983 we began a phase-II study to evaluate the effectiveness of a combination of cisplatin and 5-FU on inoperable cancer of the esophagus. Each of these two drugs, used as a single agent, has been seen to produce an objective regression of the tumor in only 15%–25% of the patients, while a combination of the two appeared to be effective in about 80% of cases, appearing to confirm the possible synergistic activity already evidenced by animal data [1, 2]. This combination had already been studied with a large number of head and neck cancer patients, whereas with esophageal cancer patients there had been only a limited experience [3, 4].

Up to April 1986, 54 consecutive patients were entered into the study. Of these, 25 had locally advanced and 29 metastatic disease. Eleven patients had previously been treated with surgery, three with surgery and radiotherapy, one with radiotherapy alone, and one with a different chemotherapy. The median age was 56 (range 37–72), and the Karnofsky performance status was 70 (range 50–90). The patients received a median of three cycles (range 2–6).

The treatment schedule consisted of cisplatin at a dosage of 100 mg/m^2 on day 1 in a 2-h infusion [4]. 5-FU at a dosage of 1000 mg/m^2 per day as a 24-h infusion on days 1–5, and allopurinol at a dosage of 600 mg orally from day -2 to day $+5$. Allopurinol was given in order to reduce myelosuppression and gastrointestinal toxicity [5, 6]. The cycle was repeated on day 22. The response to the treatment was assessed by repeating the staging examinations. Of 49 evaluable patients, 17 (35%) showed an objective response (five complete and 12 partial) and 19 other patients felt a subjective improvement in their swallowing functions. Eight responding patients, after a median of three cycles (range 3–6), underwent an operation; this was radical for five and palliative for two, while for the eighth patient, in spite of the restaging findings, it was only explorative.

Of the seven resected patients, three died at 2, 5, and 13 months, whereas the remaining four are alive and without evidence of disease at 5, 16, 18, and 37 months

Recent Results in Cancer Research, Vol. 110
© Springer-Verlag Berlin · Heidelberg 1988

respectively. The median duration of the response was 9 months (range 2–37 +). The toxicity was generally moderate and in only some cases a median delay of 7 days (range 5–14) was necessary before administration of the subsequent course. Mucositis and liver enzyme changes occurred in some cases and all were reversible.

We observed one toxic death due to a septicemia during the 2nd cycle. Another patient died 36 h after the beginning of the therapy and the autopsy revealed a serious diffuse angiosclerosis which had not been clinically apparent.

In our opinion, such results show the efficacy of the combination of cisplatin and 5-FU, even though we have not been able to confirm the 80% response rate reported in literature [7]. In our previous experience with a combination of cisplatin, bleomycin, and methotrexate administered on an outpatient basis the response rate was lower (26%): there was only one complete response of short duration, and none of the patients with a locally advanced tumor were judged operable after the treatment [8]. Cisplatin and 5-FU combined with each other and with other drugs seem to be very effective, but to date no clinical controlled trials have been made to demonstrate the superiority of the combination over the single drugs [1]. In view of this we have cooperated with the EORTC Gastrointestinal Group in designing a randomized phase-II study of cisplatin and 5-FU versus cisplatin used alone in advanced esophageal cancer: this study is now going on.

References

1. Kelsen D (1984) Chemotherapy of esophageal cancer. Semin Oncol 11: 159–168
2. Schabel EM et al. (1974) Phase-I clinical trial of combined therapy with 5-FU and cisplatin. Cancer 84: 1005–1010
3. Kish J et al. (1984) Cisplatin and 5-FU infusion in patients with recurrent and disseminated epidermoid cancer of the head and neck. Cancer 53: 1814
4. Vogl SE, Zaravinos T, Kaplan BH (1980) Toxicity of *cis*-diamminedichloroplatinum II given in a 2-h outpatient regimen of diuresis and hydration. Cancer 45: 11–15
5. Fox R, Woods RL, Tattersall MHN et al. (1981) Allopurinol modulation of fluorouracil toxicity. Cancer Chemother Pharmacol 5: 151–155
6. Howell SB, Wung WE, Taetle E et al. (1981) Modulation of 5-fluorouracil toxicity by allopurinol in man. Cancer 48: 1281–1289
7. Hellerstein S, Rosen S, Kies M et al. (1983) Cisplatin and 5-FU combined chemotherapy of epidermoid esophageal cancer. Proc American Society of Clinical Oncology, no 2, 127
8. De Besi P, Salvagno L, Endrizzi L et al. (1984) Cisplatin, bleomycin and methotrexate in the treatment of advanced esophageal cancer. Eur J Cancer Clin Oncol 20: 732

Phase-II-Study with EAP (Etoposide, Adriamycin, Cis-Platinum) in Patients with Primary Inoperable Gastric Cancer and Advanced Disease

P. Preusser, H. Wilke, W. Achterrath, U. Fink, P. Neuhaus, J. Meyer, H.-J. Meyer, and J. van de Loo

Chirurgische Klinik und Poliklinik, Westfälische Wilhelms-Universität, Jungeboldtplatz 1, 4400 Münster, FRG

Introduction

In the past approximately 35% of patients with advanced gastric cancer (AJC stage 4) survived 1 year after surgery and only 4% lived 4 years [1]. Most patients died because of local recurrence and/or metastases [2]. Today, advanced gastric cancer seems to respond partly to chemotherapy. Active chemotherapy combinations achieve better results than single-agent chemotherapy [3-7]. A remission rate of approximately 20% can be achieved with 5-fluorouracil [4, 5, 8-10], adriamycin [9, 11, 12], etoposide [13], BCNU [9, 14], and mitomycin C [15, 16].

cis-Platinum induced remission in 20% [3, 17-20] of patients who had failed to respond to previous chemotherapy. Remission rates of 21% were achieved with etoposide in previously untreated patients even though the dose was $\leq 50\%$ of the maximum tolerable dose [13, 21, 22].

cis-Platinum shows a synergistic action with etoposide [23-27] and adriamycin [28, 29] in experimental tumors. There is also a lack of cross-resistance between cis-platinum and adriamycin and between cis-platinum and etoposide [29-31].

Several studies have shown reduced myelotoxicity of cis-platinum [32, 33], adriamycin [34], and cis-platinum/etoposide [35] when split doses of cis-platinum or adriamycin were given on days 1 and 7/8, compared with single application of the same dose.

The recommended dose for phase-II studies with the combination etoposide, adriamycin, cis-platinum (EAP) was evaluated in a pilot study by administering fixed doses of cis-platinum, adriamycin and escalating doses of etoposide; ten remissions in 16 previously untreated patients were achieved [36].

Patients and Methods

Patients

Fifty-two patients with histologically confirmed advanced gastric cancer (defined as primarily inoperable gastric cancer + metastases + measurable disease) have

Table 1. Patients' characteristics

Number	52
Evaluable	44
No. too early to evaluate	8
Age (years)	18–65 (mean 50)
Ratio M/F	36/16
WHO performance status	11/44 WHO 1 (26%)
	33/44 WHO 2 (74%)
Spread of metastases	
Liver ± lymph nodes	45%
Lymph nodes (not regional)	45%
Locally advanced disease (regional lymph nodes + infiltration of other organs)	5%
Bone ± lymph nodes	5%
Two localizations	34%

Table 2. Eligibility criteria

– – –	Histologically proven primary inoperable gastric cancer ± metastasis with measurable disease
– – –	No prior chemo-radio-therapy
– – –	Age ≤ 65 years
– – –	Performance status ≤ WHO 2
– – –	Normal renal, liver, and heart status and bone marrow function
– – –	No CNS metastasis

been included into the study since 1984. Patient characteristics and eligibility criteria are summarized in Tables 1 and 2. All patients had measurable disease according to WHO criteria; 66% had one and 34% had two localizations of metastases.

Staging, Follow-up, and Laboratory Control

Localization and size of tumors and metastases were measured by CT and ultrasound. Bone lesions were measured by scan and roentgenography. The measurable tumor parameters were determined prior to therapy, before every cycle, 4 weeks after the last cycle, and then every 3 months. Complete hemogram, serum creatinine and creatinine clearance, electrolytes, and heart and liver function were determined prior to therapy, prior to every cycle, and 4 weeks after the last cycle. Additionally, complete blood counts and serum creatinine were monitored weekly.

EAP

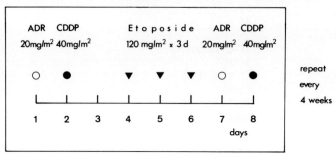

ADR: Adriamycin as short i.v. infusion over 15 min
CDDP: *cis*-Platinum – prehydration 1000 ml 0.9% saline for 2 h, then 125 ml 10% mannitol i.v., *cis*-platinum in 2000 ml 0.9% saline i.v. over 2 h, posthydration 1000 ml 0.9% saline for 1 h. Urine volume under 150 ml/h: 40 mg furosemide i.v.
Etoposide: Etoposide in 500 ml 0.9% saline i.v. over 1.5 h

NOTE! Decrease etoposide to 100 mg/m² × 3 days in patients > 60 years.

Fig. 1. EAP treatment protocol

Therapy

The treatment protocol is given in Fig. 1. EAP was administered in intervals of 22–28 days. After completion of six cycles, therapy was terminated in order to prevent neurotoxicity, which occurs more frequently after a cumulative dose of *cis*-platinum of ≥ 500 mg/m² [37]. One course of EAP had to be administered to evaluate response and toxicity. Response, remission duration, and toxicity were determined according to WHO criteria.

Results

Forty-four patients had an adequate trial and are available for evaluation of response and toxicity; eight patients are too early for evaluation because the first cycle has not yet been finished. Seven (16%) of the patients achieved complete remission and 25 (57%) patients had a partial remission, equalling an overall response rate of 73% (Table 3). Four of the seven complete remissions have been confirmed histologically by second-look surgery. Median observation time is 8 months. Sixteen of the 44 (36%) patients have survived for 3⁺–21⁺ months. Median remission duration is 7 months, median survival time for all patients is 9 months.

Two (10%) of 20 patients with liver ± lymph node metastases responded with complete remission and an additional 11 (55%) of the patients achieved a partial remission. Complete and partial remissions respectively were achieved in three (15%) and 13 (65%) of 20 patients with non-regional lymph node metastases.

Table 3. Results with EAP in gastric cancer (bulky disease) in 44 evaluable patients

	Number	(%)
Complete remission	7[a]	(16)
Complete remission plus partial remission	32	(73)
Median duration of remission (months)	7	
Median survival for all patients (months)	9	

[a] Four of seven complete remissions histologically confirmed by second-look operation.

Table 4. Response according to spread of metastases

Metastases	No. of patients	Complete remission		CR + PR	
		n	(%)	n	(%)
Liver	20	2	(10)	13	(65)
Lymph nodes	20	3	(15)	16	(80)
Locally advanced[a]	2	2	(100)	2	(100)
Bone	2	0		1	(50)
Two localizations	15	0		10	(66)

[a] Regional lymph nodes plus infiltration of other organs.

Table 5. Toxicity (WHO grading n (%))

WHO Grade	0	1	2	3	4
Nausea/vomiting	0	2 (5)	32 (73)	10 (22)	0
Alopecia	0	0	0	44 (100)	0
Serum creatinine	41 (93)	3 (7)	0	0	0
Neurotoxicity	42 (95)	0	2 (5)	0	0
Thrombocytes[a]	14 (32)	14 (32)	6 (13)	7 (16)	2 (5)
Leukocytes	4 (9)	9 (20)	15 (34)	14 (32)	2 (5)

[a] One patient with bone marrow infiltration and thrombocytopenia prior to therapy.

One of two patients with bone metastases ± lymph node metastases responded with a partial remission (Table 4). The mean number of treatment cycles was 4 (1–6). The mean number of treatment cycles until response was 2.

The dose-limiting factor was myelosuppression (Table 5). Leukocytopenia and thrombocytopenia of WHO grade 4 occurred in only 5% of the patients. Median nadir of leukocytes and thrombocytes was $2400/mm^3$ and $92\,500/mm^3$ respectively and occurred between day 11 and day 16. Bone marrow recovery was seen on days 18–26. In Table 5 other signs of toxicity are listed.

Table 6. Results of chemotherapy with 3-drug combinations in advanced gastric cancer

Chemotherapy	No. of studies	No. of patients	CR n (%)	CR+PR n (%)	mR	mS	Reference
					(in months)		
FAMe	2	55	6 (11)	15 (27)	5	6	[39, 40]
FAM	9	358	9 (3)	118 (33)	3–9+	6–9+	[12, 39,
			(0–11)	(17–47)			40–47]
FEM	1	26	0	6 (23)	nm	nm	[59]
FAMTX	4	184	21 (11)	83 (45)	9	6–8	[48–51]
			(0–15)	(0–59)			
FAMTX[a]	1	20	nm	10 (50)	5	nm	[52]
FAP	5	104	5 (5)	43 (41)	4.5–6	10	[7, 53–56]
EAP[b]	1	44	7 (16)	32 (73)	7	9	[28]

nm, not mentioned.
[a] Dose reduction for 5-FU and MTX.
[b] Primary inoperable gastric cancer + metastasis with measurable disease.

Discussion

Only patients with primary inoperable gastric cancer and bulky disease were included in the EAP study. An analysis of randomized studies shows that these patients represent a prognostically unfavorable group [10, 38]. They have a lower response rate and a significantly shorter median survival time as compared with patients with prior surgery [38].

In comparing the results of EAP with the results of FAM [12, 39–47], FAMTX [48–52], FAP [7, 53–56], FAMe [39, 40], and FAB [57, 58], patient selection is the most important factor. These studies included patients with primary inoperable gastric cancer with measurable disease as well as patients who had had prior surgery without measurable disease. EAP induces superior remission rates in prognostically unfavorable patients in comparison with other trials (Table 6). A significant median response duration and survival advantage cannot be stated yet, because the observation time is too short. An analysis of the studies with FAM, FAMe, FAB, FAMTX and FAP shows that the change from mitomycin C to MTX [48–51], *cis*-platinum [7, 53–56], BCNU [57, 58] or MeCCNU [39, 40] did not improve the results.

In view of the results of FAP [7, 53–56] and EAP, it is possible that the change from 5-FU to etoposide may be one reason for the higher response rate. A further reason for the promising results of EAP may be the split course of *cis*-platinum [32, 35]. One of the explanations to be considered concerning the comparable median remission duration and survival time is different patient selection. Finally, we feel that the promising results obtained with EAP should be confirmed in a randomized phase-III study.

References

1. Curtis RE, Kennedy BJ, Myers MH, Hankey BF (1985) Evaluation of AJC stomach cancer staging using the seer population. Semin Oncol 12: 21–31
2. Comis RL (1982) The therapy of stomach cancer. In: Carter SK, Glatstein E, Livingston RB (eds) Principles of cancer treatment. McGraw-Hill, New York, p 420
3. Lacave AJ, Wils J, Diaz-Rubio E, Clavel M, Planting A, Bleiberg H, Duez N, Dalesio O (1985) Phase-II study of cisplatin (cDDP) in chemotherapy-resistant carcinoma of the stomach. Cancer Chemother Pharmacol 14 [Suppl]: 39
4. Cocconi G, DeLisi V, DiBlasio B (1982) Randomized comparison of 5-FU alone or combined with mitomycin and cytarabine (MFC) in the treatment of advanced gastric cancer. Cancer Treat Rep 66: 1263–1266
5. Kolaric K, Potrebica V, Stanovnik M (1986) Controlled phase-III clinical study of 4-epi-doxorubicin + 5-fluorouracil versus 5-fluorouracil alone in metastatic gastric and recto-sigmoid cancer. Oncology 43: 73–77
6. Moertel CG, Mittelman JA, Bakermeier, RF, Engstrom P, Hanely J (1976) Sequential and combination chemotherapy of advanced gastric cancer. Cancer 38: 678
7. Wagener DJTh, Yap SH, Wobbes T, Burghouts JTM, van Dam FE, Hillen HFP, Hoogendoorn GJ, Scheerder H, van der Vegt SGL (1985) Phase-II trial of 5-fluorouracil, adriamycin and cisplatin (FAP) in advanced gastric cancer. Cancer Chemother Pharmacol 15: 86–87
8. Bullen BR, Giles GR, Malhotra A, Bird GG, Hall R, Bunch GA, Brown GJA (1976) Randomized comparison of melphalan and 5-fluorouracil in the treatment of advanced gastrointestinal cancer. Cancer Treat Rep 60: 1267–1271
9. MacDonald JS, Gunderson LL, Cohn I Jr (1982) Cancer of the stomach. In: DeVita VT, Hellman S, Rosenberg SA (eds) Cancer – principles and practice of oncology. Lippincott, Philadelphia, p 534
10. De Lisi V, Cocconi G, Tonato M, Di Costanzo F, Leonardi F, Soldani M (1986) Randomized comparison of 5-FU alone or combined with carmustine, doxorubicin, and mitomycin (BAFMi) in the treatment of advanced gastric cancer: a phase-III trial of the Italian Clinical Research Oncology Group (GOIRC). Cancer Treat Rep 70: 481–485
11. Moertel CG, Lavin PT (1979) Phase II-III chemotherapy studies in advanced gastric cancer. Cancer Treat Rep 63: 1863–1869
12. The Gastrointestinal Tumor Study Group (1979) Phase II-III chemotherapy studies in advanced gastric cancer. Cancer Treat Rep 63: 1871–1876
13. Kelsen DP, Magill G, Cheng E, Coonley C, Yagoda A (1982) Phase-II trial of etoposide (VP16) in the treatment of upper gastrointestinal malignancies. Proc American Society of Clinical Oncology 1, p 96, (Abstract) C-371
14. Moertel CG (1973) Therapy of advanced gastrointestinal cancer with the nitrosoureas. Cancer Chemother Rep 4: 27–34
15. Comis RL (1979) Mitomycin C in gastric cancer. In: Carter SK, Crooke ST (eds) Mitomycin C – current status and new developments. Academic, New York, p 129
16. Schein PS, Macdonald JS, Hoth D, Wooley PV (1978) Mitomycin C: experience in the United States, with emphasis on gastric cancer. Cancer Chemother Pharmacol 1: 73–75
17. Kantarjian H, Ajani JA, Karlin DA (1985) cis-Diamminodichloroplatinum (II) chemotherapy for advanced adenocarcinoma of the upper gastrointestinal tract. Oncology 42: 69–71
18. Beer M, Cocconi G, Ceci G, Varini M, Cavalli F (1983) A phase-II study of cisplatin in advanced gastric cancer. Eur J Cancer Clin Oncol 19: 717–720
19. Aabo K, Pedersen H, Rørth M (1985) Cisplatin in the treatment of advanced gastric carcinoma: a phase-II study. Cancer Treat Rep 69: 449–450
20. Leichman L, MacDonald B, Dindogru A, Samson M (1982) Platinum: a clinically active drug in advanced adenocarcinoma of the stomach. Proc Am Ass Cancer Res 110, Abstract 430

21. Aisner J, van Echo DA, Whitacre M, Wiernik PH (1982) A phase-I trial of continuous-infusion VP-16-213 (Etoposide). Cancer Chemother Pharmacol 7: 157-160

22. Greco FA, Johnson DH, Hande RK, Porter LL, Hainsworth JD, Wolff SN (1985) High-dose etoposide (VP-16) in small-cell lung cancer. Semin Oncol 12 (Suppl 2): 42-44

23. Achterrath W, Niederle N, Hilgard P (1982) Etoposide - chemistry, preclinical and clinical pharmacology. Cancer Treat Rev 9 (Suppl A): 3-13

24. Rose WC, Bradner WT (1984) In vivo experimental antitumor activity of etoposide. In: Issell BF, Muggia FM, Carter SK (eds) Etoposide (VP-16) - current status and new developments. Academic, New York, p 33

25. Mabel JA, Little AD (1979) Therapeutic synergism in murine tumors for combinations of cis-dichlorodiammineplatinum with VP-16-213 or BCNU. Proc Am Ass Cancer Res & Am Soc Clin Oncol no 20, p 230, Abstract 929

26. Schabel FM, Trader MW, Laster WR, Corbett TH, Griswold DP (1979) cis-Diamminedichloroplatinum (II): combination chemotherapy and cross-resistance studies with tumors of mice. Cancer Treat Rep 63: 1459-1473

27. Soloway MS, Masters SB, Murphy WM (1980) Cisplatin analogs and combination chemotherapy in the therapy of murine bladder cancer. In: Prestyako A, Crooke ST, Carter S (eds) Cisplatin - current status and new developments. Academic, New York, p 345

28. Preusser P, Achterrath W, Niederle N, Seeber S (1985) Cisplatin. Arzneimitteltherapie 2: 50-65

29. Schabel FM Jr, Skipper HE, Trader MW, Laster WR Jr, Griswold DP Jr, Corbett TH (1983) Establishment of cross-resistance profiles for new agents. Cancer Treat Rep 42: 905-922

30. Seeber S, Osieka R, Schmidt CG, Achterrath W, Crooke ST (1982) In vivo resistance towards anthracyclines, etoposide, and cis-diamminedichloroplatinum (II). Cancer Res 67: 4719-4725

31. Seeber S (1982) Model studies of etoposide resistance. Cancer Treat Rep 9 [Suppl A]: 15-20

32. Gandara D, Wold H, DeGregorio M, Lawrence HJ, Kohler M, George C (1986) High-dose cisplatin (200 mg/m^2) in non-small-cell lung cancer (NSCLC): reduced toxicity of a modified dose schedule. Proc American Society of Clinical Oncology, no 5, p 173

33. Panettiere FJ, Lehane D, Fletcher WS, Stephens R, Rivkin S, McCracken JD (1980) cis-Platinum therapy of previously treated head and neck cancer: the Southwest Oncology Group's two-dose-per-month outpatient regimen. Med Pediatr Oncol 8: 221-225

34. Creech RH, Catalano RB, Shah MK (1980) An effective low-dose adriamycin regimen as secondary chemotherapy for metastatic breast cancer patients. Cancer 46: 433-437

35. Wilke H, Achterrath W, Gunzer U, Preusser P (in press) Etoposide and split-dose cisplatin (CCDP) in small-cell lung cancer (SCLC) - improved results

36. Preusser P, Wilke H, Neuhaus B, Achterrath W (1986) Pilotstudie mit der Kombination Etoposid, Adriamycin, Cisplatin beim fortgeschrittenen Magenkarzinom. Tumor Diagnostik und Therapie 7: 142-144

37. Wiltshaw E (1983) Chemotherapy of ovarian malignancies at the Royal Marsden Hospital. In: Bender HG, Beck L (eds) Carcinoma of the ovary. Fischer, Stuttgart, p 169

38. O'Connell MJ (1985) Current status of chemotherapy for advanced pancreatic and gastric cancer. J Clin Oncol 3: 1032-1039

39. The Gastrointestinal Tumor Study Group (1984) Randomized study of combination chemotherapy in unresectable gastric cancer. Cancer 53: 13-17

40. Douglass HO Jr, Lavin PT, Goudsmit A, Klaassen DJ, Paul AR (1984) An Eastern Cooperative Oncology Group evaluation of combinations of methyl-CCNU, mitomycin C, adriamycin, and 5-fluorouracil in advanced measurable gastric cancer (EST 2277). J Clin Oncol 2: 1372-1381

41. MacDonald JS, Schein PS, Woolley PV, Smythe T, Ueno W, Hoth D, Smith F, Boiron M, Gisselbrecht C, Brunet R, Lagarde C (1980) 5-Fluorouracil, doxorubicin, and mito-

mycin (FAM) combination - chemotherapy for advanced gastric cancer. Ann Intern Med 93: 533-536

42. Beretta G, Fraschini P, Labianca R, Luporini G (1982) The value of FAM polychemo-therapy in advanced gastric carcinoma. Proc American Society of Clinical Oncology 23, p 103, Abstract C-400

43. Panettiere FJ, Haas Ch, McDonald B, Costanzi JJ, Talley RW, Athens J, Oishi N, Heil-brun LK, Chen TT (1984) Drug combinations in the treatment of gastric adenocarcino-ma: a randomized Southwest Oncology Group study. J Clin Oncol 2: 420-424

44. Oshima K, Yamada T, Nonaka T, Aoyama M, Hirose H, Adachi N, Kobayachi S, Udo K (1982) Treatment of advanced G. I. cancer patients with 5-FU, adriamycin, and mi-tomycin C (FAM). Proc 13th Intern Cancer Congress, Seattle, September 8-15, no 665 (Abstract 3977)

45. Haim N, Cohen Y, Honigman J, Robinson E (1982) Treatment of advanced gastric carci-noma with 5-fluorouracil, adriamycin, and mitomycin C (FAM). Cancer Chemother Pharmacol 8: 277-280

46. Beretta G, Fraschini P, Labianca R, Arnoldi E, Pancera G, Tedeschi M, Tedeschi L, Luporini G (1986) Weekly 5-fluorouracil (F) versus combination chemotherapies for ad-vanced gastrointestinal carcinomas. A prospective study program. Proc American Soci-ety of Clinical Oncology 5, p 94, Abstract 367

47. Haas C, Oishi N, McDonald B, Coltman C, O'Bryan R (1983) Southwest Oncology Group phase II-III gastric cancer study: 5-fluorouracil, adriamycin, and mitomycin-C + vincristine (FAM vs V-FAM) compared to chlorozotocin (CZT), M-AMSA, and di-hydroxyanthracenedione (DHAD) with unimpressive differences. Proc American Soci-ety of Clinical Oncology, no 2, p 122, Abstr C-478

48. Klein HO, Wickramanayake PD, Farrokh G-R (1986) 5-Fluorouracil (5-FU), adriamycin (ADM), and methotrexate (MTX) - a combination protocol (FAMTX) for treatment of metastasized stomach cancer. Proc American Society of Clinical Oncology, no 5, p 84, Abstract 325

49. Wils J, Bleiberg H, Blijham G, Breed W, Diaz-Rubio E, Mulder N, Neijt J, Planting A. Splinter T, van Toorn W, Duez N, Dalesio O (1986) An EORTC Gastrointestinal (GI) Group phase-II evaluation of sequential high-dose methotrexate (MTX) and 5-fluoro-uracil (F) combined with adriamycin (A) (FAMTX) in advanced gastric cancer. Proc American Society of Clinical Oncology, no 78, Abstract 302

50. Cunningham D, Gilchrist NL, Forrest GJ, Soukop M, McArdle CS, Carter DC (1985) Chemotherapy in advanced gastric cancer. Cancer Treat Rep 69: 927-928

51. Herrmann R, Heim M, Ho AD, Fritze D, Queißer W, Schlag P (1984) Methotrexate (M), 5-fluorouracil (F) and adriamycin (A) in metastatic or locally advanced gastric cancer. J Cancer Res Clin Oncol 107 [Suppl]: 53

52. Scherdin G, Garbrecht M, Müllerleile U, Hossfeld DK (1986) Polychemotherapy with methotrexate in medium dosage range, 5-fluorouracil and adriamycin in advanced gas-tric carcinoma. J Cancer Res Clin Oncol 111 [Suppl]: 85

53. Rougier P, Droz JP, Amiel JL, Ruffier P, Theodore C, Kac J, Chavy A (1985) Gastric car-cinoma: a phase-II trial of chemotherapy with association 5-fluorouracil (5-FU), adri-amycin (ADR) and cis-platinum (cDDP) (FAP protocol) in metastasized or inoperable patients. Preliminary results. Cancer Chemother Pharmacol 14 [Suppl]: 54

54. Moertel C, Fleming T, O'Connell M, Schutt A, Rubin J (1984) A phase-II trial of com-bined intensive course 5-FU, adriamycin and cis-platinum in advanced gastric and pan-creatic carcinoma. Proc American Society of Clinical Oncology, no 137, Abstract C-535

55. Figoli F, Galligioni E, Crivellari D, Vaccher E, Lo Re G, Tumolo S, Veronesi A, Frustaci S, Canale V, Monfardini S (1986) Cisplatin (DDP) in combination with adriamycin (A) and fluorouracil (F) (DAF) in advanced gastric cancer - a phase-II study. Proc Ameri-can Society of Clinical Oncology, no 95, (Abstract 369)

56. Wooley P, Smith F, Estevez R, Gisselbrecht C, Alvarez C, Boiron M, Machado C, Lagarde C, Schein P (1981) A phase-II trial of 5-FU, adriamycin and cisplatin (FAP) in

206   P. Preusser et al.

advanced gastric cancer. Proc American Association for Cancer Research and of the American Society of Clinical Oncology, no 22, p 455, Abstract C-481

57. Schnitzler G, Queißer W, Heim ME, König H, Katz R, Fritze D, Herrmann R, Arnold H, Henss H, Trux FA, Bloch R, Keymling M, Wolkewitz KD, Fritsch H, Hanisch I, Brumen L, Edler L (1986) Phase-III study of 5-FU and carmustine versus 5-FU, carmustine, and doxorubicin in advanced gastric cancer. Cancer Treat Rep 70: 477–479

58. Levi JA, Dalley DN, Aroney RS (1979) Improved combination chemotherapy in advanced gastric cancer. Br Med J 2: 1471–1473

59. Queißer W, Flechtner H, Heim ME, Henß H, Arnold H, Fritze D, Herrmann R, Fritsch H, Penzkofer F, Trux FA, Kabelitz K, Edler L (1986) 5-Fluorouracil, 4-epidoxorubicin, and mitomycin C (FEM) for advanced gastric carcinoma. A phase-II trial. J Cancer Res Clin Oncol 111 [Suppl]: 85

60. Miller AB, Hoogstraaten B, Staquet M, Winkler A (1981) Reporting results of cancer treatment. Cancer 47: 207–214

Background for and Progress of an Ongoing EORTC Phase-II Study in Metastatic Gastric Cancer

G. H. Blijham

Interne Geneeskunde, Academisch Ziekenhuis Maastricht, Postbus 1918, 6201 BX Maastricht, The Netherlands

This paper presents old and published data on the chemotherapy of advanced and metastatic gastric cancer in a somewhat unusual format in order to put response rates in this disease in the context of their impact on survival and to provide a justification for our decision to perform uncontrolled phase-II studies in untreated patients with this disease. It also briefly presents the rationale and outline of the ongoing EORTC gastric cancer trial with sequential methotrexate (MTX) and 5-fluorouracil (5-FU); only some very general progress data are discussed.

In gastric cancer, 5-FU as a single agent has shown very moderate activity, with no indications that this drug alters the natural history of the disease. Therefore, other drugs have been added to 5-FU, resulting in regimes such as FA(driamycin)M(itomycin-C), FA-nitrosurea and FAM-nitrosurea [1]. Results of uncontrolled phase-II-type studies with these regimens are summarized in Table 1. Response rates appear superior to those with 5-FU alone and, as was stressed in many of these reports, responders lived considerably longer. Such results, of course, can be regarded only as promising; patient selection may play a part in the higher response rates, and it is now generally recognized that making deductions from survival curves of responding compared with non-responding patients may be very misleading [2].

Therefore, large-scale phase-III trials with similar regimens were undertaken, and the cumulative response rates are summarized in Table 2. Response rates were generally lower than those observed in phase-II trials, and with very few exceptions no particular regimen consistently improved survival. In fact, in one of the latest trials survival curves for 5-FU and FAM appeared to be very similar, summarizing 10 years of phase-III testing as being essentially negative.

In general, phase-III trials are undertaken on the basis of results from non-randomized phase-II or pilot studies. These results should be considered promising enough to make superiority over standard or no treatment likely or at least possible. The experience in gastric cancer shows that such evaluations are difficult and, in effect, have been poor. How can this be improved, so that overextended expectations are prevented and negative phase-III trials with a waste of patients and resources avoided? To address this issue, we asked how, in these trials, response rates relate to the survival of the patients treated. Ten large randomized trials with

Table 1. Non-randomized trials in gastric cancer with combinations of 5-fluorouracil, adriamycin, mitomycin C, and/or nitrosureas

	Median response rate (range)	Median survival time (range)
FAM[a]	43% (8–55)	6 months (6–10)
FA-BCNU[b]	51%	10 months
FAM-nitrosurea[c]	27% (26–34)	7 months (3–7)

[a] Five trials, 175 patients.
[b] One trial, 35 patients.
[c] Three trials, 76 patients.

Table 2. Randomized trials in gastric cancer with combination of 5-fluorouracil, adriamycin, mitomycin C, and/or nitrosureas

	Median response rate (range)	Median survival time (range)
FAM[a]	25% (17–38)	7 months (6–8)
FA-nitrosurea[b]	28% (17–47)	7 months (6–8)

[a] Five trial arms, 116 for response evaluable patients.
[b] Five trial arms, 104 for response evaluable patients.

a total of 30 treatment arms from cooperative groups were used for this analysis. With two exceptions (AMSA and mitoxantrone) the drugs used were 5-FU, adriamycin, mitomycin C, nitrosureas, and two or three combinations thereof. We plotted, for each treatment arm within each trial, response rate versus median survival time, as depicted in Fig. 1. We then calculated the best-fitting line in order to answer two questions: Is there a significant relationship between response rate and survival obtained in this disease and with these treatments, and if so, how is this relationship quantitatively? The answers can be formulated as follows: the relation between response rate and survival is rather poor ($r = 0.564$) though statistically significant ($P < 0.001$); the slope of the regression line is very flat (0.045), so that if the response rate rises from, for instance, 5% to 30%, median survival time increases only from 5 to 6 months.

The same response-survival (R/S) curve was constructed for nine non-randomized studies using combinations of the same three or four drugs, as shown in Fig. 2. The response rates in these trials tend to be higher and median survival times only a little longer.

The curve is virtually identical to that in Fig. 1 but with an extension to the right. This strongly suggests that non-randomized studies describe the same phenomena, but include mainly patients who belong to the "better" side of those enrolled in randomized trials. It is of interest to note that the EORTC study with FAMTX, which is not represented in these curves, projects exactly on the line with a 35% response rate and 6 months' median survival time; it fits nicely between the results of the various FAM trials.

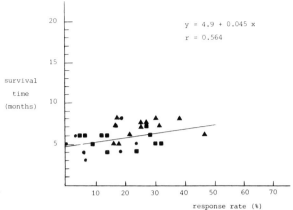

Fig. 1. Correlation of survival time to response rate in ten randomized trials

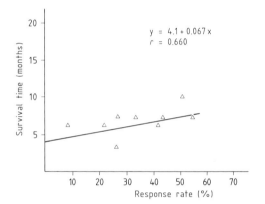

Fig. 2. Correlation of survival time to response rate in nine non-randomized studies

From this type of analysis it appears that in gastric cancer median survival and response rate each have, to a considerable extent, their own variability which can be explained by factors such as patient selection and response criteria. In as much as the variability in survival is not explained by treatment-independent factors, chemotherapy-induced responses are of such poor quality that median survival is only minimally improved. From these data it becomes apparent that the chances to obtain survival differences of any significance or magnitude by comparing chemotherapeutic regimens each with response rates lower than 50% – say 20% versus 40% – should be considered to be very small.

Unless response rates clearly exceeding 50% or a response-survival association clearly not fitting into this response-survival curve are obtained, gastric cancer can best be studied by developing and testing new drugs or regimens in a standard phase-II setting.

With regard to the phase-II study we started in 1985, during the past 10 years several approaches have been developed and tested in an attempt to increase the efficacy of 5-FU by interfering with its metabolism [3]. Modulation of the activity of 5-FU may involve several things: increased incorporation into RNA, increased binding to the target enzyme thymidilate synthetase (TS), changes in the catabolism of the drug, and possibly increased incorporation into DNA. MTX had been shown to increase the cytotoxicity of 5-FU in several in vitro tumor systems, possibly by increasing PRPP levels and/or by improving the binding of 5-FU to TS. In colorectal cancer cell lines as well as patients it has been suggested that this synergy occurs only with MTX/5-FU intervals exceeding 3 h. Kemeny and co-workers [4] compiled data from a number of trials with a less than 3-h or a more than 3-h interval between the drugs. With the short interval, a cumulative response rate comparable to that with 5-FU alone was obtained. Intervals exceeding 3 h were more promising, with response rates of around 30%. We decided to perform an MTX/FU-5 study in gastric cancer using the schedule employed by Herrmann et al. [5] in colorectal cancer. This schedule, apart from having a response rate exceeding 30%, appeared to be associated with a very low toxicity. Therefore, if it could be shown to be effective in gastric cancer, this combination would be an attractive one to build upon with other active drugs.

With this rationale, a phase-II trial was initiated; the protocol is depicted in Table 3. The precautions to be taken include the maintenance of an adequate urinary output and urinary pH. As indicated by the timetable, the schedule can be used for outpatients, which is important since it is given every 2 weeks.

As of May 1986, 23 patients had been entered. It is of course too early to show data regarding response rates and quality of response, but there have been two patients with major toxicity. Both experienced severe neutropenic septicemia despite leucovorin rescue according to the protocol. One patient had pleural fluid which was evacuated before treatment. Both patients appeared to have minor ascites detected by echography, which may very well have contributed to delayed clearance of MTX and associated toxicity as shown by MTX levels in one patient. Gastric cancer is a disease in which clinically unsuspected ascites may well be present; therefore, even this only moderately high dose of MTX may be associated with unexpected toxicity. Patients with effusions are excluded from the protocol except when the effusion can be evacuated, MTX levels can be determined, and the rescue will be adjusted to these levels. The results of this phase-II study are expected to be available in the fall of 1987.

Table 3. Protocol GI 40854: sequential MTX and 5-FU in locally advanced and metastatic gastric cancer

8:00–10:00	NaHCO$_3$ 1.4% 500 ml
10:00–10:15	MTX 150 mg/m$_2$ 100 ml 0.9% NaCl
10:15–14:15	MTX 150 mg/m$_2$ 500 ml 0.9% NaCl
14:15–17:00	0.9% NaCl 1000 ml
17:00–17:15	5-FU 900 mg/m^2 in 250 ml dextrose

Plus: NaHCO$_3$ 1 g p.o. × 4
     minimally 500 ml fluids p.o.
     diuresis ⩾ 2500 ml
     pH urine ⩾ 7.0

References

1. O'Connell MJ (1985) Current status of chemotherapy for advanced pancreatic and gastric cancer. J Clin Oncol 3: 1032–1039
2. Anderson JR, Chain KC, Gelber RD (1983) Analysis of survival by tumor response. J Clin Oncol 1: 710–713
3. Shilsky RL, Jolivet J, Chabner BA (1981) Antimetabolites. In: Pinedo HM (ed) Cancer chemotherapy. Excerpta Medica, Amsterdam, pp 8–14
4. Kemeny NE, Ahmed T, Michaelson RA, Harper HD et al. (1984) Activity of sequential low-dose methotrexate and fluorouracil in advanced colorectal carcinoma: attempt at correlation with tissue and blood levels of phosphoribosylpyrophosphate. J Clin Oncol 2: 311–315
5. Herrmann R, Spehn J, Beyer JH et al. (1984) Sequential methotrexate and 5-fluorouracil: improved response rate in metastatic colorectal cancer. J Clin Oncol 2: 591–594

5-Fluorouracil Versus a Combination of BCNU, Adriamycin, 5-FU and Mitomycin C in Advanced Gastric Cancer: A Prospective Randomized Study of the Italian Clinical Research Oncology Group

V. De Lisi[1], G. Cocconi[1], M. Tonato[2], F. Di Costanzo[3], F. Leonardi[1], and M. Soldani[2]

[1] Medical Oncology Service, University Hospital, Via Gramsci 14, 43100 Parma, Italy
[2] Medical Oncology Division, University Hospital, Perugia 26100, Italy
[3] Oncology Service, Terni 05100, Italy

Introduction

In the past 10 years, the superiority of combination chemotherapy over single-drug treatment has been proven with several solid tumors. This possibility is still questionable in advanced gastric carcinoma, where no combination of multiple agents has succeeded in demonstrating superiority in response rate over 5-FU alone, which continues to be used as the standard treatment [1-3]. A significant survival advantage using 5-FU plus BCNU compared with 5-FU alone was reported in a study from the Mayo Clinic [4].

More recently, combinations containing two or three agents, especially those including adriamycin, have seemed to yield better results than any single agent. In particular, the combination of 5-FU, adriamycin, and mitomycin (FAM), has been extensively tested in advanced disease with consistently good results [5]. Recently, however, the high level of activity of FAM, as far as response rate and overall survival are concerned, has been called into question by the results of a prospective randomized study [1]. On the other hand, the combination of BCNU, adriamycin, 5-FU, and mitomycin (BAFMi) has been reported to yield a 50% response rate in a rather low number of patients [6]. The purpose of the present multi-institutional prospective randomized study is to compare the efficacy of 5-FU alone with that of the BAFMi combination in advanced gastric carcinoma.

Materials and Methods

Patient Characteristics

Between October 1979 and December 1983, 85 consecutive patients with histologically proven gastric carcinoma were entered in this study from five participating institutions. All patients had either advanced disease beyond the possibility of a surgical excision or a recurrence following primary surgical treatment. At least one measurable or evaluable parameter of disease, evidenced either directly or by instrumental examination, was required. Patients with an expected survival of

Table 1. Clinical characteristics of patients in the study

Characteristics	Number of patients	
	5-FU	BAFMi
Evaluable patients	41	41
Median age (years)	66	63
range	35–73	39–74
Sex		
Male	30	31
Female	11	10
Age		
<60	16	17
>60	25	24
Performance status (Karnofsky index)		
100–80	32	31
70–50	9	10
Prior surgery		
Resection	19	21
No resection	22	20

<1 month, with other tumors, with brain metastases, or who had been previously treated with radiation therapy and/or chemotherapy were excluded. Laboratory requirements at the start of treatment were bilirubin <1.5 mg%, creatinine <1.5 mg%, wbc >4000 mm^3, platelets >100000 mm^3. The characteristics of the 82 evaluable patients are reported in Table 1. As can be seen, treatment allocation appears to have been well balanced between the two arms. Overall, 74% of the patients were male, median age was 64 (range 35–74), and 60% were over 60 years of age; 49% had the primary tumor resected, 12% of the total group were totally asymptomatic, and another 61% were fully ambulatory with minor symptoms.

Treatment was assigned by a centralized randomization and was performed in the participating institutions.

Treatment Procedure

Patients were randomized between the two arms of treatment, 5-FU or BAFMi. They were stratified according to sex, age (< or >60 years), prior surgery (resection of primary tumor or not), and Karnofsky performance status (100–80 vs 70–50).

Drugs were given i.v. according to the following doses and schedules: Arm A – 5-FU, 13.5 mg/kg/day by bolus injection for 5 consecutive days, every 5 weeks; Arm B – BCNU 50 mg/m^2, days 1 and 29; adriamycin 25 mg/m^2, days 1, 8, 29, 36; 5-FU 400 mg/m^2, days 1, 8, 15, 29, 36; mitomycin 10 mg/m^2, day 15. This course was repeated every 9 weeks. Table 2 shows the dosages and schedule of the BAFMi combination.

Table 2. BAFMi combination, course repeated every 9 weeks

Drugs		Days					
		1	8	15	22	29	36
BCNU	50 mg/m^2	×				×	
Adriamycin	25 mg/m^2	×	×			×	×
5-FU	400 mg/m^2	×	×	×		×	×
Mitomycin	10 mg/m^2			×			

There was not an escalation plan in the protocol to increase doses of chemotherapy in patients who did not show myelosuppression. The following dose attenuation schedule for bone marrow depression was used in both arms: 100% of the dose for patients with wbc count > 4000/mm^3 and platelet count $> 100\,000$/mm^3; 50% for wbc count between 3999 and 2500/mm^3 and/or platelet count between 99\,999 and 75\,000/mm^3; suspension of treatment for wbc count < 2500/mm^3 and/or platelet count $< 75\,000$/mm^3. Adriamycin dosage was decreased by 50% for bilirubin > 1.5 mg% and/or for bromosulfthalein (BSF) retention > 9% after 45 min and by 25% for bilirubin > 3 mg% and/or for BSF retention > 15%. Hemoglobin measurements and wbc and platelet counts were performed before each dose, except on days 2–5 of the 5-FU arm.

Patients with progressive disease after two complete cycles of 5-FU received the FAM regimen in order to ensure the best possible evaluation of survival data. Patients with progressive disease after one complete cycle of BAFMi were taken off the study.

Assessment of Response

At the time of entry in the study, a clinical examination was performed to measure and record any assessable tumor parameters. Abdominal masses and liver edges that were palpable under the costal margin were measured in centimeters, and a map was drawn outlining the assessable tumor. At the same time, each patient had a routine biochemical examination, a liver scan and/or echotomographic examination and, if primary or recurrent tumor was present in the stomach, upper gastrointestinal roentgenography. Endoscopic examination was mandatory if tumor in the stomach was the only assessable parameter.

WHO criteria were used to evaluate side effects and response [7].

Direct clinical examination was performed every month to assess therapeutic effects and to record toxicity. Liver and renal function tests were periodically repeated. Radiographic, endoscopic, and radioisotopic investigations were repeated after 9 weeks to assess clinical response. If the indicator lesion was primary or a recurrent tumor in the stomach, evaluation of response required a repeated endoscopic examination, unless contrast radiography clearly showed PD.

Duration of response was calculated from the beginning of treatment until objective proof of tumor progression was obtained. Survival was calculated from the beginning of treatment until death.

Statistical comparison of responses between the two treatments was performed by the chi-square method. Duration of response and survival was evaluated by the Kaplan and Meier method [8]. Differences between distributions were determined using the Cox-Mantel test [9].

Results

Therapeutic Results

Three of the 85 patients entered in the study were considered to be non-evaluable for therapeutic response, two (one on 5-FU and one of BAFMi) because of disease-related early death 4 weeks after the initiation of chemotherapy and one (on 5-FU) because of loss to clinical controls after one cycle of treatment, before the first assessment of response was performed. A total of 41 patients who received 5-FU and 41 who received BAFMi were evaluable. The types of responses observed are summarized in Table 3. In the 5-FU arm, six of 41 patients achieved an objective remission (15%): there were one CR and five PR. The complete disappearance of assessable tumor was observed in one patient with cytologically proven left supraclavicular metastatic nodes as the only indicator lesion, and PR was noted in two patients with unresectable gastric tumor mass, in two with liver metastases, and in one patient with an abdominal mass. In the BAFMi arm, nine of 41 patients achieved an objective remission (22%); there were two CR and seven PR. The complete disappearance of lesions previously assessable by CAT was observed in one patient with abdominal mass and in another with liver and intra-abdominal metastases. The seven patients who achieved PR had objectively reduced liver metastases in three cases, significant endoscopic improvement of primary tumor and regression of liver metastases in one case, significant endoscopic im-

Table 3. Objective Responses

	Number of patients (%)	
	5-FU (41)[a]	BAFMi (41)[a]
CR	1 (3%) (15%)[b]	2 (5%) (22%)[b]
PR	5 (12%)	7 (17%)
SD	18	17
PD	17	15
Median time to progression (weeks)	14	14
Range	4–106+	4–88+
Median duration of response (weeks)	31[b]	40[b]
Range	18–106+	16–88+
Median duration of survival (weeks)	28[b]	24[b]
Range	4–180+	2–151+

[a] Forty-three patients on 5-FU and 42 on BAFMi were considered in the calculation of survival.

[b] $P > 0.05$.

provement of primary tumor in one case, and regression of assessable metastatic nodes in one case.

The difference in response rate between 5-FU (15%) and BAFMi (22%) was not statistically significant ($P = 0.6$).

The possible influence of several factors on therapeutic response was analyzed overall. The objective remission rate was similar in 63 patients with a 100–80 Karnofsky index (18%) as in 19 patients with a 70–50 index (20%). The difference in the response rate of 61 men (15%) and 21 women (29%) was not statistically significant.

Forty patients with prior surgery showed a higher objective remission rate (27%) than 42 patients with no prior surgeryy (9%) ($P = 0.06$). The observed difference in objective remission rate related to prior surgery was approximately the same in the 5-FU (resected 21%, non-resected 9%) and the BAFMi arm (33% vs 10%). Ten and seven patients on 5-FU and BAFMi respectively had only non-measurable disease parameters. In these cases, objective remission was observed in two of the ten and one of the seven. Conversely, objective remission in patients having measurable disease site was observed for four of 31 on 5-FU (13%) and eight of 34 on BAFMi (23%).

Median duration of response was 31 weeks (range 18–106+) on 5-FU and 40 weeks (range 16–88+) on BAFMi ($P = 0.74$). Median time to progression was identical, 14 weeks in both arms ($P = 0.96$). Survival was calculated for all the 85 patients who had been randomized. The median duration was 28 weeks (range 4–180+) for those on 5-FU and 24 weeks (range 2–151+) for those on BAFMi. This difference was not statistically significant ($P = 0.84$).

Toxic Effects

Non-hematologic side effects were mild to moderate in both arms. Nausea, rarely with vomiting, was present in all patients. There were no episodes of clinically significant mucositis. Alopecia was observed in all patients treated with the BAFMi regimen.

Cardiotoxicity associated with adriamycin was never observed; however, no patient received a cumulative dose of adriamycin in excess of 400 mg/m².

Analysis of hematologic toxicity showed that it was more frequent and severe with the BAFMi regimen (Table 4). While dosage reductions were rather frequent, episodes of transient suspension of treatment were rare. Leukopenia with transient reversible sepsis was observed in one case treated with 5-FU. Treatment on both arms was, on the whole, well accepted by patients and the average percent of optimal dose was 93% on 5-FU and 82% on the BAFMi arm.

Discussion

The present study showed that BAFMi induces a response rate (22%) only slightly superior to that observed using 5-FU alone (15%). The increase is so small that any statistical significance is lacking, and the response rate observed with BAFMi

Table 4. Hematologic toxicity

	5-FU (n=41) %	BAFMi (n=41) %
Leukopenia ($\times 100$)		
3.9– 3.0	17	31
2.9– 2.0	2	24
1.9– 1.0	5	2
<1.0	2	–
Thrombocytopenia ($\times 100$)		
99.0–75.0	–	17
74.0–50.0	5	17
49.0–25.0	2	7
<25.0	–	–

is absolutely on the same order as that usually reported using 5-FU alone. In addition, no difference between 5-FU and the combination was shown as regards median duration of response, median time to progression, and median duration of survival.

In the BAFMi combination, BCNU is added to the three-drug FAM combination. Considering the drugs which are present in both combinations, the doses calculated for two cycles were somewhat different, with more adriamycin ($+25\%$) and less 5-FU (-25%) on BAFMi than on FAM; even the schedule of drugs in BAFMi was slightly modified (Table 2) in comparison with that used in the FAM combination.

The activity of FAM is presently a generally accepted indication of the superiority of combination chemotherapy over single-agent activity in gastric carcinoma. However, initially high response rates using this combination were not confirmed in a subsequent study [10], and the only prospective randomized comparison of FAM with 5-FU failed to show any significant advantage as far as response rate and survival were concerned [1].

Considering the absolute value of response rates in gastric carcinoma, it would be useful to discuss the possible explanations for very high differences reported using the same single drug or the same or relatively similar combinations. One of the reasons to be considered is whether there was prior resection of primary tumor. In fact, in our series, 11 of 15 objective remissions were observed in previously resected patients and median survival was statistically superior in this group (36 vs 22 weeks; $P<0.05$).

Altogether, our report strongly indicates that any good result obtained with combination chemotherapy in gastric carcinoma should be controlled by a direct phase-III comparison with 5-FU alone.

References

1. Cullinan S, Moertel CG, Thomas MD, Fleming R, Rubin J, Krook JE, Everson LK, Windschite HE, Twito DI, Marschre RF, Foley JF, Pfeifle DM, Barlow JF (1985) Comparison of three chemotherapeutic regimens in the treatment of advanced pancreatic and gastric carcinoma. JAMA 253: 2061–2067
2. Cocconi G, De Lisi V, Di Blasio B (1982) Randomized comparison of 5-FU alone or combined with mitomycin and cytarabine (MFC) in the treatment of advanced gastric cancer. Cancer Treat Rep 66: 1263–1266
3. Moertel CG, Engstrom P, Lavin PT, Gelber RD, Carbone PP (1979) Chemotherapy of gastric and pancreatic carcinoma. A controlled evaluation of combination of 5-fluorouracil with nitrosoureas and "lactones". Surgery 85: 509–513
4. Kovach JS, Moertel CG, Shutt AJ, Hahn RG, Reitemeier RJ (1974) A controlled study of 1,3- bis (2-chloro-ethyl)-1-nitrosourea and 5-fluorouracil for advanced gastric cancer and pancreatic cancer. Cancer 33: 563–567
5. MacDonald JS, Schein PS, Woolley PV, Smythe T, Ueno W, Hoth D, Smith F, Boiron M, Gisselbrecht C, Brunet R, Lagarde C (1980) 5-Fluorouracil, doxorubicin, mitomycin C (FAM) combination chemotherapy for advanced gastric cancer. Ann Intern Med 93: 533–536
6. Bernath AM, Thornsvard CT (1979) Treatment of advanced gastric carcinoma with BCNU, adriamycin, 5-FU and mitomycin C (BAFMi). Proc American Society of Clinical Oncology, no 20, p 312
7. Miller AB, Hoogstaten B, Staquet M, Winkler A (1981) Reporting results of cancer treatment. Cancer 47: 207–214
8. Kaplan EL, Meier P (1958) Nonparametric estimation from incomplete observations. J Am Stat Assoc 53: 457–481
9. Gehan EA (1976) Statistical methods for survival-time studies. In: Staguet MJ (ed) Cancertherapy: prognostic factors and criteria of response. Raven, New York, pp 7–35
10. Haim N, Cohen Y, Honigman J, Robinson E (1982) Treatment of advanced gastric carcinoma with 5-fluorouracil, adriamycin, and mitomycin C (FAM). Cancer Chemother Pharmacol 8: 277–280

5-Methyltetrahydrofolic Acid (MFH4): An Effective Folate for the Treatment of Advanced Colorectal Cancer with 5-FU

P. La Ciura, G. La Grotta, E. Nigra, A. Comandone, G. Grecchi, G. Leria, and A. Calciati

Division of Oncology, Ospedale San Giovanni, Via Cavour 31, Torino, Italy

The standard chemotherapeutic agent for the treatment of advanced colorectal cancer is fluorouracil (5-FU). Yet the overall response rate to this drug has remained at 20%, and its use has not significantly improved the survival of patients with large-bowel cancer [1].

The mechanism of action of 5-FU is believed to be the competitive inhibition of thymidylate synthetase by the 5-FU metabolite, 5-fluoro-2'-deoxyuridine-5'-monophosphate (FdUMP), forming a ternary complex with the enzyme and a reduced folate (5-10-methylene tetrahydrofolic acid) [2, 3]. Several studies in vitro [3, 4] and in vivo [5] have shown that the administration of folates (5-d,l formyltetrahydrofolic acid) markedly increases the effectiveness of 5-FU [10–16].

Not clear is the action of 5-methyltetrahydrofolic acid (MFH4), one of the most important compounds in the pool of folates. In an attempt to confirm the effectiveness of this folate, we initiated a trial for patients with advanced colorectal cancer, using 5-FU with MFH4.

Materials and Methods

Fifty-one patients with metastatic colorectal adenocarcinoma and measurable disease were entered into this study from February 1983 to July 1985.

Patient Eligibility

Patients with histologically proven adenocarcinoma and demonstrated metastases before the treatment were included. Also required were a Karnofsky performance status of 40%, adequate bone marrow, hepatic, and renal functions determined according to the following laboratory criteria: WBC count $\geq 4000/mm^3$, platelet count $\geq 100000/mm^3$, serum creatinine ≤ 1.5, serum bilirubin ≤ 2, SGOT $\leq$ 60 I.U./dl; no second tumor; expected survival of at least 2 months; informed consent.

Recent Results in Cancer Research, Vol. 110
© Springer-Verlag Berlin · Heidelberg 1988

The pretreatment evaluation included complete history and physical examination, chest roentgenogram, abdominal sonogram and CT scan, colonoscopy, bone scan, CBC, biochemical screening profile, CEA, and ECG. This evaluation was repeated every 3 months for follow-up.

Drug Therapy

5-d,l Methyltetrahydrofolic acid (Bio Research, Milan) was given at 100 mg/m^2 in 100 ml of isotonic solution in perfusion over 10 min (light proof), 5-FU 500 mg/m^2 in 250 ml isotonic solution in perfusion over 30 min, 50 min after 5-MFH4, days 1-5, every 3 weeks.

Treatment was continued until progression of disease was noted, but in the case of complete remission the chemotherapy was maintained for two more cycles.

CBC was measured 1 or 2 days before each treatment, and for ten patients every week to determine the nadir. If the WBC count was 2000-3000 and/or the platelet count was 50000-100000/mm^3, the 5-FU dose was reduced by 25%. If the WBC count was 2000/mm^3 or the platelet count was 50000/mm^3, treatment was delayed for at least 1 week or until the blood cell count had recovered. If the creatinine rose to 1.5 mg/dl no therapy was administered until the cause had been adequately evaluated.

Response was quantitatively determined by the comparison of objectively measurable lesions and was categorized as follows: Complete remission (CR), defined as disappearance of all clinical evidence of active tumor for a minimum of 4 weeks; partial remission (PR), defined as reduction in the sum of the products of the longest perpendicular diameters of all measurable lesions by at least 50%, in the absence of any new site of malignancy (patients with massive liver metastases were required to have a 30% reduction in the sum of measurements below the costal margin, always for a minimum of 4 weeks); no change (NC), defined as tumor regression <50% or stable disease for at least 3 months; progressive disease (PD) defined as the appearance of any new lesion and/or an estimated increase of 25% or more in existing lesions.

Survival curves and response duration were evaluated by the method of Kaplan and Meier. Survival times and time to disease progression were calculated from the onset of therapy. Patients were considered adequately treated if they received three cycles of therapy.

Results

Fifty-one patients were originally entered into the study. Six patients had major protocol violations and were excluded from analysis.

Forty-five patients (29 men and 16 women) were eligible for evaluation. The median age was 57 years (range 31-73).

Five patients had received prior radiotherapy to sites other than those being evaluated for response and ten patients had received prior chemotherapy with 5-FU.

Table 1. Patients' characteristics

Characteristic	Patients (n)
Total	45
Male/female	29/16
Median age, yrs. (range)	57 (31–73)
Median Karnofsky PS (range)	70 (50–90)
Site of primary	
Sigmoid	22
Colon	11
Rectum	12
Metastases	
Liver ⎫	17
Pelvis ⎬ only one site	6
Lung ⎭	3
More than one site	19
Previous treatment	
None	3
Surgery: radical	38[a]
palliative	4
Surgery/radiotherapy	5
Chemotherapy with 5-FU	10

[a] Surgery: Miles, 9; Hartmann, 3; left colectomy, 26; palliative or derivative, 4.

Table 2. Results of treatment

	No. of patients with				
	CR	PR	CR + PR (%)	SD (%)	PD (%)
Previous chemotherapy	1	4	5	3	2
No previous chemotherapy	2	9	11	15	9
	3	13	16 (35.5)	18 (40)	11 (24.4)

Twenty-six patients had only one metastatic site while 19 had metastases at more than one site. The liver was the most common site of metastatic disease. Patients' characteristics are presented in Table 1.

The overall response rate was 35.5%, with three CR and 13 PR (Table 2).

Of the 35 patients who had not been previously treated with 5-FU, two obtained CR and nine PR, with a response rate of 31.4% in this subgroup. Among the ten patients who had been previously treated with 5-FU, one achieved CR and four PR. Eighteen patients had no significant change in their tumor measurements; the remaining 11 patients showed progressive disease. Median survival time for the 16 responders was 18 months from the onset of therapy (range: 2.3–29 +); the median survival of the 18 patients with no change was 14 months (range: 7–27 +);

the median survival of those with progressive disease (11 patients) was 9.5 months (range: 4.6–25) (Fig. 1).

The survival of responders was superior to that observed in patients with no change ($P < 0.05$) and to that for patients with progressive disease ($P < 0.05$). No statistical difference was noted between the NC group and the PD group ($P > 0.05$). Time to disease progression in responders ranged from 2.3 to 14 months

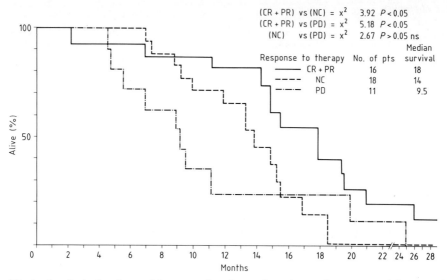

Fig. 1. Survival of patients with metastatic colorectal carcinoma from onset of therapy with 5-FU and MFH4

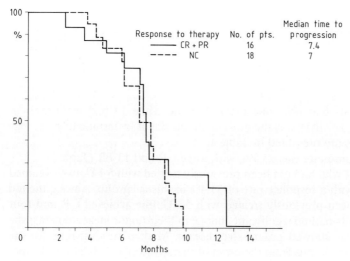

Fig. 2. Time to disease progression from the onset of therapy

(median 7.4); in the group with no change time to disease progression ranged from 3.7 to 10 months (median 7) (Fig. 2).

Gastrointestinal toxicity (stomatitis, diarrhea) was frequently encountered. All toxicities were evaluated on 393 courses of chemotherapy. Myelosuppression was characterized mainly by leukopenia (59 episodes of grade 1 and three episodes of grade 2; no episodes of grade 3 were observed); the leukocyte nadir occurred between 16 and 19 days after the cycle.

Cumulative myelosuppression was not observed, and this allowed for repeated cycles of treatment to be given at 21-day intervals. No toxic death occurred. Miscellaneous toxicity included fever, conjunctivitis, venous pigmentation, nausea and vomiting in a low percentage of patients. Alopecia was mild (11%). One episode of cardiac arrhythmia, one of transient cardiac pain, and one of laryngeal oedema were observed (Table 3).

Table 3. Overall toxicity in 45 patients treated with 5-FU and MFH4 (393 courses)

Toxic effect and degree	No. of patients with toxic effects	No. of courses with toxic episodes according to degree		
Oral mucositis	26 (57.7%)			
1		24		
2		18		
3		5		
4		–		
Diarrhea	21 (46.6%)			
1		28		
2		15		
3		5		
4		–		
Hematological toxicity	27 (60%)	WBC	Plt	Hb
1		59	10	14
2		31	3	5
3		–	1	–
4		–	–	–
Fever	10 (22%)			
1		8		
2		10		
Nausea/vomiting	5 (11.1%)			
1		7		
2		2		
Conjunctivitis	20 (44.4%)	32		
Alopecia	5 (11.1%)			
Dry skin rush	8 (17.7%)			
Venous pigmentation	26 (57.7%)			
Whole body pigmentation	7 (15.5%)			
Laryngeal oedema	1			
Cardiac arrhythmia	1			
Transient cardiac pain	1			

Table 4. Basis for use of methyltetrahydrofolate with 5-FU

- MFH4 is the form of transport of folates in plasma [7, 8].
- Formyl-FH4 must be largely converted to MFH4 before it can be utilized by tissue [7].
- The half-life of MFH4 is four times longer than the half-life of formyl-FH4 [8].
- There is a possible direct transformation of MFH4 to the active folate methylene-FH4 through a methylene-reductase blockade [4].

Discussion

The results of this study suggest an enhancement of the activity of 5-FU with the addition of 5-MFH4 acid to the daily schedule (for 5 days) and dosage administered. The response rate is superior to that generally expected with 5-FU as a single agent.

Survival of the responders, with a median of 18 months, seems to be superior to our previous experience with 5-FU alone (median 11 months). Although the toxic effects of this combination were qualitatively similar to those of 5-FU alone they appeared to be more severe in degree, indicating a possible synergistic toxicity.

The study suggests that with the increasing interest in modulation of fluoropyrimidine activity with reduced folates there is a distinct place for MFH4, the rationale for which is shown in Table 4; it is the main metabolite of formyl-FH4 and the form of transport of folates in human plasma [5–9].

It is worthy of note that the results obtained with this schedule and this dose are superimposable on those obtained with similar schedules which employ doses of formyl FH4 two or more times higher [11–16].

References

1. Friedman M, Sadée W (1978) The Fluoropyrimidines: Biochemical mechanisms and design of clinical trials. Cancer Chemother Pharmacology 1: 77–82
2. Evans M et al. (1981) Effectiveness of excess folates and deoxyinosine on the activity and site of action of 5-FU. Cancer Res 41: 3288–3295
3. Ullman B et al. (1978) Cytotoxicity of FdUrd: requirement for reduced folate co-factors and antagonism by methotrexate. Proc Natl Acad Sci USA 75 (2): 980–983
4. Waxman S et al. (1982) The enhancement of 5-FU antimetabolic activity by leucovorin, menadione and a-tocopherol. Eur J Clin Oncol 18: 685–692
5. Houghton J et al. (1984) Basis for the interaction of 5-FU and leucovorin in colon adenocarcinoma. Symposium on the current status of 5-FU–calcium leucovorin combination, New York, March 12, pp 23–32
6. Danenberg P (1984) The role of reduced folates in the enhanced binding of FdUMP to dTMP synthetase. Symposium on the current status of 5-FU–calcium leucovorin combination, New York, March 12, pp 5–12
7. Periti P (1983) Coenzimi folici. Chemioterapia vol 2 (4) Suppl
8. Mehta B, Gisolfi A, Hutchison D, Nirenberg A, Kellick M G, Rosen G (1978) Serum distribution of citrovorum factor and 5-methyltetrahydrofolate following oral and i.m. administration of calcium leucovorin in normal adults. Cancer Treat Rep 62: 345–350
9. Straw J et al. (1984) Pharmacokinetics of the diastereoisomers of leucovorin after intravenous and oral administration to normal subjects. Cancer Res 44: 3114–3119

10. Grecchi G et al. (1986) The current status of fluoropyrimidines – modulation with reduced folates. Minerva Medica. (in press)
11. Madajewicz S et al. (1984) Phase I–II trial of high-dose calcium leucovorin and 5-FU in advanced colorectal cancer. Cancer Res 44: 4667–4669
12. Machover D et al. (1985) Treatment of advanced colorectal and gastric adenocarcinomas with 5-FU combined with high-dose folinic acid – an update. Chemioterapia 4: 369–376
13. Bruckner H (1984) An efficient leucovorin–5-FU sequence: dosage escalation and pharmacologic monitoring. Symposium on the current status of 5-FU–leucovorin calcium combination. New York, March 12, pp 49–54
14. Budd GT et al. (1985) A randomized comparison of two dose schedules of 5-FU and folinic acid for the treatment of metastatic colorectal cancer. Proceedings of the American Society of Clinical Oncology, no C-318
15. Schmoll J et al. (1985) Sequential high-dose folinic acid and 5-FU in advanced colorectal cancer with measurable progressive disease. Proceedings of the American Society of Clinical Oncology, no C-365
16. Bertrand M et al. (1985) High-dose folinic acid by continuous infusion and i.v. bolus in patients with advanced colorectal cancer. A randomized study. Proceedings of the American Society of Clinical Oncology, no C-297

Intraoperative Radiotherapy in Carcinoma of the Stomach and Pancreas

W. F. Sindelar

Surgery Branch, National Cancer Institute, National Institutes of Health, Bethesda, MD, USA

Background of Intraoperative Radiotherapy

Intraoperative radiotherapy (IORT) involves delivering large single doses of radiation during surgery directly to operatively exposed tumors or to resected tumor beds at risk for residual malignancy. The rationale for the use of IORT is to maximize the dose of radiation delivered to neoplastic tissues and to minimize the radiation dose to normal tissues which may surround the neoplastic area. Normal tissues may be excluded from the irradiated area by operative displacement from the beam path or by protection with shielding materials positioned at surgery. Manipulations to protect normal tissues at the time of IORT may permit high tumoricidal doses of radiation to abdominal malignancies which otherwise might not be possible by conventional radiotherapy techniques. External-beam radiotherapy (EBRT) delivered in standard fashion may result in radiation enteritis or other toxicity when given in high doses to large abdominal fields.

Intraoperative irradiation has drawn considerable interest recently from oncologists as a potentially valuable therapeutic modality [1]. However, the concept of delivering radiation during surgery dates back to as early as 1915, when X-rays were directed to bulky unresectable gastric cancers at laparotomy, and scattered reports of the use of intraoperatively delivered radiation in the treatment of abdominal cancers were published during the first half of this century [1, 2], but the technical limitations of the available roentgenographic units permitted only shallow radiation-beam penetration and low-dose delivery rates, rendering unfeasible the routine use of intraoperative irradiation.

High-energy megavoltage radiation therapy units were introduced by 1960, which permitted the delivery of large doses of external-beam radiation to deep-seated tumors. Megavoltage treatment to the abdomen, however, resulted in frequent toxicity to the gastrointestinal tract.

The intraoperative use of high-energy megavoltage radiotherapy was explored during the 1960s and 1970s in Japan, with much of the early work performed at Kyoto University [3-5]. The Japanese experience demonstrated that intraoperative radiation was feasible for the treatment of various intra-abdominal malignancies, and doses as high as 4000 cGy appeared to be capable of being delivered with

Recent Results in Cancer Research, Vol. 110
© Springer-Verlag Berlin·Heidelberg 1988

safety. During the 1970s and 1980s, the use of megavoltage intraoperative irradiation became widespread in Japan. By 1986, over 30 Japanese institutions had regularly utilized IORT, and the accumulated Japanese experience with IORT has grown to be in excess of 2000 patients.

In the United States investigations of IORT were initiated in the middle and late 1970s at Howard University [6, 7], the Massachusetts General Hospital (MGH) [8, 9], the National Cancer Institute (NCI) [10], and the Mayo Clinic [11]. Various pilot clinical trials of IORT have been undertaken, with preliminary results suggesting acceptable toxicity, enhanced local tumor control, and possible survival prolongation in gastrointestinal cancers [1]. At present, approximately 50 institutions in the United States are utilizing IORT in some measure.

Rationale for the Use of Intraoperative Radiotherapy in Gastric and Pancreatic Carcinoma

Intraoperative irradiation may have clinical utility by providing a method of delivering radiation to areas where conventional techniques of radiotherapy produce severe dose-limiting toxicity in normal tissues. Conventional fractionated radiotherapy is poorly tolerated in the upper abdomen and results in gastrointestinal toxicity at high doses. Consequently, the use of IORT appears to be potentially valuable for the treatment of malignancies of the upper gastrointestinal tract, since IORT techniques potentially enable the delivery of tumoricidal doses of radiation to the neoplasm while sparing radiation exposure to surrounding normal abdominal viscera. Advanced cancers of the stomach and pancreas typically are extensively locally infiltrative and involve regional lymph nodes. Advanced gastric and pancreatic cancers are rarely cured by surgical resection. However, the use of IORT might enable local control of upper abdominal tumors with a low degree of treatment toxicity. Consequently, attention has been directed to both gastric and pancreatic carcinoma as appropriate diseases in which to investigate the efficacy of IORT, both in the treatment of unresectable tumors and in combination with the surgical excision of gross disease.

Clinical Techniques of Intraoperative Radiotherapy

Patients currently considered for intraoperative irradiation of gastric or pancreatic cancers at institutions utilizing IORT are surgically explored for staging of the extent of malignant disease. At most institutions, patients who are found at exploration to have peritoneal or visceral metastases are not candidates for IORT treatment, since localized radiotherapy is unlikely to affect patient survival in the presence of disseminated disease. Patients with local disease only comprise the population most likely to benefit from IORT.

Whenever feasible, surgical resection is carried out. In gastric cancers, gastrectomy should be performed even if the resection is incomplete because of bulky or infiltrative disease. Gastrectomy is performed prior to irradiation to remove tumor bulk and to provide access to the gastric bed and regional nodal basins. In pancreatic cancers, resection should be performed if possible, but resectable lesions form only a small percentage of all cases of pancreatic carcinoma. In the treatment of either pancreatic or gastric carcinomas, surgical mobilizations of the tissue in the vicinity of the tumor are performed to provide access for direct irradiation of the neoplasm or of the resected tumor bed. For gastric or pancreatic tumors where portions of the gastrointestinal tract must be resected, reconstruction is performed following IORT.

After exploration, tissue mobilization, and resection if possible, careful evaluation is made of the extent of disease, and the IORT field to be intraoperatively irradiated is defined. Typically, the field includes all gross tumor and areas of potential direct extension or nodal spread. After the field to be irradiated is defined, trial IORT treatment applicators, or cones, are selected to cover the treatment portal. A variety of sizes and shapes of applicators may be utilized, including circular and rectangular. Most institutions delivering IORT utilize circular applicators in treating gastric and pancreatic fields [1]. A pentagonal cone which fits over the celiac axis and extends under the costal margins is frequently used at Japanese institutions following gastrectomy [12]. A horseshoe-shaped applicator, which allows positioning on sloping surfaces and matching of multiple fields, often is employed at the National Cancer Institute [13]. Stainless-steel shields around the applicator can practically eliminate scatter radiation transmitted through the walls of the IORT applicator [13].

After the treatment field has been planned, patients are taken to the radiation unit for IORT. Dedicated IORT facilities exist in only a few institutions, where combined operating and radiation therapy rooms permit surgery and irradiation to be performed in the same area. In dedicated IORT facilities, patients are positioned under the radiation treatment unit immediately after surgical exposure or resection is completed. Figure 1 illustrates a portion of the IORT facility at the NCI, including the radiation unit, treatment cone and docking apparatus, television field verification system, and operating-radiation treatment table.

Most centers performing IORT do not possess dedicated units and must transport patients under anesthesia between the operating and radiotherapy rooms. Prior to patient transport, the operative incision is temporarily closed with retention sutures to prevent evisceration, and the operative field is covered with sterile protective sheets. Patients are then transferred from the operating table to a mobile cart for transport to the radiation treatment room. Portable anesthesia, ventilation, monitoring, and resuscitation equipment must accompany the patients at all times during transport, while anesthesiologists continually ventilate the patients and assess vital signs. After arrival in the radiotherapy room, patients are transferred to the radiation treatment table.

The radiation treatment room must function in the capacity of an operating room, with adequate lighting, sterile instruments and supplies, suction, anesthetic gases, and monitoring equipment. Supplies must be present for controlling surgical emergencies which might arise in the radiation treatment area, such as sudden hemorrhage or gastrointestinal leakage. Preparation of the radiation treatment room must be completed in advance of patient transfer.

After patient positioning in the radiation treatment room, the operative incision is opened, and the treatment field is exposed. Self-retaining retractors are utilized

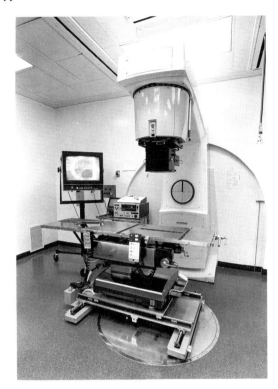

Fig. 1. Facility utilized for intraoperative irradiation at the National Cancer Institute. Illustrated are the linear accelerator used for IORT, the docking adaptor with a treatment applicator or cone, and the operating-radiation treatment table

to maintain exposure during irradiation, when patients must be left physically unattended in the treatment room but remotely monitored. The sterile radiation treatment cone and surrounding stainless-steel shield are positioned over the treatment volume, and all radiosensitive normal tissues are mobilized and displaced from the beam path. The applicators serve both to collimate the radiation beam and to retract normal tissues to prevent their falling into the treatment volume. Sterile lead wafers may be used to shield normal tissues which are not able to be physically moved from the beam path. Figure 2 illustrates the IORT field utilized in the treatment of an unresectable carcinoma in the head of the pancreas. After positioning of the treatment applicator, the cone is docked to the head of the radiation unit. Suction is maintained continuously in the treatment volume to prevent accumulation of blood or serum which could alter the depth of radiation beam penetration into tissues. After docking, the treatment volume is verified by viewing devices, such as periscopes or television monitors, to ascertain that the field has not shifted or that no normal viscera has slipped into the treatment volume during docking. Sterile drapes are placed around the docked treatment applicator, and the room is evacuated for the treatment. Irradiation is delivered, and the patients are remotely monitored through closed-circuit television and through electronic devices for recording electrocardiogram, pulse, blood pressure, and respiratory status. The total treatment time averages under 15 min and is dependent upon the total radiation dose and rate of dose delivery.

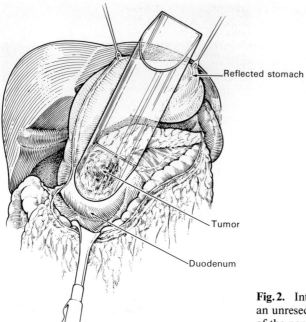

Reflected stomach

Tumor

Duodenum

Fig. 2. Intraoperative irradiation of an unresectable carcinoma of the head of the pancreas

After irradiation, the treatment applicator is undocked from the radiation unit and is removed from the patient. After hemostasis and clinical stability are established, the surgical procedure is completed. Simple closure may be completed in the radiation room. For complex closures or reconstructions, patients may have the operative incision temporarily closed and may be transported back to the operating room for completion of surgery. Because gastrointestinal anastomoses are usually located in positions that cannot be easily displaced from the irradiation volume, and since IORT delivered to areas of anastomoses may lead to significant complications, anastomosis and reconstruction of the gastrointestinal tract are typically performed after the completion of IORT.

Results of Intraoperative Radiotherapy in Gastric Cancer

Japanese clinical experiences had established by the early 1970s that intraoperative irradiation performed in the treatment of gastric carcinoma was technically feasible and frequently produced favorable treatment results [5, 12]. Abe and colleagues [12] at Kyoto University reported upon 38 patients with advanced carcinomas of the stomach treated with IORT in doses ranging from 1800 to 4000 cGy. Table 1 summarizes the results of the Kyoto trial. Gastrectomy with IORT was utilized in 24 patients while 14 patients with metastatic disease received intraoperative irradiation of the primary tumor without resection. In the unresected patient group the median survival was six months, there were no reported serious complications, and most patients experienced significant palliation of pain. Widespread

Table 1. Kyoto University experience with intraoperative irradiation in gastric carcinoma during the late 1960s and early 1970s [12]

Clinical status	No. of patients	Median survival (months)
Unresected	14	6
Palliative resection	7	16
Complete resection	17	> 44

Table 2. Five-year survival of patients with gastric carcinoma treated at Kyoto University with gastrectomy alone or with gastrectomy and intraoperative irradiation [5]

Stage	Disease extent	Gastrectomy alone		Gastrectomy + IORT	
		No.	Survival (%)	No.	Survival (%)
I	Mucosa	43	93	20	87
II	Muscularis	11	62	18	77
III	Local nodes	38	37	19	45
IV	Through serosa	18	0	27	20

destruction of the primary tumor was observed pathologically at autopsy in patients receiving IORT at doses of 4000 cGy, but viable tumor was regularly found within irradiated fields at lower doses. Seven patients underwent palliative gastrectomy, leaving gross residual nodal disease, and received IORT in doses of 2000–3500 cGy. No complications were reported. In the palliatively resected patient group the median survival was 16 months, and two patients survived more than 5 years. Seventeen patients underwent gastrectomy with curative intent (all disease resected) and received IORT in doses ranging from 2500 to 4000 cGy. The actuarial median survival of the completely resected patient group receiving IORT was in excess of 44 months, and no surgical or radiation-related complications were reported.

A nonrandomized trial of IORT in gastric cancer has been carried out at Kyoto University since the mid 1970s [5]. Patients with carcinoma of the stomach scheduled for surgical exploration on the particular days of the week when IORT procedures were performed received combined surgery and intraoperative irradiation. Patients operated upon on days when IORT was not performed received surgery alone. IORT doses ranged from 2800 to 4000 cGy, with 3000 cGy being the typical dose used in combination with gastrectomy. Results of the Kyoto University experience are summarized in Table 2. Five-year survival rates were similar for gastrectomy alone (93%) and gastrectomy with IORT (87%) in patients with stage-I gastric carcinoma confined to the mucosa. In stage-II disease within the gastric wall, the 5-year survival for patients receiving IORT (77%) was superior to that for patients undergoing surgery alone (62%). Stage-III patients with perigastric lymph nodal involvement demonstrated a 5-year survival somewhat superior (45%) to that for patients not irradiated (37%). Patients with advanced stage-IV disease denoting extragastric tumor extension without visceral metastases showed a 20% 5-year survival rate after resection with IORT, while no (0%) 5-year survivors were among the patient group undergoing surgery alone. Serious complications associated with intraoperative irradiation were not reported, and the overall complication rates were reported to be similar in the gastrectomy alone and gastrectomy with IORT groups for all stages of disease.

The experience with IORT in gastric cancer at Kyoto University has suggested that intraoperative irradiation of the gastric bed and regional lymph nodal basins following resection can improve survival in locally advanced malignancies of the stomach. The use of IORT for gastric cancer has become frequent in several major Japanese oncologic centers where facilities exist for the delivery of intraoperative irradiation. Abe (M. Abe, personal communication) at Kyoto University currently advocates the use of IORT whenever the primary tumor can be grossly removed, whenever the tumor occurs in the corpus or antrum, and whenever direct invasion, if present, occurs from the posterior gastric wall into the retroperitoneum. Patients with tumors occurring in the cardia or fundus are not considered to be IORT candidates by the Japanese because the pentagonal IORT applicators routinely utilized in many Japanese institutions cannot be positioned over the diaphragm in the region of the proximal stomach and esophageal hiatus. Similarly, areas of direct tumor extension outside of the gastric bed, such as extension to the abdominal wall, generally are not amenable to coverage by the single Japanese IORT portal. Abe requires that all lymph nodal basins harboring tumor be covered by a single celiac axis IORT portal.

Currently, Abe recommends IORT at the time of gastrectomy whenever a curative resection is not possible. A curative resection is defined as gastrectomy performed in the absence of nodal involvement or serosal penetration. Gastrectomy alone is advocated following complete extirpation of gastric cancer in the absence of regional lymph nodal involvement or direct tumor extension, but IORT is utilized whenever microscopic residual remains in nodal areas or in the resection bed following gastrectomy (usual IORT dose 2800 cGy) or whenever gross tumor remains following resection (IORT dose 3000-3500 cGy). At Kyoto University, patients with gastric cancers that are deemed inoperable on the basis of clinical evaluation are typically treated with chemotherapy and conventional EBRT. Gastric carcinomas which are considered resectable are taken to surgery with the intention of resection; if gastrectomy is possible IORT is given in conjunction with resection, while postoperative chemotherapy and conventional radiotherapy are given if the operative findings preclude gastric resection.

In 1980 the National Cancer Institute initiated a prospectively randomized protocol study of resectable carcinoma of the stomach, comparing IORT with conventional treatment in an attempt to evaluate the overall efficacy and toxicity of IORT. Patients with adenocarcinoma of the stomach who have no evidence of disseminated disease after clinical evaluation have been randomly allocated to an experimental treatment arm which receives gastrectomy with IORT or to a control arm which receives standard therapy. Patients who at exploration have been found to have visceral metastases have been excluded from the protocol, but all patients who have been found to have only local disease have been retained in the study even if all gross tumor was unable to be extirpated. All patients have received resection appropriate for the location and stage of disease: esophagogastrectomy for proximal tumors, subtotal gastrectomy for distal tumors, or total gastrectomy for lesions involving large portions of the stomach. Extended resections, including partial pancreatectomy, hepatic lobectomy, or excision of portions of the diaphragm have been performed in the event of local extragastric tumor invasion.

All patients in the experimental therapy group have received IORT electron beam irradiation (11-14 MeV) at a dose of 2000 cGy to the gastric resection bed, to regional lymphatic drainage basins, and to areas of potential contiguous tumor spread. All patients who received IORT have been treated with the hypoxic cell sensitizer misonidazole (3.5 g/m^2 in a single intravenous dose) immediately prior to irradiation.

Patients randomized to the standard therapy treatment arm have received gastrectomy alone for early-stage gastric cancer confined to the mucosa or muscularis. Advanced-stage patients with penetration of the gastric serosa, extragastric extension, or lymph nodal involvement have received gastrectomy followed by conventional fractionated postoperative radiotherapy to the upper abdomen (5000 cGy EBRT delivered in 175-200 cGy/day fractions over 5-6 weeks). Patients in both experimental and control arms have been followed up for the time to disease recurrence, for the pattern of disease recurrence and local tumor control, for overall survival, and for the incidence and type of treatment-related complications.

The NCI trial of IORT in gastric carcinoma is ongoing, and present results are preliminary. Table 3 summarizes the patient characteristics and results as of 1986. Thirty patients have been placed on study, 11 in the IORT arm and 19 in the standard therapy arm. Eleven patients had tumors of the esophagogastric junction, cardia, or fundus; six patients had tumors of the corpus or antrum; and 13 patients had linitis plastica lesions involving the bulk of the stomach. Three patients had stage-I disease confined to the mucosa, no patients had stage-II disease confined to the muscularis, 17 patients had stage-III disease involving the serosa or regional lymph nodes, and ten patients had stage-IV disease involving direct spread of tumor to neighboring extragastric organs without visceral metastases. The tumor sites and stages were similar in both the experimental and control arms of the study.

Treatment complication rates have been similar in both IORT and conventional therapy arms and have not differed statistically. Seven of 11 patients (64%) receiving gastrectomy with IORT have suffered complications, including two with gastrointestinal fistulae, one with sepsis, one with a myocardial infarction, and three with mild anastomotic strictures. Two patients died in the postoperative period following gastrectomy with IORT, one of a myocardial infarction and the other with septic complications of a gastrointestinal fistula. Thirteen of 19 patients (68%) receiving conventional treatment developed complications, including six with fistulae, two with sepsis, two with radiation enteritis, one with intestinal obstruction, and two with anastomotic strictures. No postoperative deaths have occurred in the conventional therapy group. At present, no significant differences have developed between the IORT and the conventional therapy groups in the median disease-

Table 3. Current status of a trial of intraoperative irradiation in gastric carcinoma at the National Cancer Institute

Category	Treatment arm	
	IORT	Standard therapy
No. of patients randomized	11	19
Disease stage		
I	1	2
II	0	0
III	6	11
IV	4	6
Disease location		
Proximal stomach	4	7
Distal stomach	1	5
Linitis plastica	6	7
Treatment complications		
Postoperative death	2	0
Fistula	2	6
Sepsis	1	2
Cardiopulmonary	1	0
Stricture	3	2
Other	0	3
Survival data (median)		
Overall	24 months	27 months
Disease-free	12 months	8 months
Time to local failure	14 months	8 months

free interval (IORT 12 months, conventional therapy 8 months), in the median time to local disease recurrence (IORT 14 months, conventional therapy 8 months), or in the median overall survival (IORT 24 months, conventional therapy 27 months). In advanced-stage cancers extending beyond the mucosa, an early suggestion of improvement in local disease control has developed among patients receiving IORT (Fig. 3), but the improvement in local control at present has not been translated into an enhancement of overall survival in the IORT group as compared with the standard therapy patients (Fig. 3). Patients with advanced-stage proximal cancers (esophagogastric junction, cardia, or fundus) treated with resection and either IORT or EBRT have shown survival (median survival 26 months combining both IORT and standard treatment arms) superior to that for patients with advanced distal lesions (corpus or antrum; median survival 8 months in combined IORT and standard treatment arms) or with linitis plastica (median survival 4 months in combined IORT and standard treatment arms) treated with resection and IORT or EBRT. Survival was improved among advanced-stage proximal-lesion patients treated with IORT compared with advanced proximal-lesion patients treated with standard therapy. No significant survival differences have developed in advanced-stage distal lesion or linitis plastica patients treated with IORT or with conventional therapy.

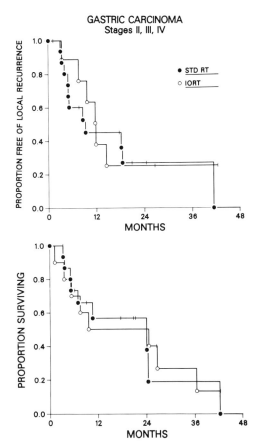

Fig. 3. Current results in a National Cancer Institute randomized trial of gastrectomy combined with intraoperative or standard external-beam radiotherapy in carcinoma of the stomach which extends through the muscularis, involves regional lymph nodes, or extends into extragastric tissues in the retroperitoneum. *Upper panel* shows time to local disease recurrence; *lower panel* shows survival

Results of Intraoperative Radiotherapy in Pancreatic Cancer

Intraoperative irradiation in pancreatic carcinoma was utilized in Japan in the late 1960s and early 1970s [5]. Most patients underwent explorative surgery and palliative biliary or gastric bypasses for unresectable pancreatic malignancies and had the primary pancreatic tumor intraoperatively irradiated with doses ranging from 1500 to 4000 cGy. The Japanese experience demonstrated that IORT can be utilized with acceptable morbidity in patients with pancreatic cancer. In 108 patients with unresectable pancreatic carcinoma treated with IORT by various Japanese institutions and reported on in combined series, the resulting observed median survival of 6 months appeared to be only modestly enhanced over the survival which would be expected from conventional therapy [5]. Only five patients were alive more than 1 year following treatment, and the longest survival was 43 months. However, IORT appeared to be of significant palliative benefit, reducing or eliminating pain in a large proportion of patients. Tumor necrosis was consistently found within IORT fields in patients subjected to postmortem examination.

Howard University reported a pilot series utilizing IORT in 19 patients with advanced carcinoma of the pancreas, including ten patients with hepatic metastases [14]. The median survival was 6 months. Evidence of tumor necrosis was present in some patients, and the trial confirmed the Japanese observation that utilizing IORT was feasible in the treatment of patients with pancreatic cancer.

The combination of IORT with preoperative or postoperative conventional EBRT has been utilized at the MGH since 1978 in patients with unresectable pancreatic carcinoma [9, 15, 16]. Shipley et al. [16] reported the MGH experience of 29 patients with localized unresectable carcinomas of the pancreas treated by electron-beam IORT in combination with palliative surgical biliary or gastric bypass and with additional photon EBRT (see Table 4).

Patients treated at the MGH received 1000–2000 cGy conventional external-beam fractionated radiotherapy over 1–6 weeks, finishing 1–10 days prior to surgery. IORT to the primary tumor was given to a dose of 1500–2000 cGy. Thirteen patients received the hypoxic cell sensitizer misonidazole at the time of IORT. Following surgery, 27 patients received additional EBRT (3000–4000 cGy postoperatively to a total EBRT dose of 5000 cGy). Chemotherapy consisting of 5-fluorouracil (5-FU) was given to 23 patients during the period of postoperative EBRT; 15 patients received combination chemotherapy consisting of 5-FU, doxorubicin, and mitomycin after an initial course of 5-FU administered at the time of EBRT.

Table 4. Massachusetts General Hospital experience with intraoperative irradiation in unresectable pancreatic carcinoma [16]

Category	Number
Patient characteristics	
Treated with IORT	29
Completed IORT and EBRT	27
Chemotherapy given	23
Misonidazole given with IORT	13
Complications	
Early	3
Fistula	1
Sepsis	1
Ileus	1
Late	22
Gastrointestinal hemorrhage	7
Gastric or biliary obstruction	3
Vascular occlusion	1
Exocrine insufficiency	10
New diabetes	1
Survival results (median)	
All patients	17 months
Patients completing IORT and EBRT	17 months
Patients receiving chemotherapy	17 months
Patients receiving misonidazole	> 12 months

Median survival for the MGH group of patients with unresectable pancreatic carcinoma was 17 months. The actuarial local control rate at 1 year for all patients was 64%. Ten patients progressed with regional disease, and eight of the ten regional progressions recurred within the IORT field. Distant metastases developed in 12 patients, including five patients failing both regionally and distantly. Of 16 patients presenting with abdominal pain at the time of treatment, eight patients experienced complete and lasting resolution of pain, while four other patients had transient pain relief.

Treatment-related complications occurred early in three patients (10%) and included a gastric fistula in one patient, a fungal pancreatic abscess in one, and prolonged gastric atony in one. Late treatment complications occurred in 22 patients (76%) and included late upper gastrointestinal hemorrhage in seven, late gastric outlet or biliary obstruction in two, mesenteric vascular occlusion in one, progressive exocrine insufficiency in ten, and the onset of diabetes in one patient.

The preliminary impression of the MGH group has been that IORT promotes local tumor control, palliates pain, and may prolong survival in selected patients with locally advanced pancreatic cancers [16].

The Mayo Clinic has utilized IORT in unresectable carcinoma of the pancreas since 1981 [11]. Patients with unresectable local pancreatic cancer, in the absence of visceral or peritoneal metastases, have been treated with IORT (1750–2000 cGy) to the primary tumor at the time of surgical exploration and with additional postoperative photon fractionated EBRT (4500–5000 cGy in 180 cGy/day fractions). Many patients received chemotherapy with 5-FU at the time of EBRT, and some patients received intraperitoneal 5-FU postoperatively. Forty-six patients with primary unresectable carcinoma of the pancreas have been treated utilizing IORT at the Mayo Clinic by Gunderson and colleagues, with the current treatment results summarized in Table 5 (L. L. Gunderson, personal communication).

At the time of last analysis, 32 of the 46 pancreatic cancer patients treated at the Mayo Clinic with IORT and EBRT had died, with 25 (54% of total) having shown clinical evidence of disease progression, one (2%) having no disease evident on autopsy, and six (13%) having uncertain clinical evidence of disease progression. Of the 14 patients alive at the time of analysis, three (7% of the total) had clinically

Table 5. Mayo Clinic experience with intraoperative irradiation in unresectable pancreatic carcinoma (L. L. Gunderson, personal communication)

Category	Number
Patients treated	46
Median survival	11 months
Patterns of disease failure	
All sites	70%
Central (within IORT field)	5%
Regional (within EBRT field)	8%
Peritoneum	28%
Distant metastases	48%

progressive disease while 11 (24%) had no evidence of tumor progression. The median survival of the Mayo patient group has been 11 months, with an actuarial 1-year survival rate of 46% and a 2-year survival rate of 8%.

The pattern of disease failure was evaluable in 40 of the pancreatic cancer patients treated at Mayo. Twenty-eight patients demonstrated clinical progression of tumor, with 19 (48% of the total population evaluable) showing distant visceral metastatic spread and 11 (28%) showing peritoneal metastases. Five patients (13%) demonstrated clear clinical evidence of local disease progression, and tumor progression within the IORT field was documented in only two patients (5%). It must be recognized that it is difficult to clinically assess with certainty local disease control in the pancreas, and reported local control figures must be regarded as estimates. The Mayo results suggest that IORT may enhance local control. However, since systemic disease progression typically occurs in pancreatic cancer, enhanced local control at present appears to have a limited impact on overall survival.

The use of intraoperative irradiation as an adjunct to surgical resection in pancreatic carcinoma has been studied in only a limited fashion. Hiraoka (personal communication) of Kumamoto University has collected a series of seven patients who at the time of pancreatectomy for carcinoma were treated with IORT (3000 cGy) to the resection bed and regional lymph nodes. The 18-month median survival observed in the patients receiving pancreatectomy with IORT was superior to the 8-month median survival seen in eight patients treated with pancreatectomy alone at Kumamoto University. The early 1-year survival was superior in the IORT group of patients, with 71% of the patients receiving pancreatectomy and IORT alive at 1 year while only 35% of the pancreatectomy-alone patients survived 1 year. The late 2-year survival, however, showed no major differences between the patients receiving IORT with pancreatectomy (0% alive beyond 2 years) and patients undergoing pancreatectomy alone (25% alive beyond 2 years).

A prospectively randomized trial evaluating IORT in pancreatic cancer has been underway at the NCI since 1980, comparing IORT with conventional treatment in both resectable and nonresectable carcinomas of the pancreas. Patients with resectable lesions have been randomly allocated to an experimental or to a standard therapy group. The experimental group has received pancreatectomy with intraoperative electron-beam irradiation (8-14 MeV) delivered to a dose of 2000 cGy to the resection bed and to regional nodal basins or to areas of potential contiguous tumor spread. The conventional therapy group has received pancreatectomy alone for early-stage disease (confined to the pancreas) or, for advanced stages (extending through the pancreatic capsule or involving regional nodes), pancreatic resection followed by conventional external-beam irradiation (5000 cGy in 175-200 cGy/day fractions) after recovery from surgery.

Patients with unresectable pancreatic cancers who have no evidence of visceral metastases on preoperative evaluation have received palliative biliary (cholecystojejunostomy or choledochojejunostomy) and gastric (gastrojejunostomy) bypasses at exploration and have been randomized to receive experimental or conventional therapy. All patients explored have been retained in the study, even if unexpected peritoneal or visceral metastatic disease was present. Experimental therapy has consisted of IORT to the primary tumor (2500 cGy utilizing 22 MeV electrons) with postoperative EBRT (5000 cGy in 175-200 cGy/day fractions) combined with monthly 5-FU (500 mg/m^2 daily intravenously for 3 consecutive days), beginning at the time EBRT was initiated and continuing for 12 cycles. Conventional therapy has consisted of EBRT (total dose of 6000 cGy in cycles of 2000 cGy given over 2 weeks in 200 cGy/day fractions, with each cycle separated by a 2-week rest) combined with monthly 5-FU (500 mg/m^2 daily intravenously for 3 consecutive days) initiated at the time of EBRT and continuing for 12 cycles.

All patients receiving IORT for both resectable and nonresectable pancreatic cancers have been given the hypoxic sensitizer misonidazole (3.5 g/m^2 in a single intravenous dose) immediately prior to IORT. Both resectable and nonresectable patients have been followed up for overall survival, for the time to disease progression, for the pattern of disease failure, and for the incidence of treatment-related complications.

At present, 26 patients with resectable carcinomas of the pancreas have been randomized and entered in the NCI study, 13 receiving IORT and 13 receiving conventional therapy (see Table 6). More patients with early-stage disease have been included in the control group than in the IORT group, and more advanced-stage patients have been entered into the IORT group than into the conventional-treatment group: stage-I disease (confined to the pancreas) patients included six receiving conventional treatment but none receiving IORT, stage-II (extension into the duodenum) patients included one receiving IORT and one receiving EBRT conventional therapy, stage-III (nodal involvement) patients included eight receiving IORT and four receiving EBRT, and stage-IV (peritoneal disease or gross re-

Table 6. Current status of trial of intraoperative irradiation in pancreatic carcinoma at the National Cancer Institute

Category	Resectable lesions		Unresectable lesions	
	IORT	Standard therapy	IORT	Standard therapy
No. of patients randomized	13	13	11	12
Disease stage				
I	0	6	0	0
II	1	1	0	0
III	8	4	5	4
IV	4	12	6	8
Treatment complications				
Postoperative death	5	2	1	0
Fistula	1	2	0	2
Sepsis	4	3	0	1
Haemorrhage	0	0	3	1
Cardiopulmonary	1	0	1	0
Other	0	2	0	0
Survival data (median; operative deaths excluded)				
Overall	18 months	10 months	8 months	9 months
Time to progression	11 months	8 months	7 months	7 months
Time to local failure	18 months	9 months	7 months	6 months

sidual after resection) patients included four receiving IORT and two receiving conventional EBRT.

The incidence of treatment-related complications has been similar in both the IORT and the conventional-therapy group. Seven of 13 patients (53%) in the IORT arm have experienced complications, including four with septic complications, one with a gastrointestinal fistula, one with cardiac failure, and one with chronic chylous ascites. Five patients receiving IORT have died of operative complications. Six of 13 patients (46%) in the conventional treatment arm have developed complications, including three with septic complications, two with gastrointestinal fistulae, and one with chronic chylous ascites. Two patients in the control treatment arm died postoperatively of complications.

When all patients with resectable pancreatic cancer on the protocol are considered, due to the high perioperative surgical mortality characteristic of pancreatic resections, no statistically significant differences have developed at present between the IORT and standard therapy arms with respect to overall survival, disease-free interval, and local disease control. If operative deaths are excluded, then IORT at present appears to prolong overall survival (IORT group, median survival 18 months; control group, median survival 10 months), disease-free interval

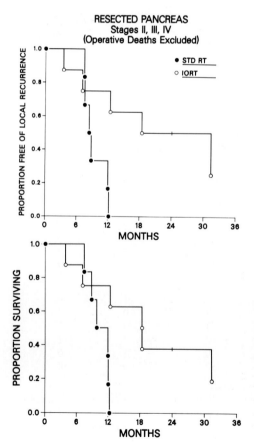

Fig. 4. Current results in a National Cancer Institute randomized trial of pancreatectomy combined with intraoperative or standard external-beam radiotherapy in resectable carcinoma of the pancreas which extends through the pancreatic capsule, involves regional lymph nodes, or extends into extrapancreatic tissues in the retroperitoneum. *Upper panel* shows time to local disease recurrence; *lower panel* shows survival

(IORT median 11 months, control median 8 months), and local disease control (IORT median 18 months, control median 9 months). Survival and local tumor control have been enhanced in advanced-stage patients (stages II, III, and IV) who have been treated with pancreatectomy and IORT, as compared with patients who have been treated with pancreatectomy and conventional EBRT (see Fig. 4).

Twenty-three patients with unresectable pancreatic carcinoma have been entered at present into the NCI randomized trial, 11 receiving IORT and 12 receiving conventional therapy (see Table 6). Nine patients had local disease only, while 14 patients had visceral metastatic disease discovered at laparotomy. The distribution of local-disease and metastatic-disease patients was similar in both experimental and control groups.

Complication rates were similar in both experimental and control treatment arms. Four of 11 IORT patients (36%) developed complications, including three with late upper gastrointestinal hemorrhage and one with pulmonary failure. One postoperative death occurred in the IORT group. Four of 12 conventional-therapy patients (33%) experienced treatment-related complications, including one with acute hemorrhage, two with gastrointestinal fistulae, and one with sepsis.

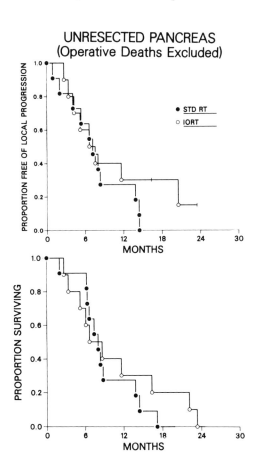

Fig. 5. Current results in a National Cancer Institute randomized trial of intraoperative with external-beam irradiation and chemotherapy compared with external-beam irradiation and chemotherapy in unresectable carcinoma of the pancreas. *Upper panel* shows time to local disease progression; *lower panel* shows survival

Current analysis of the unresected pancreatic carcinoma patients in the NCI study has shown no significant differences between IORT and conventional therapy patients in overall survival (IORT median 8 months, control median 9 months; see Fig.5) and in the time to disease progression (IORT median 7 months, control median 7 months). The time to local disease progression tended to be somewhat longer in the IORT group (median 7 months) as compared with the conventional-therapy group (median 6 months), but the difference has failed to achieve statistical significance at present (see Fig.5).

Current Status of Intraoperative Radiotherapy in Gastric and Pancreatic Cancer

Intraoperative irradiation has been demonstrated to be a feasible adjunct in the treatment of carcinomas of the stomach and pancreas. IORT can be performed without apparent significant increases in complication rates over the rates expected with conventional therapy.

In gastric carcinoma, the Japanese experience suggests that IORT with gastrectomy offers survival superior to that with gastrectomy alone in advanced lesions. The National Cancer Institute experience suggests that IORT may be superior to conventional fractionated external-beam radiotherapy in promoting local control of advanced gastric cancers.

For carcinoma of the pancreas, the early experience at the Massachusetts General Hospital in selected patients with localized unresectable disease suggested that IORT in combination with conventional radiotherapy can promote local disease control and survival. Subsequent experiences with patients suffering from unresectable pancreatic cancer at the Mayo Clinic and the NCI have failed at present to convincingly demonstrate improvements in survival in patients treated by IORT as compared with conventional therapeutic techniques. However, IORT does appear to have enhanced the local control of primary unresectable pancreatic cancers. The experience with the use of IORT as an adjunct to pancreatectomy for resectable pancreatic carcinomas is limited, but the NCI trial has suggested that IORT may enhance both local control and overall survival following pancreatic resection.

References

1. Gunderson LL, Tepper JE, Biggs PJ, Goldson A, Marin JK, McCullough EC, Rich TA, Shipley WU, Sindelar WF, Wood WC (1983) Intraoperative ± external beam irradiation. Curr Probl Cancer 7: 1–69
2. Eloesser L (1937) The treatment of some abdominal cancers by irradiation through the open abdomen combined with cautery excision. Ann Surg 106: 645–652
3. Abe M, Takahashi M, Yabumoto E, Onoyama Y, Torizuka K, Tobe T, Mori K (1975) Techniques, indications and results of intraoperative radiotherapy of advanced cancers. Radiology 116: 693–702
4. Abe M, Takahashi M, Yabumoto E, Adachi H, Yoshii M, Mori K (1980) Clinical experiences with intraoperative radiotherapy of locally advanced cancers. Cancer 45: 40–48

5. Abe M, Takahashi M (1981) Intraoperative radiotherapy: the Japanese experience. Int J Radiat Oncol Biol Phys 7: 863–868
6. Goldson A (1978) Preliminary clinical experience with intraoperative radiotherapy. J Natl Med Assoc 70: 493–495
7. Goldson AL (1981) Past, present, and prospects of intraoperative radiotherapy (IOR). Semin Oncol 8: 59–64
8. Gunderson LL, Cohen AM, Welch CE (1980) Residual, inoperable or recurrent colorectal cancer. Interaction of surgery and radiotherapy. Am J Surg 139: 518–525
9. Gunderson LL, Shipley WU, Suit HD, Epp ER, Nardi G, Wood W, Cohen A, Nelson J, Battit G, Biggs PJ, Russell A, Rockett A, Clark D (1982) Intraoperative irradiation. A pilot study combining external-beam photons with "boost" dose intraoperative electrons. Cancer 49: 2259–2266
10. Sindelar WF, Kinsella T, Tepper J, Travis EL, Rosenberg SA, Glatstein E (1983) Experimental and clinical studies with intraoperative radiotherapy. Surg Gynecol Obstet 157: 205–219
11. Gunderson LL, Martin JK, Earle JD, Byer DE, Voss M, Fieck JM, Kvols LK, Rorie DK, Martinez A, Nagorney DM, O'Connell MJ, Weber FC (1984) Intraoperative and external-beam irradiation with or without resection: Mayo pilot experience. Mayo Clin Proc 59: 691–699
12. Abe M, Yabumoto E, Takahashi M, Tobe T, Mori K (1974) Intraoperative radiotherapy of gastric cancer. Cancer 34: 2034–2041
13. Fraass BA, Miller RW, Kinsella TJ, Sindelar WF, Harrington FS, Yaekel K, van de Geijn J, Glatstein E (1985) Intraoperative radiotherapy at the National Cancer Institute: technical innovations and dosimetry. Int J Radiat Oncol Biol Phys 11: 1299–1311
14. Goldson AL, Ashaveri E, Espinoza MC, Roux V, Cornwell E, Rayford L, McLaren M, Nibhanupudy R, Mahan A, Taylor HT, Hemphil N, Pearson O (1981) Single high-dose intraoperative electrons for advanced-stage pancreas cancer: phase-I pilot study. Int J Radiat Oncol Biol Phys 7: 869–874
15. Wood WC, Shipley WU, Gunderson LL, Cohen AM, Nardi GL (1982) Intraoperative irradiation for unresectable pancreatic carcinoma. Cancer 49: 1272–1275
16. Shipley WU, Wood WC, Tepper JE, Warshaw AL, Orlow EL, Kaufman D, Battit GE, Nardi GL (1984) Intraoperative electron-beam irradiation for patients with unresectable pancreatic carcinoma. Ann Surg 200: 289–296

Is There a Role for Hyperthermia in Gastrointestinal Tract Cancer?*

J. Overgaard and M. Overgaard

Danish Cancer Society, Department of Experimental Clinical Oncology, Radiumstationen, Nörrebrogade 44, 8000 Aarhus C, Denmark

The question about a potential role of hyperthermia in the treatment of gastrointestinal cancer will have to be separated into at least two parts: first, an analysis of the course of failure to achieve sufficient tumor control, second, whether this failure can be diminished by adding hyperthermia to the treatment.

Hyperthermia alone has only a minor role, if any, in curative cancer treatment [17], and the attention will therefore be given to various situations where hyperthermia is used in conjuction with other modalities. This paper will deal especially with the interaction between heat and radiation, although hyperthermia may be beneficial in improving the effect of chemotherapy. However, this is mainly a palliative procedure and is not likely to result in improved persistent tumor control.

If one analyzes the reasons for unsuccessful cancer treatment it becomes apparent that lack of sufficient local control is a major cause of death from cancer. Thus, in most advanced tumors insufficient local-regional cancer therapy contributes heavily to the failure of treatment [25, 26]. Insufficient local-regional control in turn may increase the risk of developing distant metastases. An improved local control is thus likely to improve survival. Also in the treatment of recurrent or inoperable colorectal disease it has been shown that local control is fundamental to having a chance of surviving the disease [6, 7, 10, 20, 21, 26, 27] (Fig. 1).

Radiotherapy is a major modality in improving local control, but most gastrointestinal tumors require high doses of radiation to be controlled [20, 27]. Thus, the amount of radiation which can be given without causing too extensive complications in normal tissue is frequently not sufficient.

Hyperthermia has been shown to markedly improve the effect of radiotherapy; furthermore, this effect can be used almost selectively. The major indication for hyperthermia in gastrointestinal cancer at the moment, therefore, seems to be as an adjuvant to radiotherapy in order to improve the treatment of locally advanced tumors.

---

* Supported by the Danish Cancer Society.

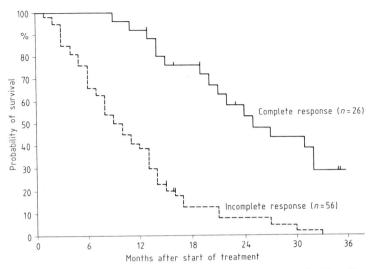

Fig. 1. Actuarial survival as a function of local tumor control in patients treated with radiotherapy for recurrent or inoperable colorectal carcinoma. (From Overgaard et al. [20])

Table 1. Interaction between hyperthermia and radiation

A. Hyperthermic radiosensitization
1. Direct radiosensitization (decreased D_0)
2. Reduced repair of sublethal damage
3. Increased sensitivity of cells in radioresistant phases of the cell cycle
4. Reduced repair of potential lethal damage
(Maximal with simultaneous treatment)

B. Hyperthermic cytotoxicity
Increased under environmental conditions such as:
1. Nutritional deprivation
2. Chronic hypoxia
3. Acidity (most important)
(Independent of sequence and interval)

Interaction Between Hyperthermia and Radiation

The interaction between hyperthermia and radiation is based on two principles of independent mechanism [3, 4, 12, 14, 15, 16, 19]. First, hyperthermia has a direct radiosensitizing effect. This implies that adding heat to radiotherapy will quantitatively increase the effect of radiation by various modifications of the radiation response, but the qualitative expression of damage will be unaltered (Table 1). This hyperthermic radiosensitization occurs equally in normal tissue and tumor and is most pronounced when the treatment is given simultaneously.

Second, hyperthermia modifies the effect of radiation on malignant tumors due to the so-called hyperthermic cytotoxicity, i.e., a direct effect of hyperthermia on

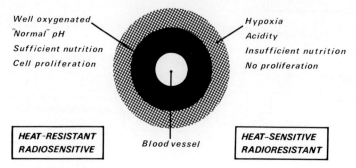

Fig. 2. Schematic illustration of the microenvironment in tumors due to insufficient vascularization and its influence on the sensitivity to heat and radiation

malignant cells. A high dose of heat given to a malignant tumor or to a normal tissue will result in a destruction of all cells, the most extreme situation being a burn. However, a moderate-heat treatment will tend to destroy certain areas of malignant tumors selectively. These areas can easily be identified histopathologically and are those at the greatest distances from the blood vessels (Fig. 2). Although this could be a phenomenon related to vascular cooling of the other parts of the tissue, it has been shown to be due to variation in tumor environment. Thus, cells situated closest to a blood vessel are characterized by a normal physiological environment with sufficient oxygen and normal pH. These cells are the most sensitive to radiotherapy due to the presence of oxygen and their active proliferation, but they are relatively resistant to hyperthermia. On the other hand, cells situated further away from blood vessels have less access to oxygen, which makes them hypoxic and radioresistant. The same lack of oxygen causes the metabolism to become more anaerobic and thereby produce increasing amounts of, for instance, lactic acids, which accumulate (due to the long diffusion distances to the blood vessels). The environment will therefore become more acidic and an increased acidity strongly increases the sensitivity for hyperthermic destruction. Cells in this area wil consequently be destroyed selectively by hyperthermia at heat doses which do not cause damage to normal tissue or tumor cells in a normal environment. Because these deprived cells are the most resistant to radiotherapy there exists a situation in which the most radioresistant cells are destroyed by hyperthermia whereas the radiosensitive cells are relatively resistant to heat. This phenomenon occurs only in tumors and the effect may be utilized selectively to enhance the damage to malignant tumors.

These two different mechanisms of interaction give two rationales for applying hyperthermia as an adjuvant to radiotherapy: one is to increase the biological effect of the given radiation dose by using the principles of hyperthermic radiosensitization; the other is to destroy radioresistant cells by direct hyperthermic cytotoxicity.

The problem is how to distinguish between these two principles. It is evident that subjecting only the tumors to hyperthermia would be beneficial to achieve the highest amount of thermal damage. Current technique does not generally allow application of hyperthermia selectively to tumors, but in many instances such a se-

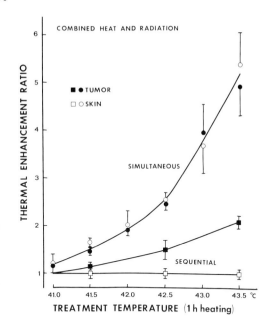

Fig. 3. Thermal enhancement ratio after simultaneous or sequential treatment at various temperatures. Note that the normal tissue is also enhanced with simultaneous treatment. See Fig. 4 for definition of simultaneous and sequential heating. (Modified from [12])

lective enhancement of the radiation damage can be achieved by biological manipulation. To further understand this phenomenon of interaction it will be necessary to define the so-called thermal enhancement ratio (TER), i.e., the dose of radiation alone to achieve an end point relative to the dose of radiation with heat to achieve the same amount of damage. The highest thermal enhancement ratios are achieved with a simultaneous treatment and depend on the temperature and the heating time (Fig. 3). Any interval between heat and radiation will tend to decrease the TER. If hyperthermia is supplied prior to radiation this will cause a reduction in TER but still give an enhancement in both normal tissue and tumors. If hyperthermia is supplied after radiation the response is similar in the tumor, with a gradual decrease until it reaches a lower but stable plateau level in TER. In normal tissue treatment this sequence will result in a rapid decrease in TER, which completely vanishes within 3–4 h in contrast to the persistent level in the tumor (Fig. 4). This results in a therapeutic gain if tumor and normal tissues are heated to the same extent. The higher enhancement after simultaneous treatment is due to the hyperthermic radiosensitization, whereas the persistent damage in the tumor is a consequence of the hyperthermic cytotoxicity, which occurs selectively in malignant tumors because normal tissue does not contain areas with deprived environmental conditions.

So far, it can be concluded that hyperthermia enhances the effect of ionizing irradiation. This effect depends on temperature and time. Simultaneous treatment causes the highest TER but to the same extent in tumor and normal tissue. Therefore, no therapeutic gain will be present if tumor and normal tissue are given the same amount of heat treatment. The effect seen with simultaneous treatment is due to the hyperthermic radiosensitization.

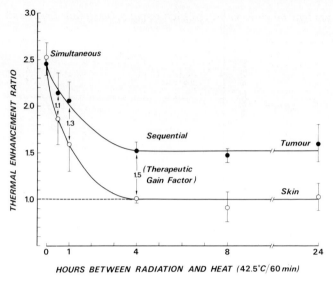

Fig. 4. Thermal enhancement ratio as a function of the time interval between hyperthermia and radiation treatment of a mouse adenocarcinoma and its surrounding skin. The different decay of TER in tumor and skin with increasing interval results in an increased therapeutic gain factor

Sequential treatment, where heat is given 3–4 h after radiation, results in a lower TER. However, with such an interval no enhancement persists in normal tissue whereas it will be present in the tumor due to the selective hyperthermic destruction of radioresistant tumor cells in a deprived environment characterized by increased acidity. Therefore, an improved therapeutic ratio is obtained despite a general decrease in TER (Fig. 4).

These principles create the basis for the use of hyperthermia as an adjuvant to radiotherapy [17, 19]. Although the use of fractionated treatment schedules makes the biological rationale more complex, a discussion of these problems is beyond the scope of the present paper; it has been dealt with in detail elsewhere [17, 18].

The described biological principle has been confirmed clinically [14, 17], and in general there is a very good correlation between experimental data and clinical observations with regard to the interaction between hyperthermia and radiation. Although clinical results have been achieved mainly in superficial tumors owing to the problems of achieving proper heating in deep-seated tumors, it is evident that hyperthermia results in a significant improvement of the tumor response (Table 2). Furthermore, it has been shown that in a specific tumor type where dose-response curves for radiation damage can be constructed there is a significant shift in the curves when hyperthermia is added and TERs between 1.5 and 2 are likely to be achieved [16, 17]. Although the data on gastrointestinal cancers are very sparse, it is likely that they will respond in a manner similar to other tumors.

Biologically, there seem to be obvious indications for applying hyperthermia in the treatment of inoperable or recurrent colorectal carcinoma. These are unfortunately frequent, and although radiotherapy can provide frequent palliation and

Table 2. Effect of adjuvant hyperthermia on the radiation response (Data from Overgaard [17])

Study	No. of tumors	Frequency of complete response	
		Radiation alone (%)	Radiation + heat (%)
Arcangeli et al.	163	38	74
U et al.	7	14	85
Overgaard	62	34	67
Johnson et al.	14	36	86
Kim et al.	159	33	80
Bide et al.	76	0	7
Hiraoka et al.	33	25	71
Kochegarov et al.	161	16	63
Lindholm et al.	85	25	46
Corry et al.	33	0	62
Scott et al.	44	64	86
Li et al.	124	29	54
van der Zee et al.	71	5	27
Steeves et al.	75	23	61
Dunlop et al.	86	50	60
Gonzalez et al.	46	33	50
Valdagni et al.	78	36	73
Li et al.	64	36	64

occasional tumor control, the radiation dose required is so large that this therapy is limited by normal tissue tolerance [20]. Currently there are significant technical problems related to the heating of tumors in the pelvis, but the continuous development of regional deep hyperthermia makes it reasonable to expect that such treatment can be achieved in the near future [5, 22, 24].

There is reason to expect that the TER achieved in colorectal cancer will be of the same magnitude as in advanced breast or head and neck nodes. As seen in Fig. 5, a crude estimate of tumor control with radiation alone can be presented in a dose-response fashion. A theoretically calculated dose-response curve with a TER of 1.5 has been added, indicating the extent of improvement which is expected to be achieved if hyperthermia is given together with radiotherapy, mainly in a sequential treatment approach.

If this prediction holds, it will certainly bring many recurrent tumors within the range of local control and hopefully result in a better survival. This would be an important indication for clinical hyperthermia.

Based on present knowledge it appears reasonable to conclude (a) that local control is a significant problem in most cases of gastrointestinal cancer, (b) that radiotherapy may improve local control but requires very high doses, and (c) that hyperthermia markedly improves the effect of radiation and can biologically be almost selectively directed against solid tumors. The final question is therefore: Can gastrointestinal tumors be heated sufficiently?

The major experience with hyperthermia has been in superficial tumors, which have been treated by a variety of techniques using ultrasound, microwaves, RF-ca-

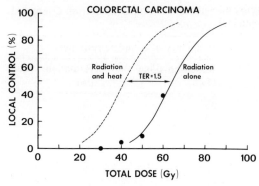

Fig. 5. Dose-response relationship for radiation-induced local control of inoperable or recurrent colorectal carcinoma. *Dashed line* indicates the theoretically expected dose-response relationship for similar radiation treatment given combined with hyperthermia. (Data for radiation alone from Overgaard et al. [20])

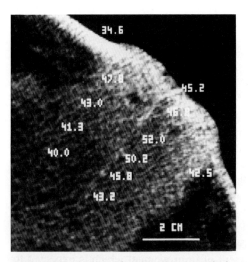

Fig. 6. CT-scanning of a gluteal metastasis from a rectal carcinoma treated with superficial hyperthermia using 144 MHz RF-inductive heating. Note the heterogeneous temperature distribution with high central and low peripheral temperatures. One of the multi-thermocouples used for temperature measurement is seen centrally in the tumor

pacity, or RF-inductive heating [15, 24]. Although a decent heating pattern has been achieved in many superficial tumors there is a significant heterogenicity in the heat distribution in most instances (Fig. 6). Especially the peripheral areas are subjected to less heating than central (more necrotic) parts of the tumor, probably due to a relatively higher vascularization. However, in a combined approach the periphery will be the area where radiotherapy will be most effective, whereby this problem is diminished. Heat treatment of deep-seated tumors is more complex. At

Table 3. Effect of radiation alone or combined with hyperthermia in patients with inoperable esophageal carcinoma [11]

Treatment	Number of patients	Local response (CR)	Survival (3-year)
Radiation alone (60–70 Gy)	83	16%	0%
Radiation (40–60 Gy) + heat (3–4 treatments)	78	63%	15%

present it requires the use of multiple applicators, preferably in a phased-array system, a technique which is still at the developmental stage [5, 15, 22, 24]. Although there are a number of commercial apparatuses available and several investigations have been performed, the problems of sufficiently heating pelvic tumors, for example, are still substantial and must by and large be solved before sufficient biological questions can be answered. At present, practical use of hyperthermia has shown that a certain amount of heat can be delivered to deep-seated tumors if patients are reasonably slim, and some promising experience has been gained in this field in recent years [2, 8]. The sparse clinical information is not sufficient to act as a guideline, but there is no indication that the biological promise will not hold if the treatment can be applied sufficiently. The two commercial types of equipment which currently dominate the market apply different approaches, namely an annular phased-array system or a direct-capacity heating principle. The latter, which is used in the Japanese Thermatron [8] machine, has shown some ability to heat deep-seated abdominal and pelvic tumors [2, 8], but mainly in slim Japanese patients who have a thin layer of subcutaneous fat. Whether such a technique is generally suitable for more well fed Europeans and Americans needs to be demonstrated. However, early Japanese studies have shown optimistic results which should be followed carefully [2,8].

While abdominal and pelvic tumors may be difficult to heat there is an option of treating esophageal tumors by means of intracavitary hyperthermia. This has been utilized in several studies applying various intracavitary heating techniques. One of the most extensive investigations is a Soviet trial by Kochegarov et al. [11], which showed a significant improvement in both local recurrence and survival in cases where hyperthermia was added to radiotherapy in the treatment of advanced esophageal cancer (Table 3). Similar results from China and Japan have been published where combined hyperthermia, radiotherapy, and chemotherapy have been used preoperatively in patients with advanced esophageal tumors [2, 9, 15, 23].

A special situation in which hyperthermia may be advantageous is in association with interoperative radiation [1]. A single heat treatment is likely to result in significant tumor damage if given properly, and this provides a rationale for using hyperthermia in the treatment of macroscopically persistent tumors during an interoperative procedure. The heating techniques in this situation will be much easier and can be performed by an external applicator, using microwaves, or RF heating, or by interstitial hyperthermia with implanted electrodes. Since hyperthermia in this situation can be given almost selectively to tumors, relatively high temperatures can be applied [16, 19]. If such treatment in association with radiotherapy is further combined with a hypoxic sensitizer (e.g., misonidazole) is it likely that significant improvement will be achieved [13]. Experimentally, this treatment principle has shown a remarkable effect. In a study with a mouse adenocarcinoma, which requires 56 Gy to be controlled by a single dose of radiation alone, this dose could be reduced to below 4 Gy (an enhancement ratio of about 15) if simultaneous hyperthermia at 43.5 °C was supplied for 1 h together with a dose of misonidazole [13]. This certainly is a treatment schedule which deserves further clinical investigation. It should be understood that this treatment schedule can be optimally applied only under circumstances where either radiotherapy or hyperthermia is given selectively to the tumor area, since it otherwise risks increasing damage to normal tissue as well, although to a far lesser extent. This situation exists with "intraoperative" radiotherapy and the increased use of hyperthermia as an adjuvant in gastrointestinal cancer is a challenge which should be met.

In conclusion, there is a biological rationale for using hyperthermia to improve the local control of advanced gastrointestinal tumors. The early clinical trials have established that the biological rationale can be transferred to the clinical situation, but the technical difficulties related to heat treatment of pelvic and abdominal tumors need to be solved before a final answer to the question raised in the title of this paper can be given. Although this is not likely to occur within a short time, the possibility of adding hyperthermia to the armamentarium of the gastrointestinal oncologist appears so advantageous that it should indeed be further explored. Such investigation should include an attempt to identify the role of hyperthermia in interoperative radiotherapy.

References

1. Abe M (1984) Intraoperative radiation therapy for gastrointestinal malignancy. In: Decosse JJ, Sherlock P (eds) *Clinical management of gastrointestinal cancer*. Nijhoff, Boston, pp 327–349
2. Abe M, Takahashi M, Sugahara T (eds) (1984) *Hyperthermia in cancer therapy*. Proceedings of the first annual meeting of the Japanese Society of Hyperthermia Oncology, Tokyo
3. Dewey WC, Freeman ML, Raaphorst GP, Clark EP, Wong RSL, Highfield DP, Spiro IJ, Tamasovic SP, Denman DL, Coss RA (1980) Cell biology of hyperthermia and radiation. In: Meyn RE, Withers HR (eds) Radiation biology in cancer research. Raven, New York, pp 589–621
4. Field SB, Bleehen NM (1979) Hyperthermia in the treatment of cancer. Cancer Treat Rev 6: 63–94
5. Gibbs FA (1984) Regional Hyperthermia: a clinical appraisal of noninvasive deep-heating method. Cancer Research [Suppl] 44: 4765s–4770s
6. Gunderson LL, Sosin H (1974) Areas of failure found at re-operation (second or symptomatic look) following "curative surgery" for adenocarcinoma of the rectum: clinicopathologic correlation and implications for adjuvant therapy. Cancer 34: 1278–1292
7. Gunderson LL, Martin JK, O'Connell MJ, Beart RW, Kvols LK, Nagorney DM (1986) Local control and survival in locally advanced gastrointestinal cancer. *Int J Radiat Oncol Biol Phys* 12: 661–665
8. Hiraoka M, Jo S, Takahashi M, Abe M (1984) Thermometry results of RF capacitive heating for human deep-seated tumors. In: Overgaard J (ed) *Hyperthermic oncology, vol 1*. Taylor and Francis, London, pp 609–612

9. Kai H, Ueo H, Sugimachi K, Inokuchi K, Shiragami T, Kawai Y (1985) Hyperthermo-chemo-radiotherapy and esophageal carcinoma. In: Abe et al. (eds) *Hyperthermia in cancer therapy*. Proceedings of the first annual meeting of the Japanese Society of Hyperthermia Oncology, Tokyo

10. Kapp DS (1986) Site and disease selection for hyperthermic clinical trials. Int J Hyperthermia 2: 139–156

11. Kochegarov AA, Muratkhodzhaev NK, Alimnazarov ShA (1980) Hyperthermia in the combined treatment of esophageal cancer patients. Vopr Onkol 26: 19–24

12. Overgaard J (1980) Simultaneous and sequential hyperthermia and radiation treatment of an experimental tumor and its surrounding normal tissue in vivo. *Int J Radiat Oncol Biol Phys* 6: 1507–1517

13. Overgaard J (1980) Effect of misonidazole and hyperthermia on the radiosensitivity of a C3H mouse mammary carcinoma and its surrounding normal tissue. Br J Cancer 41: 10–21

14. Overgaard J (1981) Fractionated radiation and hyperthermia. Experimental and clinical studies. Cancer 48: 1116–1123

15. Overgaard J (ed) (1985) *Hyperthermic oncology,* vols 1, 2. Taylor and Francis, London

16. Overgaard J (1985) Hyperthermia and radiation – an update of biological and clinical experience. Proceedings of the XVI international congress of radiology, pp 211–217

17. Overgaard J (1987) The design of clinical trials in hyperthermic oncology. In: Franconi C, Field SB (eds) *Physics and technology of hyperthermia*. Nijhoff, Dordrecht, pp 598–620

18. Overgaard J, Nielsen OS (1983) The importance of thermotolerance for the clinical treatment with hyperthermia. Radioth Oncol 1: 167–178

19. Overgaard J, Nielsen OS, Lindegaard JC (1987) Biological basis for rational design of clinical treatment with combined hyperthermia and radiation. In: Franconi C, Field SB (eds) *Physics and technology of hyperthermia*. Nijhoff, Dordrecht, pp 54–79

20. Overgaard M, Overgaard J, Sell A (1984) Dose-response relationship for radiation therapy of recurrent, residual, and primarily inoperable colorectal cancer. Radiother Oncol 1: 217–225

21. Rich T, Gunderson LL, Galdabini J, Cohen, AM, Donaldson G (1983) Clinical and pathologic factors influencing local failure after curative resection of carcinoma of the rectum and rectosigmoid. Cancer 52: 1317–1329

22. Sapozink MD, Gibbs FA, Egger MJ, Stewart JR (1986) Regional hyperthermia for clinically advanced deep-seated pelvic malignancy. *Am J Clin Oncol (CCT)* 9(2): 162–169

23. Sha Y-H, Li D-J, Qui S-L, Hou F-X, Li Z-C, Zhao Y-Z (1984) The combined treatment of esophageal cancer – a clinical pathological study of 42 cases. In: Overgaard J (ed) *Hyperthermic oncology,* vol 1. Taylor and Francis, London, pp 371–374

24. Strohbehn JW (1985) Summary of physical and technical studies. In: Overgaard J (ed) *Hyperthermic oncology 1984,* vol 2. Taylor and Francis, London, pp 353–369

25. Suit HD (1982) Potential for improving survival rates for the cancer patient by increasing the efficacy of treatment of the primary lesion. Cancer 50: 1227–1234

26. Suit HD, Westgate SJ (1986) Impact of improved local control on survival. *Int J Radiat Oncol Biol Phys* 12: 453–458

27. Tepper JE (1986) Adjuvant irradiation of gastrointestinal malignancies: impact on local control and tumour cure. *Int J Radiat Oncol Biol Phys* 12: 667–671

Intraperitoneal Chemotherapy and Immunotherapy

B. E. Wolf and P. H. Sugarbaker

Health Science Center, University School of Medicine, 1327 Clifton Road N.E., Atlanta, GA 30322, USA

Introduction

Treatment failures following putatively curative resections for circumscribed neoplasms are well recognized and the recurrence patterns have been analyzed. These observations compel us to reshape our conceptual model, for such cancers, from one of malignancy as a localized process to that of a regionalized process. Consequently, treatments should evolve to include not only the primary cancer (removed by surgery) but also the entire anatomic region (peritoneal cavity). Regionalized processes command a combined-modality approach to effect cure or, at least, to favorably alter the natural history of the disease. It follows, then, that if for a given neoplasm the available agents are not ideal and, furthermore, that no new agents have been developed in the recent past that offer a hope of improved survival; we must exploit the agents at hand in the most effective manner.

The intraperitoneal administration of chemotherapy is such a strategem, and is the focus of this review. We will discuss the theoretical models for transperitoneal drug distributions that have been the impetus for pharmacokinetic and clinical investigations and then discuss the natural history of gastrointestinal and ovarian malignancies in order to establish an anatomic pattern of treatment failure that is suited to I.P. therapy.

Finally, we will examine the experience with traditional chemical therapeutics administered by the i.p. route and consider future prospects that may utilize biologic response modifiers and monoclonal antibodies.

The Models

The peritoneal cavity behaves, pharmacokinetically, similarly to the pleural and pericardial cavities and the cerebrospinal fluid space [1–3]. These third spaces possess membranous boundaries that are diffusion barriers to the systemic release of directly instilled drugs.

Much of the work on i.p. therapy derives from the insights of Chabner and Young [2]. While investigating the effects of large-volume pleural effusions and peritoneal ascites upon intravenous drug pharmacokinetics and toxicology, they found that immediately following dosing, when plasma levels were high, the third-space fluid was accumulating drug, and, in fact, that eventually the "ascitic" fluid drug concentration exceeded that of the plasma. They deduced that a diffusion barrier associated with the limiting boundary of the third space was responsible for the observations.

The Compartmental Model

Dedrick and colleagues then created mathematical models describing the concentration gradients to be expected across body compartments [4–9]. Their elegant mathematics appear in Appendix A. Many experimental data have subsequently been accumulated which support the validity of the models. The initial model is a (two-) compartment analysis of the kinetics of drug exchange between the peritoneal fluid and plasma (Fig. 1).

In the model:

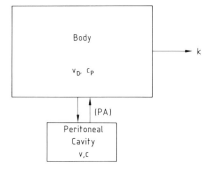

Fig. 1. Two-compartment open model for peritoneal pharmacokinetics. V_D, volume of distribution; C_P, drug concentration; A, area; P, permeability; PA, intercompartmental transport; V, volume; C, concentration. (Reprinted with permission [4])

For the moment, we will ignore the transport process. When $K >> PA$, at a steady state, $Cp < C$.

This is borne out in experiments in which mannitol was injected i.p. in rats: peritoneal concentrations exceed plasma concentrations by an order of magnitude in the steady state [10]. Such a pattern is to be expected with molecules that distribute evenly in the fluid phases (Fig. 2). Therefore, such a model has broad implications for traditional chemotherapeutic drugs, as they are almost exclusively hydrophilic [3].

This simple model understates the pharmacokinetic advantage of i.p. administration. Significant metabolism of drug in a "first-pass" phenomenon would markedly reduce bioavailability, greatly increasing the advantage of i.p. administration.

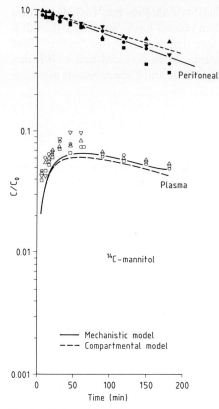

Fig. 2. Peritoneal-to-plasma transport of [^{14}C] mannitol. Dimentionless concentration vs time (min). Plasma concentrations are denoted by *open symbols* and peritoneal concentrations by *solid symbols*. *Solid lines* represent distributed model output, *dashed lines* represent compartmental model output.

Studies suggest that as much as 80% of drug absorbed into plasma passes initially through the portal system [11, 12]. The prospects of very high peritoneal drug concentrations with subtoxic plasma concentrations is an exploitable advantage.

To calculate concentration with respect to time (drug activity), we need to know the clearances and other pharmacokinetic parameters. PA in the human can be estimated by either (a) extrapolating from experimental systems or (b) estimating from chemical measurements of various molecules and then making correlations with specific molecular properties. Such an analysis has been shown for the clearance of urea and insulin in rats, rabbits, dogs, and human beings [13]. The linear, almost parallel relationship has a slope of two thirds, which tells us that the area of the peritoneum varies as two thirds the power of body weight (Fig. 3). A similar exponential relationship exists for body surface area vs. body weight. Hence, the two area measurements are proportional. Measurements in human beings show that PA (clearance) of drug from the peritoneal cavity decreases in proportion to

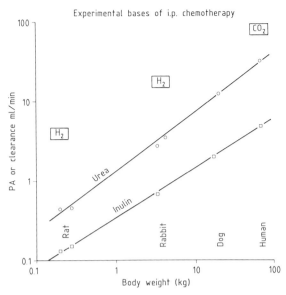

Fig. 3. Mass transfer coefficient of clearance for urea and insulin in several species. For reference, dissolved gas clearance is shown for hydrogen in the rat and the rabbit and for carbon dioxide in man.

the one-half power of molecular weight [13]. In other words, after i.p. drug instillation, the larger the drug molecule, the slower it crosses the peritoneal membrane and the greater the difference in drug concentration between the peritoneal cavity and plasma.

The model predicts that the best circumstances and drugs for attainment of a kinetic advantage from i.p. administration are:

1. Drugs with a high ratio of plasma to peritoneal clearance
2. Administration in a large volume without any concomitant drugs that might lower plasma clearance (complete for hepatic and/or renal excretion)
3. Use for tumors with a minimal thickness (volume)

It is assumed that the drug is well mixed in the intraperitoneal fluid and that this fluid is in contact with the entire peritoneal surface; this implies sufficient intra-abdominal fluid to cause distention. In the simplicity of this model lie its limitations [14]. The consequences of significant lipid solubility, which might greatly increase transcellular transport, are not considered, nor is the issue of tissue penetration addressed.

The Distributed Model

The compartmental analysis of generalized "lumped parameters" is utilitarian, but it fails to describe all the phenomena that have been recorded. Thus, Dedrick et al.

Table 1. Absorption of intraperitoneally administered antineo-plastic agents in the rat [21]

Drug	% Absorbed[a]	MWT	K (heptane)
Asparaginase	9	133.000	0.1
Doxorubicin[b]	10	544	...
Bleomycin	12,3	1.400	0.002
Methotrexate	15	472	0.001
Actinomycin D[b]	21	1.255	0.23
cis-DDP	24.6	300	<0.001
Melphalan	25.0	323	0.1
5-FU	28.4	130	0.09
Ara C	29.5	243	0.006
Thiotepa[b]	74.4	188	0.21
Hexamethylmelamine[b]	91.7	210	11.2

[a] Percent absorbed over 1 h.
[b] Drugs whose lipid solubility caused significant increase in percent absorved over 1 h.

developed a spatially distributed model of solute transport between the peritoneal cavity and the plasma [5–10]. Drug penetration into tumor, defined by the concentration gradient from peritoneum into the tissue, is predicted by this theory. The actual tissue drug-concentration gradient is a function of the rates of diffusion and convection through the tissue and the rates of removal by chemical reaction and uptake into capillaries or lymphatics.

There are three exits from the peritoneum: (a) diffusion through the parietal peritoneal surfaces, (b) diffusion through visceral peritoneal surfaces, (c) absorption through lymphatics. Lymphatic drainage is a significant mode of egress for particles the size of small proteins or larger, such as India ink, colloidal chromic 32p-phosphate, red blood cells, and tumor cells [15, 16]. Absorption occurs through intracellular pores and transcellularly. The former is governed by the sign of the molecule (Stokes-Einstein radius). Transcellular movement is through a bilayer lipid membrane and is a function of lipid solubility. The permeability constants for antineoplastic drugs for lipids are given in Table 1. Excepting hexamethylmelamine, most antineoplastic agents are hydrophilic with a pKa of approximately 0.02 or less. Therefore, molecular weight is the determinant of peritoneal absorption for these drugs.

The peritoneal surface has both a parietal and a visceral component. In general, the venous drainage of the parietal layer is to the systemic circulation, that of the visceral to the portal circulation [3].

Because of the redundancy of the visceral peritoneal surface, the surface area is much greater than the parietal peritoneal surface area. Outside of the peritoneum, capillary flow, local metabolism, and tissue binding are the constituents of whole-body clearance. The former exhibits first-order kinetics, the latter two may be saturable processes bringing to bear on a non-linear relationship for drug clearance. In a simple analysis, we assume the capillaries to be uniformly distributed and that

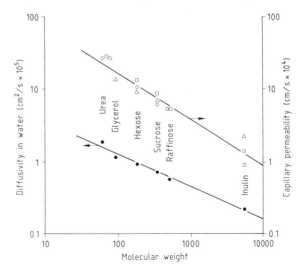

Fig. 4. Capillary permeability and agneous diffusitivty of marker molecules vs. molecular weight. ◯, cat leg; ☐, human forearm; △, dog heart.

metabolism, convection, and lymphatic uptake are negligible. Then, in the steady state, the drug concentration in the tissue will approach its peak concentration exponentially [10]. Penetration is related to the ratio of capillary permeability to intratissue diffusivity.

Experimentally, we find that capillary permeability is inversely related to the 0.6 power of molecular weight and diffusivity in water to the 0.5 power (Fig. 4). Now, if we describe our tissue as water, then our model predicts, perhaps surprisingly, that larger molecules penetrate more deeply. However, for very large molecules our initial analysis must be expanded to incorporate convection and lymphatic transport. Depth of penetration of small and large molecules have been studied using quantitative autoradiography. Flessner studied radioisotopically labelled EDTA and human serum albumin [6, 7]. He found that for the small molecule, tissue concentration decreased rapidly with distance from surface, reaching 10% within 400–500 µm (Fig. 5). Findings for protein molecules were surprisingly different. Over the visceral tissues concentration decreased with distance, though more slowly; over the parietal tissues the concentration was both high and constant (Fig. 6). There are two explanations:

1. Peritoneal pressure is expressed across the entire abdominal wall. Therefore, the transabdominal wall pressure is the peritoneal minus atmospheric pressure. This is the driving force for convection through the parietal component. The visceral surface has little transmural pressure; convection forces are low [10].
2. The lymphatic drainage of the visceral tissue is rich, that of the parietal comparatively poor. Lymphatic drainage as a constituent of whole-body clearance is less effective in the parietal tissues.

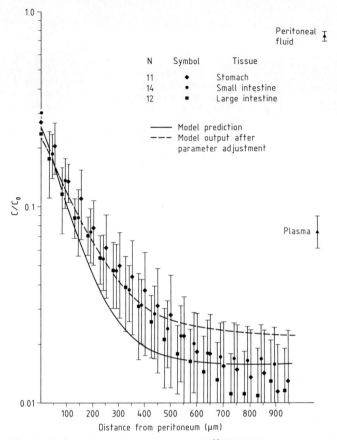

Fig. 5. Peritoneal-to-plasma transport of [^{14}C] EDTA: gastrointestinal tract tissue concentration gradients (concentration in wet tissue divided by Co vs. distance in μm from peritoneum). Dialysis solution is Inpersol (1.5% dextrose). *Solid line* represents distributed model prediction, *dashed line* represents model output with a doubled intratissue diffusion adjustment. (Reprinted with permission [8])

To summarize, the compartment model very adequately predicts peritoneal and plasma drug concentrations following i. p. administration. In order to consider the subtleties of solute transport, and tissue penetration in particular, a distributed model is used. The ramifications of the distributed theory remain to be fully explored.

Technical Considerations

The first principle of i. p. drug administration is to use sufficient volumes of fluid. Empirically, 1500–2000 ml is usually needed to obtain uniform distribution of solute within the abdominal cavity. Computed tomography of the abdomen after instillation of 50–100 ml of 25% hypaque per liter of instillate reveals uniform distribution even in patients with extensive peritoneal carcinomatosis or adhesions [17].

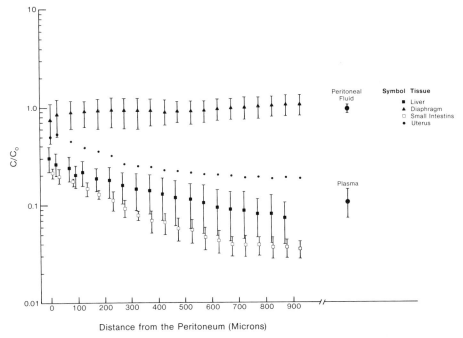

Flessner et al, Am J Physiol, 1985

Fig. 6. Peritoneal-to-plasma transport of ^{125}I-labeled human serum albumin. Tissue concentration (based on wet tissue wt.) divided by initial peritoneal concentration vs. distance in μm from peritoneum. Duration of dialysis, 185 min. (Reprinted with permission [7])

Small-volume instillation tends to pool near the site of injection and is therefore ineffective [14].

Peritoneal access for i. p. administration borrows from the experience of continuous ambulatory peritoneal dialysis for chronic renal failure [18–20] Tenckhoff [19] developed a simple fenestrated silastic catheter with an acceptable incidence of complications. There are three principle methods of access in use: Tenckhoff catheters and variants thereof, implantable Port-a-Cath systems, and repeated paracentesis and instillation. Preferences are individual and complications are not dissimilar [21].

The Tenckhoff catheter may be the gold standard, but it is associated with high maintenance requirements and poor patient acceptability (Table 2). The Port-a-Cath is, in effect, maintenance free and has a higher patient acceptability; however, it does not allow the rapid inflow and outflows possible with the Tenckhoff (Fig. 7). Use of single use catheters run the risks of repeated peritoneal punctures.

Placement of semipermanent catheters, such as a Tenckhoffs catheter, is performed in the operating room with a sterile technique [22–25]. The catheter is placed through the anterior abdominal wall, just lateral to the m. rectus abdominus, usually at the level of the umbilicus (Fig. 8). The peritoneum/fascia is secured about the catheter and the catheter is then tunneled subcutaneously 5–7 cm later-

Table 2. Complications of Tenckhoff catheter function in 143 patients [21]

	NCI (n=71)	Amsterdam (n=53)	NYU (n=19)	Total no (%)
Partial outflow obstruction	12	15	2	29 (20)
Total inability to drain	14	10	10	34 (23)
Total inflow obstruction	3	3	0	6 (4.1)
Infections				
exit site	3	6	0	9 (6.2)
intra-abdominal	3	4	1	8 (5.5)
Respiratory difficulty	1	0	1	2 (1.3)
Discomfort, irritation	14	NA	2	>16 (>11.1)

NCI, National Cancer institute; *Amsterdam,* Netherlands Cancer Institute; *NYU,* New York University Medical Center; *NA,* not available.

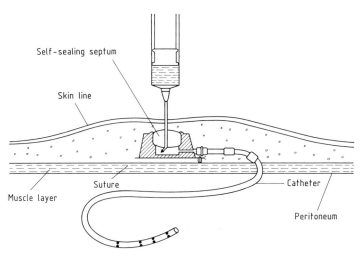

Fig. 7. Port-A-Cath i. p. system, consisting of an implanted portal and a Tenckhoff catheter. (Reprinted with permission [12])

ally before exiting the skin. Placement of the catheter through the linea alba has a higher incidence of leakage.

Following insertion, catheters are maintained by the strict aseptic techniques used for dialysis patients. A relaxed method of Tenckhoff maintenance after the wounds have healed, consisting of daily shower of catheter and skin with soap and water, followed by the application of an occlusive sterile dressing, resulted in no differences in the incidence of catheter removal for infection when compared with the strict technique [22]. This may not be true in a compromised host.

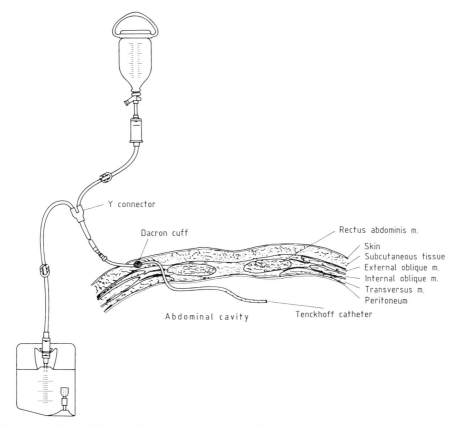

Fig. 8. Position of Tenckhoff catheter. Catheter is placed through the anterior abdominal wall just lateral to the m. rectus abdominis. The Dacron cuff is infiltrated by fibrous tissue from the surrounding subcutaneous fat. A Y connector and clamps allow fluid to run into the abdominal cavity, dwell, then drain out. (Reprinted with permission of *Surgery, Gynecology & Obstetrics* [22])

Natural History of Gastrointestinal and Ovarian Malignancies

Initial investigations with intraperitoneal chemotherapy were derivative of the observation that ovarian cancer is predominantly an intraperitoneal disease [26]. Though malignant tumors of the ovary may arise from epithelial, stromal, or germinal cells, 85% are of epithelial origin and are termed "ovarian cancer" for the purposes of intraperitoneal considerations. Table 3 shows the FIGO staging with 5-year survivals. Symptoms tend to appear late [27, 28]; on presentation only 25% of patients are in stage I or stage II.

Primary surgery permits staging, histopathologic grading, and optimal cytoreduction. Aggressive debulking of disease, which reduces residual tumor to nodules of less than 2 cm, may result in improved survival and quality of life. It is this small-volume residual disease in the peritoneum for which our theoretical foundation predicts successful drug penetration into tumor [29–37].

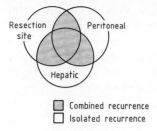

☐ Combined recurrence
☐ Isolated recurrence

Fig. 9. Treatment failure in large-bowel cancer patients. A small percentage have isolated recurrence as peritoneal carcinomatosis, hepatic metastases, or loco-regional disease. A large majority have combined recurrence. Successful adjuvants must be designed to treat all sites of treatment failure

Table 3. Staging scheme of the International Federation of Gynecology and Obstetrics for ovarian cancer and survival rates following surgery ± irradiation and/or single-agent chemotherapy

Stage	Five-year survival (%)
I. Growth limited to ovaries	60
A. Growth limited to one ovary; no ascites	
B. Growth limited to both ovaries; no ascites	
C. Tumor stage I A or I B plus ascites or malignant cells in peritoneal washings	
II. Growth involving one or both ovaries with pelvic extension	39
A. Extension or metastases or both to uterus or tubes or both	
B. Extension to other pelvic tissues	
C. Tumor stage II A or II B plus ascites or malignant cells in peritoneal washings	
III. Growth involving one or both ovaries with intraperitoneal metastases outside the pelvis or positive retroperitoneal nodes, or both; tumor limited to true pelvis with histologically proven malignant extension to small bowel or omentum	6
IV. Growth involving one or both ovaries with distant metastases; pleural effusion must contain malignant cells to indicate stage-IV disease; parenchymal liver metastases indicates stage-IV disease	4

The anatomic sites of recurrence for colon and rectal cancer following primary surgery have been defined by several series [12, 38]. Accurate determination of peritoneal carcinomatosis requires direct inspection, given the current limitations of imaging technology. Tong found peritoneal disease in 44% of patients explored with curative intent as a second-look surgical procedure [39]. Consideration of these several studies leads to the conclusion that the common sites of treatment failure after surgical resection of large-bowel adenocarcinomas are (a) the resection site and adjacent lymph nodes, (b) the liver, and (c) the peritoneal surfaces, and that most patients eventually develop a mixed pattern of recurrence (Fig. 9).

Gastric cancer, classically linked with the metastatic Krukenberg tumor implants upon ovaries, would seem to be another disease process in which i.p. chemotherapy may be advantagenus [40–42]. Likewise, any intra-abdominal cancer extending to the overlying serosa can result in peritoneal carcinomatosis.

In particular, then, there are select patient populations in which the predisposition to peritoneal carcinomatosis is increased. These include patients with perforated large-bowel cancer, mucinous large-bowel cancer, and ovarian cancer and those in whom there has been intra-abdominal spillage of tumor cells. These are the classes of patients for whom i.p. chemotherapy may favorably alter the natural history of the disease.

Chemotherapies

Clinical trials with i.p. chemotherapy have recently been reviewed by Brenner [43]. Experience with 5-FU, methotrexate, cisplatin, doxorubicin, melphalan, and cytosine arabinoside are presented.

Intraperitoneal 5-FU has been used in controlling malignant ascites for several decades [44–46]. Dedrick's compartment model predicts a significant peritoneal-to-plasma concentration ratio. Work by Speyer et al. at the NCI revealed: (a) a PA of 14 ml/min and a concentration gradient of 298; (b) a sharp dose-response curve, demonstrating saturable kinetics; (c) high portal vein drug concentrations; and (d) dose limited by systemic toxicity [47]. 5-FU clearance is rate limited by the enzyme dihydrouracil dehydrogenase. This enzyme is found in the liver and the lung. Dose-limiting toxicities are myelosuppression, nausea, vomiting, chemical peritonitis, and mucositis. Sugarbaker et al. reported the results of a prospective randomized trial of 66 patients with advanced primary colorectal cancer, each receiving 5-FU, either i.v. or i.p. [12]. No difference was found in survival or disease-free interval. What was found was that in the i.p. group the incidence of first recurrence in the peritoneum was decreased, while the incidence of extraperitoneal recurrence increased. The dose-limiting factor in this study was abdominal pain from chemical irritation of peritoneal surfaces.

Methotrexate has been well studied [48, 49]. Furthermore, we know that leucovorin is an effective blocking agent against methotrexate and that when administered systemically, it tends to stay in the plasma [50]. Howell studied i.p. methotrexate using i.v. leucovorin to limit the systemic toxicity of myelosuppression. He found that when leucovorin administration was adjusted to keep plasma methotrexate levels below 50 mmol, toxicity was expressed primarily by thrombocytopenia, which was well tolerated. Intraperitoneally, the limiting toxicity is chemical peritonitis. A 100-fold concentration advantage was measured. One of 18 patients with ovarian cancer responded.

Cisplatin is one of the most effective drugs in the ovarian cancer armamentarium [51, 52]. When administered in hypertonic saline dialysate, with concomitant systemic thiosulfate, its nephrotoxicity is abated [53, 54]. Data from studies by ten Bokkel-Huinink et al. [55] and by Cohen [35] suggest that i.p. cisplatin may be able to salvage some patients with small-volume residual disease. Pretorius et al. found that three patients who had previously failed to respond to i.v. cisplatin responded to i. p. administration [56]. Responses in this refractory group are encouraging.

Doxorubicin, though appropriate for i. p. chemotherapy from a kinetic stance, is limited in its usefulness because of the frequency of chemical peritonitis at modest doses [57].

Melphalan, like cisplatin, appears to be effective in the treatment of ovarian cancer. Furthermore, the compartment analysis predicts a quantitative pharmacokinetic advantage for i. p. administration [58]. Perhaps most intriguing is the fact that melphalan uptake by cells requires active transport by the amino-acid transport system. This uptake is inhibited by glutamine. Therefore, Holcenberg et al. co-administered glutaminase i. p. to patients, utilizing the enzyme as a local "cytotoxic enhancer" [59]. Fortuitously, glutaminase is rapidly cleared from the systemic circulation. Use of enhancement agents may prove invaluable in the delivery of cytotoxic doses of antineoplastic drugs.

Cytosine arabinoside has been studied as a single-agent chemotherapy. It offers an i. p. concentration advantage of 300–1000. Studies by King et al. resulted in two responses in a group of ten patients with advanced ovarian cancer [60].

Multiple-agent i. p. studies with cisplatin-cytosine arabinoside with or without the addition of doxorubicin have been evaluated by Markman et al. [61, 62]. The addition of doxorubicin increased the incidence of abdominal pain but did not improve efficacy. Responses were noted in 21 of 56 patients with ovarian cancer. The effect upon survival is not clear.

Selection of cytotoxic agents for use in i. p. chemotherapy is dependent upon a kinetic advantage for the route and the effectiveness of the drug. The former is predictable on the basis of molecular characteristics; the latter is an empirical determination. Furthermore, individual patient responses for the cancers we are treating by the i. p. route differ. Ideally, we can individualize the selection of agents to the partricular characteristic of a given tumor, recognizing that within each tumor there is some variation of the cellular population. The human clonogenic assay (HCTA) developed by von Hoff provides a technique analogous to the microbiology technique of antibiotic sensitivity testing [63]. At this time, in vitro predictions of in vivo activity are quite accurate for drug resistance but not as well attuned to sensitivity. Potentially, the HTCA is an invaluable tool for chemotherapeutic selection.

Ovarian carcinoma is an entity almost exclusively confined to the peritoneum during its natural progression. Colon and rectal carcinoma recurrence patterns following primary surgical resection reveal failure at the resection site, the liver, and the peritoneal surfaces. A similar pattern of treatment failure with regard to anatomic distribution is seen in other gastrointestinal cancers. One would infer that antineoplastic drug administration i. p., into the cavity confinement of recurrent cancer, would be most effective in the treatment of these cancers.

The ideal mechanical delivery system for i. p. administration does not exist. There are advantages as well as disadvantages to each of the principle systems.

In the clinical trials that have been carried out to date, the pharmacokinetic advantage of i. p. administration of antineoplastic drugs has not translated into a survival advantage. Experience with 5-FU in colorectal cancer suggest that i. p. administration prolongs the time course to intracavity recurrence, while extracavity recurrence is unaffected. Combined trials with i.p. cisplatin and cytosine arabinoside hold some promise.

Future prospects for intraperitoneal treatments include the sequential use of antineoplastic treatments to all sites of treatment failure. In addition, new therapeutic agents need to be critically tested locoregionally. Biological response modifiers (interleukin-2 and interferon gamma) and monoclonal antibodies are considered potentially valuable treatment options for intra-abdominal malignancy.

Intraperitoneal Immunotherapy

Another agent to be tested i.p. in patients with recurrent cancer confined to the abdominal cavity is interferon gamma. When exposed to peripheral blood monocytes, this biological response modifier causes monocyte activation so that fresh tumor cells are lysed in vitro. To test the feasibility of the adoptive transfer of large numbers of interferon gamma-activated monocytes in patients with intra-abdominal recurrence of colon cancer, a trial was begun at the NCI [64]. We treated six patients with the adoptive transfer of peripheral blood monocytes given every 2 weeks. Patients were treated with cytoreductive surgery prior to the initiation of monocyte therapy. These trials showed that i.p. adoptive transfer of autologous monocytes is possible. No survival benefit was possible to discern in this non-randomized trial, but results are encouraging and suggest the need for further studies.

Some surprisingly good preliminary results with interferon alpha have been reported by Berek et al. with Eastern Cooperative Oncology Group (ECOG) [64]. They used interferon alpha i.p. in patients with recurrent ovarian cancer; the patients showed complete response. Pharmacokintic data showed two orders of magnitude concentration differences in the peritoneal cavity over the plasma. These interesting studies need to be vigorously pursued.

Predictions from the distributed model for i.p. chemotherapy suggest that larger molecules may give higher tissue levels than small molecules. Antibodies bearing radioactive iodine or chemotherapy drug labels may be used to selectively treat tumor nodules with high concentrations of antineoplastic agents. Time of exposure, concentration of antibody, and its specificity for tumor antigens may all be important in determining a therapeutic effect.

Lotze and colleagues studied the i.p. administration of IL-2 (interleukin-2) [65]. They found peritoneal concentrations two orders of magnitude greater than serum levels and also measured greater than 100-fold increases in the i.p. mononuclear cell populations. These observations are consistent with our theoretical model predictions for large molecules and suggest that combined i.p. IL-2 and lymphokine-activated killer cells may be a fruitful area for further investigation.

Conclusions

Two models exist for predicting the pharmacokinetics of antineoplastic drugs instilled into the peritoneal cavity. The simpler compartmental model assumes that the changes in drug distribution are solely dependent upon movement across a peritoneal membrane. This model fails to consider changes in drug distribution that may occur as a result of lipid solubility, molecular size, and anatomic variations within the abdominal cavity (parietal vs. visceral peritoneal surfaces). The distributed model takes these variables into account but does so by markedly complicating the mathematical formula by which drug concentrations are predicted. A contrast may exist between drug effects in tumors of different vascularity when drug delivery is by the i.v. or i.p. route. Response are not expected with i.v. drug administration in tumors with minimal vascularity. Just the opposite may occur with i.p. drug delivery and minimally vascularized tumors. The distributed model predicts better drug penetration into poorly vascularized tumor than into vascularized tissue for i.p. administration. This is because drug enters the avascular tissue and is not removed by capillaries or lymphactics.

Concentration differences between peritoneal fluid and plasma of one to three orders of magnitude are predicted and observed. The clinical implications of this concentration difference are markedly improved locoregional drug delivery. Also, a greater proportion of clinical responses from increased concentration-over-time (area under the curve) should be evident.

Summary

1. The predictive model is validated empirically; a kinetic advantage for i.p. administration of certain antineoplastic drugs exist.
2. The concentrations achieved in the peritoneum are orders of magnitude greater than those found in the plasma, so rate-limiting systemic toxicities may be avoided.
3. The aspirin principle – if one is good, two are better – may not be applicable unless we can utilize this advantage to improve survival.

Appendix. Mathematical model describing the concentration gradients to be expected across body compartments [5]

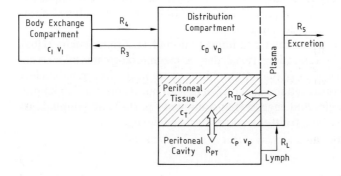

Mass balances on the various compartments yield the following equations

$$\frac{d(C_pV_p)}{dt} = -(R_L + R_{PT}) \tag{1}$$

$$\frac{\partial C_T^x}{\partial t} = D_{EFF}\frac{\partial^2 C_T}{\partial x^2} - \frac{\partial(fJ_vC_T)}{\partial x} - J_aa \tag{2}$$

$$\frac{d(C_DV_D)}{dt} = R_{TD} + R_L + R_4 - (R_3 + R_5) \tag{3}$$

$$\frac{d(C_IV_I)}{dt} = R_3 - R_4 \tag{4}$$

where

C_I concentration in compartment i (g/ml)
V_I volume of compartment i (ml)
t time (s)
x   distance coordinate (cm from peritoneum)
D_{EFF} effective tissue diffusivity (cm²/s)
f   retardation factor
$J_v(x)$ local volume flux through tissue (cm³·cm⁻²·s⁻¹)
J_aa effective solute transfer per unit volume of tissue (g·s⁻¹·ml⁻¹)
R_L rate of mass transfer via lymphatics (g/s)
R_{PT} rate of mass transfer between peritoneal cavity and the tissue (g/s)
R_{TD} rate of mass transfer between peritoneal tissue and the distribution compartment (g/s)
R_3, R_4 intercompartmental mass transfer (g/s)
R_5 rate of excretion of tracer (g/s)

A balance on the volume in the peritoneal cavity yields

$$\frac{dV_P}{dt} = -[F_L + (J_aa)AX_1] \tag{5}$$

where

F_L effective rate of lymph flow (ml/s)
J_aa local transcapillary volume transport (ml·ml⁻¹·s⁻¹)
A apparent peritoneal surface area (cm²)
X_1 thickness of tissue (cm)

Positive values of F_L and J_aa correspond to flow from the cavity.
   Volumes of the other two compartments have been assumed constant

$$\frac{dV_1}{dt} = \frac{dV_D}{dt} = 0 \tag{6}$$

The rate law defining the rate of mass transfer via lymphatics is

$$R_L = F_LC_P \tag{7}$$

The rate of mass transfer from the peritoneal cavity to the tissue cand be obtained as a boundary condition to the tissue space

$$R_{PT} = -D_{EFF}A\frac{\partial C_T}{\partial x}\Big|_{x=0} + fJ_vAC_T\Big|_{x=0} \tag{8}$$

The local volume flux in tissue can be modeled as

$$J_v(x) = (J_c a) - (J_c a)x \tag{9}$$

where

$J_c a$ $L_P a[P_T - P_D - \Sigma\sigma_c (\Pi_T - \Pi_D)]$
$L_P a$ capillary hydraulic permeability ($ml \cdot ml^{-1} \cdot mmHg^{-1}$)
c   capillary reflection coefficient for osmotic solute
Π_i osmotic pressure of osmotic solute in compartment i (mmHg)
   The macromolecular transcapillary solute flux can be modeled as

$$J_a a = - K_a(C_D) \tag{10}$$

The rate of mass transfer into the plasma (or into the well-mixed distribution compartment) may now be found. At any time it is the integral of *Eq. 10A* within the tissue space

$$R_{TD} = \int_0^{X_1} (J_a a) A \, dx \tag{11}$$

The rate expressions governing the masss transfer between the body exchange compartment and the distribution compartment and the excretion rate are

$$R_3 = K_3 C_D V_D; \quad R_4 = K_4 C_1 V_1; \quad R_5 = K_5 C_D V_D \tag{12}$$

Boundary conditions are as follows

at $t = 0$, $C_P = C_0$; $C_D = C_1 = C_T(x, 0) = 0$
or $C_D = C_0$; $C_P = C_1 = C_T(x, 0) = 0$ $\tag{13}$
and at $x = X_1$, $\partial C_T / \partial x = 0$

References

1. Clarkson B, O'Connor A, Wilson L et al. (1964) The physiologic disposition of 5-fluorouracil and 5-fluoro-2(1)-deoxyuridine in man. Clin Pharmacol Ther 5: 581–610
2. Chabner BA, Young RC (1973) Threshold methotrexate concentration for in vivo inhibition of DNA synthesis in normal and tumorous target tissues. J Clin Invest 52: 1804–1811
3. Myers CE, Collins JM (1983) Pharmacology of intraperitoneal chemotherapy. Cancer Invest 1 (5): 395–407
4. Dedrick RL, Myers CE, Bungay PM, DeVita VT (1978) Pharmacokinetic rationale for peritoneal drug administration in the treatment of ovarian cancer. Cancer Treat Rep 62: 1–11
5. Flessner MF, Dedrick RL, Schulte JS (1984) A distributed model of periotoneal plasma transport: theoretical considerations. Am J Physiol 246: R597–R607
6. Flessner MF, Fenstermacher JD, Blasberg RG, Dedrick RL (1985) Peritoneal absorption of macromolecules studied by quantitative autogradiography. Am J Physiol 248: H26–H32
7. Flessner MF, Fenstermacher JD, Blasberg RG (1985) A distributed model of peritoneal-plasma transport: tissue concentration gradients. Am J Physiol 248: F425–F435
8. Flessner MF, Dedrick RL, Schulte JS (1985) A distributed model of peritoneal-plasma transport: analysis of experimental data in the rat. Am J Physiol 248: F413–F424
9. Flessner MF, Dedrick RL, Schltz JS (1985) Exchange of macromolecules between peritoneal cavity and plasma. Am J Physiol: H15–H25

10. Dedrick RL (1985) Theoretical and experimental bases of intraperitoneal chemotherapy. Semin Oncol 12 (3): 1–6
11. Speyer JL, Sugarbaker PH, Collin JM, Dedrick RL, Kleeker RW, Meyers CE (1981) Portal levels and hepatic clearance of 5-fluorouracil after intraperitoneal administration in humans. Cancer Res 41: pp 1916–1922
12. Sugarbaker PH, Gianola FJ, Speyer JL, Wesley R, Barofsky I, Meyers CE (1985) Prospective randomized trial of intravenous v intraperitoneal 5-FU in patients with a primary colon or rectal cancer. Semin Oncol 12 (3): 101–111
13. Dedrick RL, Flessner MF, Collins JM et al. (1982) Is the peritoneum a membrane? ASAIO 5 (1): 1–8
14. Dunnick NR, Jones RB, Doppman JL, Speyer J, Myers CE (1979) Intraperitoneal contrast infusion for assessment of intraperitoneal fluid dynamics. AJR 133: 221–223
15. Feldman GB, Knapp RI (1974) Lymphatic drainage of the peritoneal cavity and its significance in ovarian cancer. Am J Obstet Gynecol. 119: 991–994
16. Leichner PT, Rosenshein NB, Leibel SA et al. (1980) Distribution and tissue dose of intraperitoneally administered radioactive chromic phosphate in New Zealand white rabbits. Radiology 134: 729–734
17. Rosenshein N, Blake D, McIntyre P et al. (1978) The effect of volume on the distribution of substances instilled into the peritoneal cavity. Gynecol Oncol 6: 106–110
18. Teckhoff H, Schecter H (1968) A bacteriologically safe peritoneal access device. ASAO 12: 181
19. Tenckhoff H (1974) Manual for chronic peritoneal dialysis. University of Washington School of Medicine, Seattle
20. Twardowski ZJ (1985) Intraperitoneal therapy in renal failure. Semin Oncol 12 (3): 81–89
21. Piccart MJ, Speyer JL, Markman M, ten Bokkel-Huinink WW, Alberts D, Jenkins J, Muggia F (1985) Intraperitoneal chemotherapy: technical experience at five institutions. Semin Oncol 12 (3): 90–96
22. Jenkins J, Sugarbaker PH, Gianola FJ, Myers CE (1982) Technical considerations in the use of intraperitoneal chemotherapy administered by Tenckhoff catheter. Surg Gynecol Obstet 154: 858–864
23. Jenkins J (1983) Managing intraperitoneal chemotherapy: a medical, nursing and personal challenge. Semin Oncol 12 (3): 97–100
24. Davis AS, Reed WP (1983) A leak-free technique for open insertion of peritoneal dialysis catheters. Surg Gynecol Obstet 157: 579–580
25. Cerilli J, Walker J, Bay W (1983) A new technique for placement of catheters for peritoneal dialysis. Sur Gynecol Obstet 156: 663–664
26. Ozols RF, Myers CE, Young RC (1984) Intraperitoneal chemotherapy. Ann Intern Med 100: 1 118–120
27. Longo DL, Young RC (1981) The natural history and treatment of ovarian cancer. Annu Rev Med 32: 475–490
28. Buchsbaum HJ, Lifshitz S (1984) Staging and surgical evaluation of ovarian cancer. Semin Oncol 11 (3): 227–237
29. Kavanagh JJ (1985) Investigational therapies for epithelial ovarian cancer. Clin Obstet Gynec 28 (4): 846–852
30. Young RC (1984) Ovarian cancer treatment: progress of paralysis? Semin Oncol 11 (3): 327–329
31. Ozols RF, Young RC (1984) Chemotherapy of ovarian cancer. Semin Oncol 11 (3): 251–263
32. Thigpen JT, Vance RB, Lodovico B, Khansur TF (1984) New drugs and experimental approaches in ovarian cancer treatment. Semin Oncol 11 (3): 314–326
33. Hamilton TC, Young RC, Ozols RF (1984) Experimental model systems of ovarian cancer: applications to the design and evaluation of new teatment approaches. Semin Oncol 11 (3): 285–298

34. Ozols R (1985) Intraperitoneal chemotherapy in the management of ovarian cancer. Semin Oncol 12 (3): 75–80
35. Cohen CJ (1985) Surgical considerations in ovarian cancer. Semin Oncol 12 (3): 53–56
36. Thigpen T, Blessing JA (1985) Current therapy of ovarian carcinoma: an overview. Semin Oncol 12 (3): 47–52
37. Alberts DS, Young L, Mason N, Salmon SE (1985) In vitro evaluation of anticancer drugs against ovarian cancer at concentrations achievable by intraperitoneal administration. Semin Oncol 12 (3): 38
39. Tong D, Russell AH, Dawson Le et al. (1983) Second laparotomy for proximal colon cancer. Am J Surg 145: 382–386
40. Speyer JL (1985) The rationale behind intraperitoneal chemotherapy in gastrointestinal malignancies. Semin Oncol 12 (3): 23–28
41. Douglass HO (1985) Gastric cancer: overview of current therapies. Semin Oncol 12 (3): 57–62
42. Wilson RE (1985) Surgical considerations in gastric cancer. Semin Oncol 12 (3): 63–68
43. Brenner DE (1986) Intraperitoneal chemotherapy: a review. J Clin Oncol 4 (7): 1135–1147
44. Higgins GA Jr, Lyndon EL, Dwight RW, Keeher RJ (1978) The case of adjuvant 5-fluorouracil in colorectal cancer. Cancer Clin Trials, Spring: 35–41
45. Christophidis N, Vajda FJE, Lucas I, Drummer O, Moon WJ, Lornis WJ (1978) Fluorouracil therapy in patients with carcinoma of the large bowel: a pharmacokinetic comparison of various rates and routes of administration. Clin Pharmacokin 3: 33–336
46. deBruijn EA, VanOosterom AT, Tjaden UR, Recuwijk HJEM, Pinedo HM (1985) Pharmacology of 5-deoxy-5-fluorouridine in patients with resistant ovarian cancer. Cancer Res 45: 5931–5935
47. Speyer JL, Collins JM, Dedrick RL, Brennan MF, Buckpitt AR, Londer H, DeVita VT, Myers CE (1980) Phase-I and pharmacological studies of 5-fluorouracil administration intraperitoneally. Cancer Res 40: 567–572
48. Jones RB, Collins JM, Myers CE, Brooks AE, Hubbard SM, Balow JE, Brennan MF, Dedrick RL, DeVita VT (1981) High-volume intraperitoneal chemotherapy with methodtrexate in patients with cancer. Cancer Res 41: 55–59
49. Howel SB, Chu BB, Wung WE et al. (1981) Long-duration intracavitary infusion of methotrexate with systemic Leucovorin protection in patients with malignant effusions. J Clin Invest 67: 1161–1170
50. Howell SB (1985) Intraperitoneal chemotherapy: the use of concurrent systemic neutralizing agents. Semin Oncol 12 (3): 17–22
51. Ozols RF, Young RC (1985) High-dose cisplatin therapy in ovarian cancer. Semin Oncol 12 (4): 21–30
52. Lopez JA, KrisKorian JG, Reich SD, Smyth RD, Lee FH, Isseil BF (1985) Clinical pharmacology of intraperitoneal cisplatin. Gynecol Oncol 20: 1–9
53. Makman M, Cleary S, Howells SB (1985) Nephrotoxicity of high-dose intracavitary cisplatin with intravenous thiosulfate protection. Eur J Cancer Clin Oncol 21 (9): 1015–1018
54. Howell SB, Pfeifle CE, Wung WE, Olshen RA (1983) Intraperitoneal cis-diamminedichloroplatinum with system thiosulfate protection. Cancer Res 43: 1426–1431
55. ten Bokkel-Huinink WW, Bubbelman R, Aartsen E, Franklin H, McVie JG (1985) Experimental and clinical results with intraperitoneal cisplatin. Semin Oncol 12 (3): 43–46
56. Pretonius RG, Hacker NF, Berek JS, Ford LC, Hoeschele JD, Butler TA, LaGasse LD (1983) Pharmacokinetics of i.p. cisplatin in refractory ovarian carcinoma. Cancer Treat Rep 67 (12): 1085–1092
57. Ozols RF, Young RC, Speyer JL et al. (1982) Phase-I and pharmacologic studies of adriamycin administered intraperitoneally to patients with ovarian cancer. Cancer Res 42: 4265–4269

58. Howell SB, Pfeifle CE, Olshen, RA (1984) Intraperitoneal chemotherapy with melphalan. Ann Int Med 101: 14-18
59. Holcenberg J, Anderson T, Ritch P et al. (1983) Intraperitoneal chemotherapy with melphalan plus glutaminase. Cancer Res 43: 1381-1388
60. King ME, Pfeifle CE, Howell SB (1984) Intraperitoneal cytosine arabinoside therapy in ovarian carcinoma. J Clin Oncol 2: 662-669
61. Markman M, Cleary S, Lucas WE, Howell SB (1985) Intraperitoneal chemotherapy with high-dose cisplatin and cytosine arabinoside for refractory ovarianm carcinoma and other malignancies principally involving the peritoneal cavity. J Clin Oncol 3: 7
62. Markman M (1985) Melphalan and cytarabine administered intraperitoneally as single agents and combination intraperitoneal chemotherapy with cisplatin and cytarabine. Semin Oncol 12 (3): 33-37
63. Weiss G, Von Hoff DD (1985) Human tumor cloning assay: clinical applications for ovarian, gastric, pancreatic and colorectal cancers. Semin Oncol 12 (3): 69-74
64. Berek JS, Hacker NF, Lichtenstein A, Jung T, Spina C, Knox RB, Brady J, Greene T, Ettinger LM, Lagasse LD, Bonnem EM, Spiegel RJ, Zigheboim J (1985) Intraperitoneal recombinant a-interferon for "salvage" immunotherapy in stage-III epithelial ovarian cancer: a Gynecologic Oncology Group Study. Cancer Res 45: 4447-4453
65. Lotze MT, Custer MC, Rosenberg SA (1987) Intraperitoneal administration of interleukin-2 in patients with cancer. Arch Surg (in press)

Predictive Assays for the Therapy of Rectal Carcinoma

C. Streffer[1], D. van Beuningen[1], M.-L. Mlynek[2], E. Gross[3],
and F.-W. Eigler[3]

[1]Institut für Medizinische Strahlenbiologie; [2]Institut für Pathologie; [3]Klinik für Allgemeine
Chirurgie, Universitätsklinikum Essen, Hufelandstraße 55, 4300 Essen 1, FRG

Introduction

The decision about the therapeutic treatment of an individual tumor is made on
the basis of the localization and the clinical as well as the histopathological staging. However, very different responses to such a treatment are observed for tumors
with the same clinical and histopathological stage. From this general clinical experience it can be concluded that these tumors differ very much in their individual
biological characteristics, which are relevant for the therapeutic response, and
more biological data are needed in order to improve the selection of the appropriate therapeutic modality on an individual basis as well as to obtain better prognostic factors [1, 2].

Radiobiological experiments have demonstrated that the DNA content as well
as cell proliferation, cell loss, and cell repopulation are important parameters
which determine and modify the radiosensitivity of cell populations and tissues [3,
4]. Furthermore, it is general experience that tissues and cells are more radioresis-
tent when they are irradiated in the absence of oxygen or under low oxygen pressure [3, 4]. It therefore appears of great interest to determine these parameters in
individual tumors and to compare the results with the clinical therapeutic response in order to establish predictive assays for a better individualization of tumor therapy.

For the determination of the DNA content and cell proliferation, pulse cytometry after staining of the cells with ethidium bromide has been used [5, 6]. For cell
loss the micronucleus assay has been established. Micronuclei are identical with
chromatin material which can be observed in the cytoplasm. The micronuclei are
formed from acentric chromosome fragments or whole chromosomes which
are not taken up into the daughter cell nuclei during or after mitosis [7, 8]. Cells
with micronuclei have lost their clonogenic ability. Such cells are observed in
tumors without treatment [5, 6]. They increase after irradiation in correlation to
cell death [9–11]. It may be possible, therefore, to obtain from the micronucleus
test a semiquantitative measure of cell loss before treatment as well as of the
radiation response during and after radiotherapy. In order to obtain data about
the oxygenation of rectal carcinomas, the density of arterial capillaries was

Recent Results in Cancer Research, Vol. 110
© Springer-Verlag Berlin·Heidelberg 1988

determined in the tumors and in the normal rectal epithelium by a histochemical method [12].

Methods and Materials

Biopsies were obtained from rectal carcinomas after surgical resection; in some cases it was possible to obtain biopsies before and after preoperative radiotherapy. The histopathological diagnosis was performed at the Institute of Pathology, Universitätsklinikum Essen. Single cell suspensions were obtained by mechanical treatment of the biopsies. Micronuclei were counted after staining with ethidium bromide [6].

For DNA measurements the cell suspensions were stained with ethidium bromide and the analysis was performed with an ICP 22 (Biophysics, Phywe, Göttingen). Under the assumption that the peaks of G_1 phase as well as of G_2 phase cells show a Gaussian distribution in the histograms, the distribution of the cells within the generation cycle was calculated [6].

For the determination of the vascularity cryosections were made from the biopsies. After diazotization of alkaline phosphatase in the endothelial cells of the blood vessels, the sections were stained with triamino-tritolyl-methane cloride (TTMC) and the number of vessels were counted in defined areas [12]. From each tumor or from the normal mucosa of each patient up to five sections from different areas were analyzed.

Results and Discussions

The DNA content was measured by cytometry in the rectal carcinomas of 129 patients. From the DNA histograms obtained it can easily be seen whether the tumor cell line has a diploid (DNA index = 1.0) or hyperploid (DNA index > 1.0) DNA content. In case of a hyperploid cell line within the tumor a second peak appears in the histogram, which is separated from the diploid cells. In all studied rectal carcinomas only one tumor cell line was observed, although in some cases samples were taken from various regions of the resected tumor [5, 6]. About 45% of the rectal carcinomas had only diploid cells. In these cases no distinction between tumor cells and normal cells was possible. In some cases it was possible to measure the DNA content not only in the primary tumor but also in a metastasis. In most of these cases the DNA content of the tumor cell line was identical in both localizations (Table 1). In this respect, rectal carcinomas apparently differ from other tumor entities, in which several tumor cell lines are found in one individual tumor more frequently.

About 55% of the tumor cell lines had a hyperploid DNA content; most of them were found between diploid and tetraploid DNA contents (DNA index 1.0-2.0). The survival of patients with a diploid tumor was significantly longer than that of patients with a hyperploid tumor [6]. From these data it can be concluded that the cellular DNA content is apparently a prognostic factor for the tu-

Table 1. DNA content (diploid = 1.0) and number of S-phase cells (percent) in primary rectal carcinomas (DNA$_P$; S$_P$) and in metastases of the same carcinomas (DNA$_M$; S$_M$)

Pat.	DNA$_P$	S$_P$	DNA$_M$	S$_M$	Localization of metastases
Di	1.7	36	1.7	24	Liver
Ho	1.5	23	1.5	20	Liver
Ga	1.0	19	1.0	16	Liver
Ba	1.9	52	1.9	37	Liver
Is	2.0	29	2.0	23	Liver
Br	2.5	39	2.8	21	Liver
We	1.0	22	1.0	23	Retroperitoneal body wall
Sch	1.7	28	1.5	–	Liver

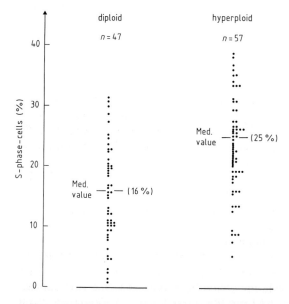

Fig. 1. Number of S-phase cells (percent) in individual human rectal carcinomas

mor patient. Similar data have been reported for other tumor entities, e.g., bladder carcinomas [13].

In contrast to the constant DNA content of the cell line in various tumor regions, the percentage of S-phase cells showed a higher variability in different tumor regions of the same tumor [5]. Also, the number of S-phase cells varied considerably from tumor to tumor (Fig. 1). In general, the number of S-phase cells was higher in hyperploid tumors (median value 25%) than in diploid tumors (median value 16%), although the calculations for diploid tumors were not quite correct, as a distinction between normal and tumor cells was not possible in these cases. Quite often, tumors with a high number of S-phase cells seem to have a worse prognosis than tumors with a low number of S-phase cells. This is quite astonishing, as one would expect tumors with a high proliferation to be more radiosensitive.

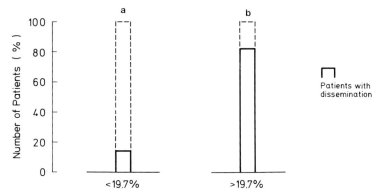

Fig. 2a, b. Percentage of patients with disseminated rectal carcinomas (disseminations to lymph nodes or distant metastases) in relation to number of S-phase cells: **a** carcinomas with number of S-phase cells below the median of 19.7%; **b** carcinomas with number of S-phase cells above the median of 19.7%

Most interesting, however was the observation that tumors with a high number of S-phase cells showed a higher degree of dissemination to lymph nodes or distant metastases (Fig. 2). The median value for the percentage of S-phase cells was 19.7% for all tumors taken together. Tumors which had a proportion of S-phase cells higher than 19.7% had a probability of 80% for dissemination, and tumors with a proportion of S-phase cells below this value had a probability for dissemination of about 20% (Fig. 2). This finding is interesting not only for tumor staging but also for the prognosis of the tumor patient. It was also interesting that the number of S-phase cells was usually higher in the primary tumor than in corresponding metastases in most cases (Table 1).

As has been pointed out earlier, cells with a micronucleus are no longer reproductive stem cells. These cells may still be able to perform cell division to a certain extent, but they are not able to form colonies. Therefore, the micronucleus test may be a useful assay to obtain semiquantitative estimates of cell loss. It was quite interesting that tumor cells can have micronuclei with a high rate before a therapeutic treatment. Apparently, a trend for a positive correlation exists between the number of S-phase cells and the number of cells with micronuclei (Fig. 3). Furthermore, it seems that patients with a bad prognosis appear in a certain region of the diagram on which the number of cells with a micronucleus is plotted against the number of S-phase cells (Fig. 3).

The number of cells with micronuclei increases among proliferating cells after radiation exposure [10, 11]. This effect was also seen in those rectal carcinomas which were treated with preoperative radiotherapy and which showed tumor regression after radiation exposure. Two fractionation schedules were used in these studies: (a) With "long-term irradiation" the patients obtained local radiotherapy with 4 fractions per week (2.0 Gy per fraction) over 3 weeks and surgery took place 10–15 days after the last radiation dose. (b) With "short-term irradiation" radiation was given in 3 fractions per day (2.1 Gy per fraction) on 3 succcessive days

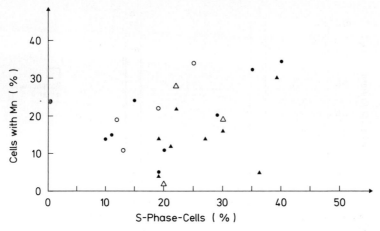

Fig. 3. Number of cells with micronuclei *(Mn)* plotted against the number of S-phase cells in individual human rectal carcinomas. *Open symbols,* living patients; *closed symbols,* dead patients; (○, ●) diploid tumors; (△, ▲) hyperploid tumors

and surgery took place 1–3 days after the last radiation dose. Micronuclei were determined before the first radiation dose and after irradiation in the tumor which was obtained from the surgical resection. With both fractionation schedules an increase of micronuclei was seen after radiotherapy for 60%–70% of the patients. These data demonstrate, especially for the short-term irradiation, that the micronucleus test can be used as an easy and fast assay to estimate radiation response in human tumors.

The number of S-phase cells was measured at the same time with the micronuclei in the same cell population. In some patients it was quite evident that the number of S-phase cells increased after irradiation. This was taken as a sign of early cell repopulation in these individual tumors. It is interesting that in these patients a local recurrence was observed within 17–31 months after surgical resection of the tumor [6].

In further experiments the density of blood capillaries was determined by a histochemical method which is characteristic for alkaline phosphatase [12]. In 32 patients the density of vessels was determined in the rectal carcinoma and in the normal mucosa of the same patient. The variability of vessel density was very high from tumor to tumor but in all cases but one, fewer capillaries were found in the rectal carcinomas than in the corresponding mucosa; therefore, the ratio (vascularization index) was smaller than one in these cases (Fig. 4). These data suggest that the oxygen supply is smaller in tumors than in the normal tissue. This phenomenon was shown for human rectal carcinomas earlier [14]. However, it was the aim of these studies not only to measure the vascularity of the tumors but also to see whether the radiosensitivity was dependent on this vascularization index.

Therefore, micronuclei were determined in the tumors of the same patients for whom the vascularization index was measured, before and after preoperative radiotherapy. The data were obtained from 12 patients and it could be demonstrated

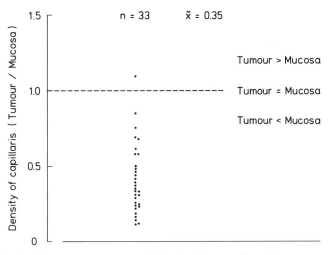

Fig. 4. Ratio of vascularization in tumors over vascularization in normal rectal mucosa (vascularization index) for individual patients with rectal carcinomas

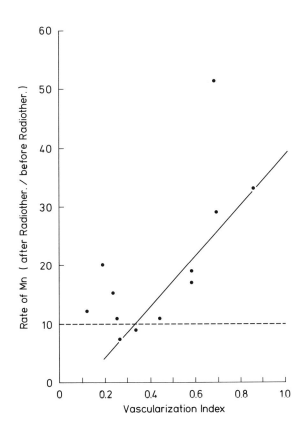

Fig. 5. Ratio of number of micronuclei after radiotherapy over number of micronuclei before radiotherapy plotted for individual patients with rectal carcinomas against vascularization index (see Fig. 4)

that a tendency existed for an increase of micronuclei after radiotherapy. This effect correlated in a positive manner with the vascularization index. The higher the density of capillaries in the tumor, the greater the radiation response was increased (Fig. 5). These data demonstrate that the vascularization index can be used to predict the radiosensitivity of the tumor.

Conclusions

1. Diploid tumors have a better prognosis than hyperploid tumors.
2. From determinations of S-phase cells before and after radiotherapy tumors with high repopulation rates and risk for local recurrences can be selected.
3. High rates of S-phase cells give a high risk for dissemination of the tumor to lymph nodes and distant metastases.
4. Radiation response can be determined early through the measurement of micronuclei.
5. Radiosensitivity of rectal carcinomas increases with density of vascularization. These measurements can be used as predictive assays for tumor therapy.

References

1. Mitchell JS, Feinendegen LE (1984) Research on the biological individualisation of cancer radiotherapy including the problems of developing countries. Report of meeting of experts, 26–30 April 1982. Strahlentherapie 160: 641–653
2. Peters LJ, Brock W, Johnson T (1985) Predicting radiocurability. Cancer 55: 2118–2122
3. Alper T (1979) Cellular radiobiology. Cambridge University Press, Cambridge
4. Streffer C (1980) Biologische Grundlagen der Strahlentherapie. In: Scherer E (ed) Strahlentherapie. Springer, Berlin Heidelberg New York, pp 197–266
5. Streffer C, van Beuningen D, Bamberg M, Eigler F-W, Gross E, Schabronath J (1984) An approach to the individualization of cancer therapy. Determination of DNA, SH-groups and micronuclei. Strahlentherapie 160: 661–666
6. Streffer C, van Beuningen D, Gross E, Schabronath J, Eigler F-W, Rebmann A (1986) Predictive assays for the therapy of rectum carcinoma. Radiother Oncol 5: 303–310
7. Schmid W (1975) The micronucleus test. Mutat Res 31: 9–15
8. Heddle JA (1973) A rapid in vivo test for chromosomal damage. Mutat Res 18: 187–198
9. Midander J, Revesz L (1980) The micronucleus (MN) in irradiated cells as a measure of survival. Br J Cancer 41: 204
10. Molls M, Streffer C, Zamboglou N (1981) Micronucleus formation in preimplanted mouse embryos cultured in vitro after irradiation with X-rays and neutrons. Int J Radiat Biol 39: 307–314
11. van Beuningen D, Streffer C, Bertholdt G (1981) Mikronukleusbildung im Vergleich zur Überlebensrate von menschlichen Melanomzellen nach Röntgen-, Neutronenbestrahlung und Hyperthermie. Strahlentherapie 157: 600–606
12. Mlynek M-L, van Beuningen D, Leder L-D, Streffer C (1985) Measurement of the grade of vascularization in histological tumor tissue sections. Br J Cancer 52: 945–948
13. Tribukait B, Gustafson H (1980) Impulscytophotometrische DNS-Untersuchungen bei Blasenkarzinomen. Onkologie 6: 278–288
14. Wendling P, Manz R, Thews G, Vaupel P (1984) Heterogeneous oxygenation of rectal carcinomas in humans. A critical parameter for preoperative irradiation? Adv Exp Med Biol 180: 293–300

Therapy of Carcinoid Tumors
with [131I] Meta-Iodo-Benzyl-Guanidine

J. Adolph, B. Kimmig, M. Eisenhut, and P. Georgi

Zentrum Radiologie, Strahlenklinik Ruprecht-Karls-Universität Heidelberg, Voßstraße 3, 6900 Heidelberg, FRG

Meta-iodo-benzyl-guanidine (MIBG) is a pharmaceutical with structural similarity to norepinephrine. It was introduced by Sisson et al. in 1981 as a pheochromocytoma scanning agent [8]. The intense and highly selective uptake of MIBG in chromaffin cells is the result of an active concentration process due to a specific cell membrane carrier. MIBG uptake has been found in pheochromocytomas, neuroblastomas, glomus tumors, and some medullary thyroid carcinomas [7]. All of these tumors are thought to belong to the neoplasms of the APUD series, according to their common neuroectodermal origin and based on histochemical criteria.

Iodine 131 is a radionuclide with a physical half-life of 8.1 days and emission of beta and gamma irradiation. Labeling of MIBG with ^{131}I yields a radiopharmaceutical agent suitable for both diagnostic and therapeutic purposes: External detection of [131I]MIBG by a gamma camera is possible because of the gamma radiation of the radionuclide, while the beta component of radiation exerts local therapeutic effects in concentrating tumors following high-dose application [4, 7]. Therapeutic experience with [131I]MIBG has so far been restricted to pheochromocytomas and neuroblastomas. In 1984, Fischer et al. found MIBG concentration in a carcinoid [3].

Carcinoid tumors are known to be uncommon, well-differentiated, hormone-secreting neoplasms with various sites of origin. They arise from the enterochromaffin cells and are attributed to the APUD neoplasms, like pheochromocytomas and neuroblastomas. The course of disease is determined by slow tumor growth, the tendency to metastasize with increasing tumor size, and late onset of unspecific symptoms. By the time of diagnosis, there is a high incidence of metastatic disease involving liver, lung, and bone [5]. First choice of treatment is surgical resection of primary tumors, which can produce some benefit even in metastatic disease. Cytotoxic chemotherapy using several combination regimens yields response rates of 20%–35% [2, 5]. In some patients with liver metastases, palliation with relief of symptoms may be achieved by hepatic artery embolization [6]. External radiation therapy is ineffective because of radioresistance of the tumors.

Recent Results in Cancer Research, Vol. 110
© Springer-Verlag Berlin·Heidelberg 1988

Table 1. Data of patients investigated

Patient	Age	Sex	Primary tumor localization	Metastases	5-HIAA excretion (mg/24 h)
I. H.	48	F	Small bowel	–	0.74
F. B.	68	M	Small bowel	Lung, liver, peritoneum	44.1
F. K.	54	M	Ileocecal	Local lymph nodes, liver	57.2
O. H.	61	M	Bronchus	Liver, spleen, bone	41.8
R. O.	50	M	Bronchus	–	3.4

Reports from other groups indicate MIBG concentration in nine of 16 patients with carcinoid tumors investigated so far [1]. We have studied five patients suffering from carcinoid tumors to assess the value of MIBG as a possible new therapeutic tool.

Patients

All patients (four male, one female) had undergone previous surgical resection with histological evaluation (Table 1). Three patients had local recurrence, one patient presented with incomplete resection of the primary tumor because of extensive mesenteric lymph node metastases, and a another patient was free of disease after resection of a bronchial carcinoid. The primary tumors were located in the gastrointestinal tract in three cases and in the bronchial system in two cases. Distant metastases were present in three of the five patients, involving the liver in all cases and the lung, the spleen and bone in one patient each. In one case, cytotoxic chemotherapy had been tried without success.

Results

Diagnostic imaging disclosed intense and long-lasting uptake of MIBG in primary tumors and metastatic sites (Fig. 1). The only false – negative result was obtained in a patient who had both multiple concentrating bone metastases in the vertebral column, ribs, and pelvis and a nonconcentrating metastasis in the skull (Table 2). In the patient free of disease the scintigram was correctly negative.

The four patients with persisting or recurrent disease were symptomatic and incurable. Following rough estimation of achievable tumor dose, we decided to perform high-dose therapy with 250–300 mCi of [^{131}I]MIBG in three patients. In the fourth patient MIBG therapy seemed of little value because of peritoneal carcinosis.

Thus far, the three patients have received two to three courses of treatment at intervals of 3–5 months. The total amounts of applied activity are 576–862 mCi.

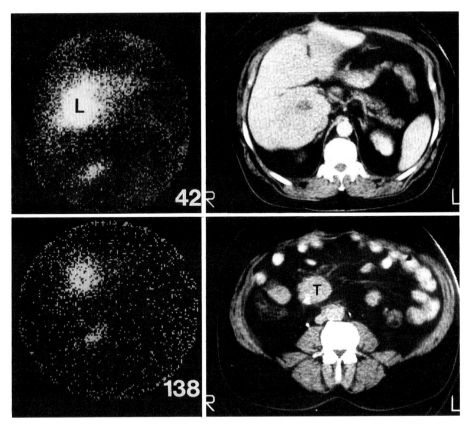

Fig. 1. *Left:* Scintigrams of the abdomen in anterior view, 42 and 138 h after injection in a patient with incomplete resection of ileocecal carcinoid and large liver metastasis. Increasing and intense MIBG concentration can be seen in the abdominal tumor and liver metastasis, while early physiological uptake in the liver *(L)* is rapidly decreasing with time. *Right:* CT cross section at level of the liver metastasis and abdominal tumor *(T)*

Table 2. Results of [^{131}I]MIBG imaging of carcinoid tumors

Patient	Primary tumor	Metastatic sites		
		Liver	Bone	Other
I. H.	+	○	○	○
F. B.	+	+	○	Lung + Peritoneum +
F. K.	+	+	○	○
O. H.	+	+	+/−	Spleen +
R. O.	○	○	○	○

Size of cross is relative to concentration of [^{131}I]MIBG and thus accumulated tumor dose of radiation.

During therapy no severe side effects were observed. The most serious side reaction was a reversible decrease of platelets to minimum values between 30000 and 80000 per μl in one patient.

The results of dosimetry during therapy with [^{131}I]MIBG are summarized in Table 3. MIBG concentration in the tumors was in the range of 0.3%–3.8% of applied activity, the effective half-life being about 61 h. The resultant therapy dose was 34 Gy on an average or – in other words – 12 Gy per 100 mCi of applied activity. Emphasis has to be put on the fact that this tumor dose in carcinoids is only one third of the values found in pheochromocytomas and neuroblastomas. Nevertheless, it is possible to achieve a total accumulated tumor dose of more than 100 Gy in carcinoids by repeated application.

In one patient we were not able to estimate the tumor volumes by computed tomography because of extensive desmoplastic reaction, which rendered impossible the definition of the borderline between tumor and surrounding tissue. Thus, the tumor dose could not be calculated in this one patient.

During the follow-up period of 8 months roentgenography, computed tomography, and ultrasound disclosed stable disease in all three patients. Two patients had symptomatic relief of flushing. In one patient with a metastatic bronchial carcinoid, calculation of tumor dose related to applied activity revealed a decrease of values between the second and third therapy cycle in a bone metastasis (Table 4). According to our experience with MIBG therapy of pheochromocytoma, this decrease is thought to be due to a reduction in the number of viable tumor cells and

Table 3. Results of dosimetry during therapy of carcinoid tumors with [^{131}I]MIBG

Patient	Tumor	Tumor mass (g)	Applied activity (mCi)	Maximum uptake (%)	Effective Half-life (h)	Tumor dose (Gy)
F.K.	Prim. Tumor	–	261	0.31	68.0	–
F.K.	Liver met.	–	261	3.75	48.5	–
I.H.	Local rec.	30	250	0.69	59.2	29.3
O.H.	Local rec.	57	300	1.28	57.9	32.5
O.H.	Bone met.	13	300	0.31	73.0	41.1

Table 4. [^{131}I]MIBG therapy of carcinoid tumor – accumulated tumor dose and tumor dose related to applied activity

Treatment course	Local recurrent bronchial tumor		Bone metastasis (vertebral col.)	
	(Gy)	(Gy/100 mCi)	(Gy)	(Gy/100 mCi)
1	32.50	10.83	41.10	13.70
2	30.12	11.60	33.45	12.87
3	29.21	9.67	30.10	9.97
Total accumulated tumor dose (Gy)	91.83		104.56	

reflects a promising effect of therapy. This effect can be expected when the total accumulated tumor dose exceeds 100 Gy. In our opinion, at least four cycles of treatment will be necessary to achieve an arrest of tumor growth or a reduction of tumor mass. However, a longer follow-up period is needed to assess the results of MIBG therapy in carcinoid tumors definitely.

Conclusion

Diagnostic imaging of carcinoid tumors with MIBG can provide information on the extent of disease. It should be performed:

1. As a pretherapeutic staging procedure in patients with suspected carcinoid tumors
2. During posttherapeutic staging and follow-up in patients with incomplete resection
3. For detection of MIBG concentration and dosimetry in case of possible therapeutic application

Therapy with [^{131}I]MIBG should be considered for surgically incurable patients with symptomatic disease. From our preliminary experience, MIBG therapy in these patients might be at least as effective as cytotoxic chemotherapy and has the advantage of substantially fewer side effects.

References

1. Adolph J, Kimmig B, Eisenhut M, Georgi P (1986) Therapie von Karzinoiden mit 131-J-Meta-Jod-Benzylguanidin. In: Höfer R, Bergmann H (eds) Radioaktive Isotope in Klinik und Forschung, vol 17/1. Egermann, Vienna, p 501
2. Engstrom PF, Lawin PT, Moertel CG, Folsch E, Douglas HO (1985) Streptozocin plus fluorouracil versus doxorubicin therapy for metastatic carcinoid tumor. J Clin Oncol 11: 1255
3. Fischer H, Kamanabroo D, Sonderkamp H, Proske T (1984) Scintigraphic imaging of carcinoid tumors with I-131-meta-iodo-benzyl-guanidine. Lancet 2: 165
4. Kimmig B, Brandeis WE, Eisenhut M, Bubeck B, Georgi P (1985) Szintigraphische Darstellung benigner und maligner Tumoren des sympathischen Nervensystems mit meta-Jod-Benzylguanidin. Röntgenblätter 38: 154
5. MacDonald JS (1982) Carcinoid tumors. In: DeVita VT, Hellman S, Rosenberg SA (eds) Cancer - principles and practice of oncology. Lippincott, Philadelphia, p 1019
6. Mitty HA, Warner RRP, Newman LH, Train JS, Parnes IH (1985) Control of carcinoid syndrome with hepatic artery embolization. Radiology 155: 623
7. Shapiro B, Fischer M (1985) Summary of the proceedings of a workshop on ^{131}I-Meta-Iodo-Benzyl-Guanidine held at Schloß Wilkinghege, Münster, Sept 29, 1984. Nucl Med Comm 6: 179
8. Sisson JC, Frager MS, Valk TW, Gross MD, Swanson DP, Wieland DM, Tobes MC, Beierwaltes WH, Thompson NW (1981) Scintigraphic localization of pheochromocytoma. New Engl J Med 305: 12

New Drug Development
in Gastrointestinal-Tract Cancer

M. R. Berger, F. T. Garzon, H. Bischoff, and D. Schmähl

Institut für Toxikologie und Chemotherapie, Deutsches Krebsforschungszentrum,
Im Neuenheimer Feld 280, 6900 Heidelberg, FRG

Introduction

GI-tract cancer continues to be a significant cause of human suffering and a leading cause of cancer mortality. The survival statistics have not changed greatly in the past 30 years [28]; however, some progress has been made in the past decade regarding techniques of radiation, combined-modality treatment, and patient care.

GI-tract cancer is a general term used for various tumors with their own biological and histologic characteristics. They share some common features, such as changing epidemiological patterns, a difficulty in establishing an early diagnosis, and a resistance to conventional chemotherapy. The latter two factors have a direct impact on the surival rate of patients with advanced disease, presenting a relatively poor prognosis.

Surgery remains the only modality with curative potential, but the majority of patients with advanced tumors are not amenable to surgical cure. Even when resection is possible, the patients remain at high risk for recurrence and metastasis; this situation leads to the concept of combined-treatment modalities, i. e., the combination of surgery with radiotherapy, which controls the locoregional recurrence, and/or in combination with chemotherapy, which in theory controls distant micrometastasis or systemic dissemination. Furthermore, the biological response modifiers, i. e., interleukin 2, interferon, and tumor necrosis factor (TNF), have emerged recently as a possible adjuvant modality in cancer treatment [21–23], with encouraging preclinical results. This treatment modality, like other approaches to cancer treatment, has better results when used for minimal neoplastic disease. Hence, the administration of systemic therapy before or after surgery of the tumor should increase the likelihood of cure when specific cytostatic agents are used [11]. However, this is only a hypothetical situation because most of the patients in the advanced state experience progressive disease in spite of conventional chemotherapy, which is characterized by being inspecific and displaying a narrow range between marginal active and toxic doses. Consequently, slight increases have been achieved in the survival time of patients with esophageal or gastric cancer [15, 26] and poor or no benefits have been obtained so far in patients with colorectal cancer [10] when mono- or combination chemotherapy has been used.

Recent Results in Cancer Research, Vol. 110
© Springer-Verlag Berlin · Heidelberg 1988

There are several continuing efforts being made to improve these results. This is the case with certain experimental approaches, such as high doses of chemotherapy to the target tissue by locoregional administration, or the use of high doses of systemic chemotherapy with subsequent bone marrow transplantation. Moreover, the value of monoclonal antibodies in cancer therapy is presently being evaluated; unfortunately, the benefit of these extended efforts is limited. Thus, new, more active drugs are urgently needed and this remains a main topic in recent cancer research.

The detection of new cytostatic agents with improved anticancer potency and the prediction of their clinical activity in GI-tract cancer depends mainly on the preclinical system which is used to evaluate the properties of the compounds being tested. Furthermore, a major difficulty in the evaluation of most anticancer agents is the lack of correlation of the animal tumor model with the drug response obtained in the respective types of human cancer [29]. In addition, the conventionally used rapidly proliferating rodent tumors have failed to identify new agents with marked activity in the treatment of large-bowel cancer [12]. The former NCI system, which was based on transplanted mouse tumors, was recently supplemented by tumors of human origin inoculated into nude mice. It was hoped at that time that xenografts derived from a certain type of human cancer, e.g., colonic cancer, would help to select active compounds against this tumor in human beings. Once again, this system showed its limitations and failed to predict or select active compounds against tumors of the GI tract [1].

Another common system of screening (Figs. 1 and 2) is based mainly on in vitro assays, with cells of human or murine origin as a first screen [25, 30]. So far, no compound derived from these systems has proven its efficacy in human beings; obvious limitations of in vitro systems are:

1. Lack of mechanisms of metabolic activation other than that exhibited by the tumor cells
2. Lack of pharmacokinetic influences or pharmacodynamic processes
3. Limited accuracy in predicting response (truly positive)
4. Established cell lines are highly selected from originally multiclonal tumors
5. Changing characteristics of tumor cells under in vitro conditions
6. Lack of heterogenicity in tumor cell culture

This situation challenges the development of new models and/or the use of rational combinations of preclinical systems which permit a more reliable selection of new compounds [6, 18].

Chemically induced autochthonous tumors have some advantages, because they are closer to the human situation than transplanted systems [32]. In fact, human GI-tract cancer is mimicked rather closely by autochthonous colorectal tumors of Sprague-Dawley rats induced with acetoxymethyl-methylnitrosamine (AMMN) [27]. The majority of these tumors are histologically well-differentiated adenocarcinomas. They are resistant to conventional chemotherapy; they show a relatively long tumor-volume doubling time and their growth within the colorectum can be diagnosed endoscopically.

Several new compounds were recently investigated in this animal model and those with antitumoral activity are briefly described: they include flavone acetic

Stage of testing

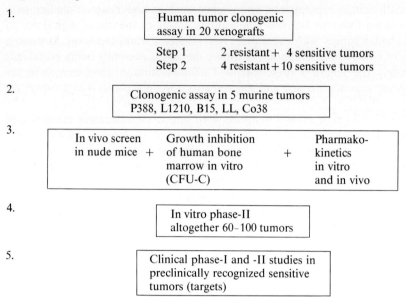

1.

Human tumor clonogenic
assay in 20 xenografts

Step 1   2 resistant + 4 sensitive tumors
Step 2   4 resistant + 10 sensitive tumors

2.

Clonogenic assay in 5 murine tumors
P388, L1210, B15, LL, Co38

3.

| In vivo screen in nude mice | + | Growth inhibition of human bone marrow in vitro (CFU-C) | + | Pharmako-kinetics in vitro and in vivo |

4.

In vitro phase-II
altogether 60–100 tumors

5.

Clinical phase-I and -II studies in
preclinically recognized sensitive
tumors (targets)

Fig. 1. Screening system currently used at the University of Freiburg Medical Department. (Adapted from Fiebig et al. [6])

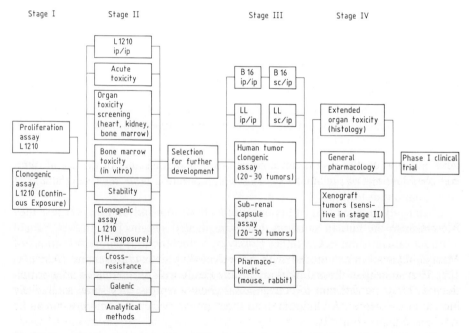

Fig. 2. Screening system currently used in the Behringwerke, Marburg, Federal Republic of Germany [18]

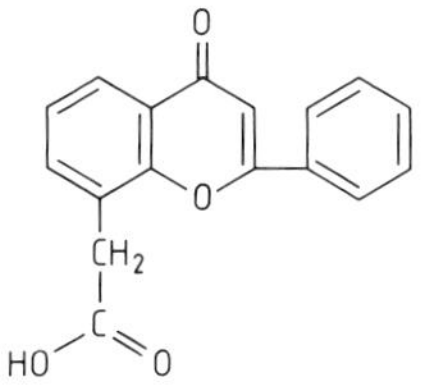

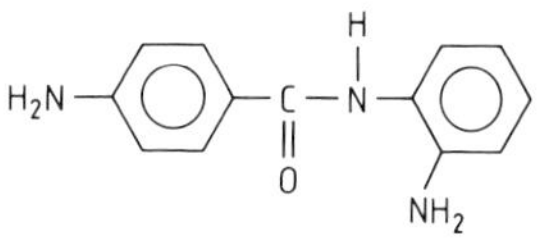

Fig. 3 *(left).* Structure of 4-oxo-2-phenyl-4H-1-benzopyran-8-acetic acid (LM975, NSC 347512, flavone acetic acid)

Fig. 4 *(right).* Structure of 4-amino-N-(2'-aminophenyl)-benzamide (GOE 1734)

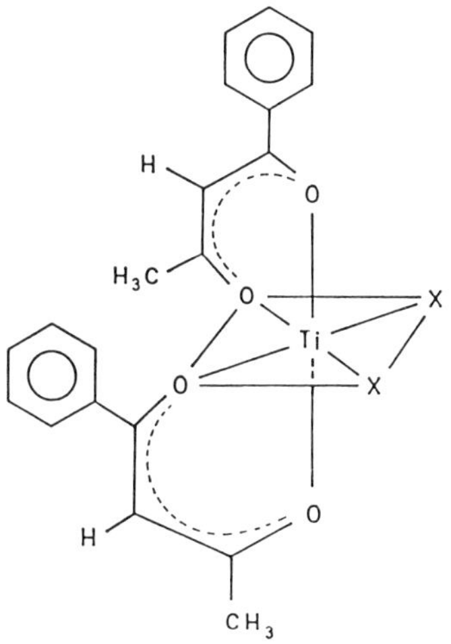

Fig. 5. Structure of diethoxybis(1-phenylbutane-1,3-dionato)titanium (IV), (Ti(bzac)$_2$(Oet)$_2$)

acid (Fig. 3) 4-amino-N-(2'-aminophenyl) benzamide (Fig. 4), an inorganic metal complex derived from titanium (Fig. 5) and ruthenium (Fig. 6), and interleukin-2.

Methodology

Male Sprague-Dawley rats (Charles River Breeding, Sulzfeld, F. R. G.) were purchased at a weight of 140–160 g and thereafter kept under conventional conditions: two rats per Macrolon III cage, tap water, and Altromin pellets and lib. The induction of colorectal carcinomas was performed using fresh 0.2% solutions of AMMN [24, 31] (Fig. 7) in physiological saline; 2 mg/kg was administered intra-rectally in weekly intervals for 10 weeks through a rectal tube, the tip of which reached the colonic flexure of rats when fully inserted.

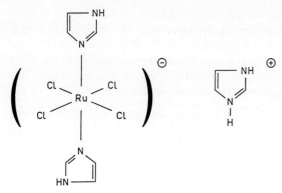

Fig. 6. Structure of imidazolium-bis(imidazole) tetrachloro-ruthenate (III), (ImH(RuIm$_2$Cl$_4$)

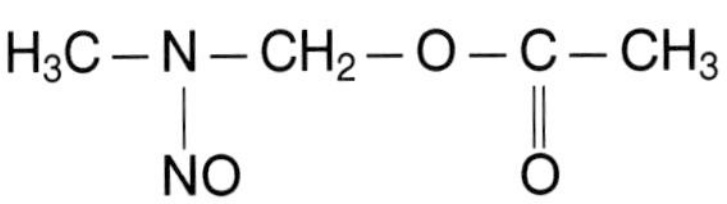

$$H_3C - N - CH_2 - O - C - CH_3$$
$$\quad\quad | \quad\quad\quad\quad\quad\; ||$$
$$\quad\; NO \quad\quad\quad\quad O$$

Fig. 7. Structural formula of acetoxymethyl-methylnitrosamine (AMMN)

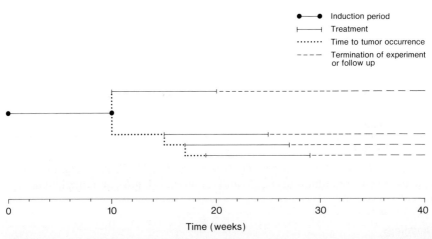

Fig. 8. Sequence of induction of colorectal cancer in SD rats with acetoxymethyl-methylnitrosamine and subsequent treatment. Treatment starts before manifestation of tumors *(top line)* or following endoscopic diagnosis of tumors *(lower three lines)*

According to the time following the end of the induction period and the diagnosis of the tumors, this animal model can be used in two modes (Fig. 8). One treatment starts immediately after the end of the induction period, normally for 10 weeks, and represents the concept of treatment for non-established tumors (Tables 1 and 3); this setting is also used to evaluate immunological approaches (Tables 5 and 6). The other treatment starts after the endoscopic diagnosis of the tumors (performed on the 5th to 9th week after the end of the induction period, normally for 10 weeks) and represents the concept of treating established tumors (Tables 2 and 4). Moreover, a double control group, one before and a second

Table 1. Therapy of AMMN-induced colorectal rat adenocarcinoma with diethoxy-bis(1-phenyl-1,3-butanedionato)titanium(IV), Ti(bzac)$_2$(Oet)$_2$

No. of animals	Treatment[a] schedule	Median tumor volume (mm^3) per rat (95% confidence limits)	T/C × 100	Median tumor number per rat (95% confidence limits)	Mortality (%)
25	Control	60 (26–102)	100	4 (2–6)	0
30	2 × 10 mg/kg Ti(bzac)$_2$(Oet)$_2$ i. v.	14 (6–27)	23	2 (2–3)	6 (20)
30	control	123 (86–164)	100	6 (5–6)	0
30	2 × 6,3 mg/kg Ti(bzac)$_2$(Oet)$_2$ i. v.	56 (33–88)	45	4 (3–5)	0

[a] Treatment was given 2 times a week for 10 weeks and started right after the end of the induction period (week 11).

Table 2. Therapy of AMMN-induced colorectal rat adenocarcinoma with imidazolium bis-imidazoltetrachlororuthenate (III), (RuCl$_4$Im$_2$)ImH

No. of animals	Treatment[a] schedule	Median tumor volume (mm^3) per rat (95% confidence limits)	T/C × 100	Median tumor number per rat (95% confidence limits)	Mortality (%)
20	Control	386 (120–683)	100	4 (2–5)	0
20	2 × 14 mg/kg (RuCl$_4$Im$_2$)ImH i. v.	80 (14–315)	21	3 (2–4)	9 (45)
12	2 × 12 mg/kg (RuCl$_4$Im$_2$)ImH i. v.	78 (4–506)	20	2 (1–3)	1 (8)
10	2 × 7 mg/kg (RuCl$_4$Im$_2$)ImH i. v.	69 (24–401)	18	4 (3–5)	0

[a] Treatment was given 2 times a week for 10 weeks and started after endoscopical diagnosis of the tumors (week 15).

Table 3. Treatment of AMMN-induced colorectal carcinomas with flavone acetic acid (*LM975*), 5'-deoxy-5-fluorouridine (*DFUR*), and the combination of both agents

Treatment schedule[a] (mg/kg)		No. of animals	Median tumor volume (mm³) (95% conf. limits)	T/C × 100	Median tumor number (95% conf. limits)	Mortality (%)
LM975	DFUR					
Control		30	123 (86–169)	–	6 (5–6)	0
100	–	20	135 (81–172)	110	5.5 (3–6)	0
200	–	20	53 (26–82)	43	4 (3–4)	10
–	300	20	85 (58–108)	69	5 (4–6)	0
–	600	20	58 (19–77)	47	3 (2–5)	10
Control		20	167 (48–589)	–	3 (2–3)	0
100	300	20	14 (3–60)	8	2 (1–3)	0

[a] Two i.p. administrations/week for 10 weeks, started right after the end of the induction period (week 11).

Table 4. Treatment of established AMMN-induced colorectal carcinomas with 4-amino-N(2' aminophenyl)benzamide (GOE 1734)

Dosage/week (mg/kg)	No. of animals	Median tumor volume (mm³) (95% conf. limits)	T/C × 100	Median tumor number (95% conf. limits)	No. of rats without tumors (%)	Mortality n (%)
Control I[a]	20	36.5 (24–74)	–	2 (1–3)	0 (0)	0 (0)
Control II[b]	20	389 (264–1046)	100	4 (3–7)	0 (0)	1 (5)
7.9; days 1–5	20	28 (12–68)	7.2	3 (2–4)	1 (5)	6 (30)
6.3; days 1–5	20	53 (19–101)	13.6	3 (2–4)	0 (0)	2 (10)
12.6; days 1, 3, 5	20	126 (33–180)	32.4	4 (3–4)	0 (0)	3 (15)

[a] Animals killed at diagnosis to establish tumor size before treatment.
[b] Controls parallel to treated groups.

group after the treatment, serves to evaluate tumor regression in this model (Table 5). In all cases the animals were randomized before the experiment into treatment and control groups.

For endoscopic examination the animals were anesthetized by intraperitoneal administration of chloral hydrate (3 g/kg diluted in physiological saline); this was followed by inspection of the colon [19, 20] using a children's bronchoscope (Olympus BF, Type 4C2, Olympūs Optical Co. Tokyo). The animals were killed after 5 (Table 5) or 10 weeks of treatment (Tables 1–4 and 6). They were dissected and the last 20 cm of the gut were removed, opened, and weighed. The number of tumors was recorded and the volume of each was estimated by measuring three diameters according to the formula axbxc/2.

Table 5. Therapy of AMMN-induced colorectal rat adenocarcinoma with interleukin 2 (IL-2)

No. of animals	Treatment schedule	Median tumor volume (mm^3) per rat (95% confidence limits)	Median tumor number per rat (95% confidence limits)	% Median weight difference (week 5- week 1)	Mortality no. (%)
10	Controls[a]	25 (3-129)	4 (3-4)	+9	1 (10)
12	10000 units/kg IL-2/weeks × 5	9 (4-27)	3 (1-5)	+4	0 (0)

[a] Animals received saline injections.

Table 6. Treatment of AMMN-induced colorectal rat adenocarcinoma with interleukin-2 (IL-2) and low-dose mafosfamide

No. of animals	Treatment schedule	Median tumor volume (mm^3) per rat (95% confidence limits)	T/C × 100	Median tumor number per rat (95% confidence limits)	Mortality no. (%)
20	Control[a]	68 (32-152)	100	2.5 (2-3)	0(0)
20	1200 U IL-2[a]	13 (5-17)	20	2 (1-2)	0(0)
20	1200 U IL-2[a] + 10 mg/kg mafosfamide i.p.	6 (1-12)	9	2 (1-3)	1(5)
20	Control[b]	62 (28-78)	100	3 (3-4)	1(5)
15	1200 U IL-2[b]	12 (4.5-69)	19	2 (2-3)	0(0)
15	1200 U IL-2[b] + 10 mg/kg mafosfamide i.p.	20 (8-72)	32	2 (2-3)	1(5)

[a] Before manifestation of the tumors.
[b] Following endoscopical diagnosis of tumors.

Results and Discussion

The titanium complex was remarkably non-toxic in preceeding experiments on transplanted tumors [13, 16], thus making it suitable for prolonged therapy. Administration of this compound started immediately after the end of the induction showed a tumor growth inhibition of 77% and 55% respective to the doses administered, and the observed toxicity was also dose related (Table 1) [3].

Preliminary experiments on ruthenium derivatives have shown promising results on transplanted tumor systems [17] and also on this animal model [9]. The growth of the colorectal tumor was inhibited to more than 80% as comparison with untreated controls with a dose-related toxicity (Table 2). Since this compound is easier to solubilize than the titanium complex, it might have some advantages in routine practice. Further experiments on this derivative and on structurally related congeners are currently being performed.

Flavone acetic acid (LM975) is a compound without activity in leukemia P388; however, it has shown a remarkably high anticancer efficacy in nine transplanted solid tumors [4]. Seven of these tumors were derived from the gastrointestinal tract, including pancreatic tissue. LM975 showed the following interesting properties: it has anticancer activity in vitro, it displays a narrow range of active doses in vivo, split doses are no better than one full dose, and its half-life is relatively long (about 7 h).

Our results in AMMN-induced colorectal carcinomas, obtained after 10 weeks of treatment immediately following the end of the induction period, confirm this activity: there was a significant antitumor effect (Table 3) at a marginal toxic dose as measured by tumor growth inhibition. A similar activity was displayed by 5'-deoxy-5-fluorouridine (5'dFUR). Interestingly, the combination of both drugs showed an additive synergistic effect at a non-toxic dose level. Therefore, this compound could easily be combined with established cytostatic therapy in the treatment of human colorectal cancer.

4-Amino-N(2'-aminophenyl) benzamide (Goe1734) shares similar characteristics with flavone acetic acid regarding its inactivity toward quickly growing leukemias [2]. There was, however, high antineoplastic effectiveness in AMMN-induced colorectal rat adenocarcinoma when the animals were treated before or after the endoscopic diagnosis of tumors. The appearance of tumors was protracted and their growth was inhibited in a dose-related manner. Moreover, a tumor growth inhibition of 95% was observed compared with the control groups before or after the treatment.. Together with the antineoplastic efficacy the toxicity was dose dependent (Table 4) [7].

Compared with these new cytostatic agents, the anticancer activity of the biological response modifier, interleukin-2 (IL-2), was modest when administered before the manifestation of tumors, in order to influence the immunological state of the animals [8]. This situation mimics that of patients with minimal residual disease [5]. In fact, a somewhat lower tumor volume and tumor number were observed following daily s.c. administration over a 5-week period (Table 5). Subsequent experiments with this agent alone and in combination with oxazaphosphorines (Mafosfamide) confirmed these results (Table 6).

Conclusions

A careful selection of suitable preclinical models should result in a more effective search for new drugs which are active against slowly growing solid tumors, especially those derived from the GI tract. Several promising new compounds having an effect on autochthonous colorectal rat adenocarcinoma have been found and preclinically characterized; however, they are still awaiting clinical evaluation. Comparison of predicted and actual clinical anticancer activity will finally draw attention to a more appropriate manner of drug selection.

References

1. Atassi G (1984) Do we need new chemosensitive experimental models? Eur J Cancer Clin Oncol 20: 1217-1220
2. Berger MR, Bischoff H, Fritschi E, Henne T, Herrmann M, Pool B, Satzinger G, Schmähl D, Weiershausen U (1985) Synthesis, toxicity and therapeutic efficacy of 4-amino-N-(2'-aminophenyl) benzamide: a new compound active in slowly growing tumours. Cancer Treat Rep 69: 1415-1424
3. Bischoff H (1986) Chemotherapie eines Nitrosamin-induzierten autochthonen Colontumors bei SD-Ratten mit β-Diketonato-Verbindungen mit Titan, Zirkonium und Hafnium, im Vergleich mit cis-Platin, Cyclophosphamid, 5-Fluorouracil und 5'-Deoxy-5-Flurouridin. Dissertation, University of Heidelberg
4. Corbett T, Bissery M, Wosniak A, Plowman J, Polin L, Tapazoglou E, Dieckman J, Valeriote F (1986) Solid tumor activity of flavone acetic acid (FAA). Proc Am Assoc Cancer Res 27: 281
5. Duncan W (ed) (1982) Colorectal cancer. Springer, Berlin Heidelberg New York (Recent results in cancer research, vol 83, pp 135-149)
6. Fiebig HH, Schmid JR, Henss H, Dentler V, Schildge J, Löhr GW (1986) Bedeutung des Kolonie-Assays als In-vitro-Verfahren zur Tumorsensibilitätstestung und für die Zytostatikaentwicklung. In: Drings P, Schmähl D, Vogt-Moykopf I (eds) Bronchialkarzinom. Zuckschwerdt, München, pp 132-161
7. Garzon, FT (1986) Versuche zur Evaluation neuer antineoplastisch wirksamer Verbindungen an autochthonen Acetoxymethyl-methylnitrosamin-induzierten kolorectalen Tumoren der SD-Ratte. Dissertation, University of Heidelberg
8. Garzon FT, Salas M, Berger MR, Kirchner H (1986) Effect of interleukin-2 on the manifestation and growth of acetoxymethyl-methylnitrosamine-induced colorectal rat adenocarcinoma. J Cancer Res Clin Oncol 111: 79-81
9. Garzon FT, Berger MR, Keppler BK, Schmähl D (1987) Comparative antitumor activity of ruthenium derivatives with 5'-deoxy-5-fluorouridine in chemically-induced colorectal tumors in SD rats. Cancer Chemother Pharmacol 19: 347-349
10. Gastrointestinal tumor group (1984) Adjuvant therapy of colon cancer – results of a prospectively randomized trial. N Engl J Med 310: 737-743
11. Goldin JH, Coldman AJ (1986) Theoretical consideration regarding the early use of adjuvant chemotherapy. In: Ragaz J, Band PR, Goldie JH (eds) Preoperative chemotherapy. Springer, Berlin Heidelberg New York, pp 30-35 (Recent results in cancer resarch, vol 103)
12. Goldin A, Venditti JM, MacDonald JS, Muggia FM, Henney JE, Devita VT (1981) Current results of the screening program at the division of Cancer Treatment, National Cancer Institute. Eur J Cancer 17: 129-142
13. Keller HJ, Keppler B, Schmähl D (1982) Antitumor activity of cis-dihalogenobis(1-phenyl-1,3-butanedionato)titanium(IV) compounds against Walker 256 carcinosarkoma. Arzneimittelforsch 32: 806-807
14. Keller HJ, Keppler B, Schmähl D (1983) Antitumor activity of cis-dihalogenobis(1-phenyl-1,3-butanedionato)titanium(IV) compounds. J Cancer Res Clin Oncol 105: 109-110
15. Kelsen DP, Bains M, Hilaris B, Chapman R, McCormack P, Alexander J, Hopfasn S, Martini N (1982) Combination chemotherapy of esophageal carcinoma using cisplatin, vindesine and bleomycin. Cancer 49: 1174-1177
16. Keppler B (1985) Synthesis and preclinical evaluation of bis-β-diketonatotitanium(IV) complexes as a new class of antitumor agents. J Cancer Res Clin Oncol 109: A43
17. Keppler B, Rupp W (1986) Antitumor activity of imidazolium-bisimidazole-tetrachlororuthenate (III). J Cancer Res Clin Oncol 111: 166-168
18. Kraemer HP, Sedlacek HH (1984) A modified screening system selects new cytostatic drugs. Behring Inst Mitt 74: 301-328
19. Merz R, Wagner I, Habs M, Schmähl D, Amberger H, Bachmann U (1981) Endoscopic

diagnosis of chemically induced autochthonous colonic tumors in rats. Hepatogastroenterology 28: 53–57

20. Narisawa T, Ching-Quo Wong DS, Weisburger JH (1975) Evaluation of endoscopic examination of colon tumors in rats. Dig Dis 20: 928–934

21. Old LJ (1985) Tumor necrosis factor. Science 230: 630–632

22. Oldham RK (1984) Biological response modifiers: the fourth modality of cancer treatment. Cancer Treat Rep 68: 221–232

23. Oldham RK, Thurman GB, Talmadge JE, Stevenson HC, Foon KA (1984) Lymphokines, monoclonal antibodies and other biological response modifiers in the treatment of cancer. Cancer 54: 2795–2806

24. Rice JM, Joshi SR, Roller PP (1975) Methyl(acetoxymethyl)-nitrosamine. A new carcinogen highly specific for colon and rectum. Proc Am Assoc Cancer Res no 16, p 32

25. Salmon SE, von Hoff DD (1981) In vitro evaluation of anticancer drugs with the human tumor stem cell assay. Semin Oncol 8 (4): 377–385

26. Schein PS, Smith FP, Dritschillo A, Stablein DM, Ahlgren JD (1983) Phase I–II trial of combined-modality FAM (5-fluorouracil, adriamycin, and mitomycin C) plus split-course radiation (FAM-RT-FAM) for locally advanced gastric (LAG) and pancreatic (LAP) cancer: a Midatlantic oncology program. Proceedings of the American Society of Clinical Oncology, no 2, 126

27. Schmähl D (1976) Utilisation of nitrosamine-induced tumours as models for cancer chemotherapy. Chemotherapy 7: 233–238

28. Silverberg E, Lubera J (1986) Cancer statistics, 1986. CA 36: 9–25

29. Venditti JM (1981) Preclinical drug development: rationale and methods. Semin Oncol 8 (4): 349–361

30. Weisenthal LM (1981) In vitro assays in preclinical antineoplastic drug screening. Semin Oncol 8 (4): 362–376

31. Wiessler M (1975) Chemie der Nitrosamine II. Synthese α-funktioneller Dimethylnitrosamine. Tetrahedron Lett 30: 2575–2578

32. Zeller J, Berger MR (1984) Chemically induced autochthonous tumor models in experimental chemotherapy. Behring Ins Mitt 74: 201–208

Sachverzeichnis